The Energy Wise Home

The Energy Wise Home

Practical Ideas for Sustainable Living

Jeff Dondero

ROWMAN & LITTLEFIELD
Lanham • Boulder • New York • London

Published by Rowman & Littlefield
A wholly owned subsidiary of The Rowman & Littlefield Publishing Group, Inc.
4501 Forbes Boulevard, Suite 200, Lanham, Maryland 20706
www.rowman.com

Unit A, Whitacre Mews, 26-34 Stannary Street, London SE11 4AB

British Library Cataloguing in Publication Information Available

Library of Congress Cataloging-in-Publication Data

Names: Dondero, Jeff, 1947– author.
Title: The energy wise home : practical ideas for sustainable living / Jeff Dondero.
Description: Lanham : Rowman & Littlefield, 2017. | Includes index.
Identifiers: LCCN 2016049121 (print) | LCCN 201604960 (ebook) | ISBN 9781442279476 (cloth) | ISBN 9781442279483 (ebook)
Subjects: LCSH: Dwellings—Energy conservation—Handbooks, manuals, etc.
Classification: LCC TJ163.5.D86 D66 2017 (print) | LCC TJ163.5.D86 (ebook) | DDC 644—dc23
LC record available at https://lccn.loc.gov/2016049121

∞™ The paper used in this publication meets the minimum requirements of American National Standard for Information Sciences—Permanence of Paper for Printed Library Materials, ANSI/NISO Z39.48-1992.

Printed in the United States of America

Contents

Acknowledgments, Dedication, and Disclaimer

The author wishes to thank the many people who assisted in the creation of this book. First, for her long-standing and patient assistance, and for being my angel in many forms, I thank Alicia Dondero. A boy's best friend really can be his mother.

Thanks to Patrick Totty for advice, confidence, encouragement, and aid in many ways, and to Chris Dondero for taking time to consume large chunks of copy in an effort to edit information and offer feedback. Likewise, my thanks go to Tammie Schmidt for wading through copy editing, and also coming to the rescue for many things computational, and to Ginja the Ninja for the exercise.

Thank you to my online editor Kathryn Knigge who, unflaggingly, and with deference and patience, was essential in getting this large undertaking in order, and to the publisher for giving me the opportunity for others to read what I write. Finally, thanks to all my pals who plied me with confidence and the occasional cocktail.

Last but not in the least, thanks to all the people who write books, put together information, struggle with statistics, make maps, create charts and tables to clarify, quantify, and illuminate the world for others.

DISCLAIMER

It is important to remember, "There are lies, damn lies, and statistics." Most of the stats here have been gathered by local, state, and federal government agencies, independent scientists and writers, power companies, universities, various water and power companies, the Internet, and other informed sources.

Consequently, I do not claim that all the statistics presented represent accurate and true statements, percentages, and facts, and I do not warrant or make any representations as to the content, accuracy, or completeness of the information, text, graphics, charts, Web links, Web sites, and other items contained in their media presentations.

Aggregating and writing information for this kind of book has its inherent problems and predicaments. When presented with questions, people use different ways to find diverse answers and conclusions. Consequently answers may vary, sometimes quite a bit. For example, prices for fuel and/or power can change not only from various utility companies, but also from state to state, and can fluctuate due to availability and demand. Opinions on how much water a family of four uses, or even an individual's survival needs, range quite a bit. Also, the results of certain criteria can be altered by many factors, depending on weather, location, cost of resources, size of home, etc. In addition, some of the facts presented might be affected by time, changing world events, or new discoveries.

Not all scientists would agree on matters such as global warming, climate change, or the fact that CO_2 is contributing to the detriment of our environment. What I have tried to do is present an informed opinion about what the future might hold for the Earth. I have also stated that there have been many doomsayers that may have made dire predictions about the fate of the Earth that have not come to pass. As in many things, opinions vary as to number, percentages, predictions, and the veracity or divergence of the results obtained by individuals using the same information. No one can completely and accurately predict the future, but what we can do is err on the side of caution and plan for a more secure, healthy, and progressive one.

Although most of the facts presented herein are defensible, I use them as literary, entertainment, and educational devices to give the reader a general perspective on the subject of resources and energy used in our homes. In an effort to communicate more easily and effectively I have taken averages, mean numbers, sometimes common sense, and have modified statements to reflect more than one, set opinion and/or I have updated them. However, we have tried to make this book as clear and concise as possible.

Legally it would be put in another way: Neither the writer, the publisher, nor any of their employees makes any warranty, or guarantee, express or implied, or assumes any legal liability or responsibility for the accuracy, completeness, or usefulness of any information, percentage, apparatus, product, device, or process disclosed, or represents that its use would not infringe privately owned rights. Reference herein to any specific commercial copyright, product, process, or service by trade name, trademark, manufacturer, or otherwise, does not necessarily constitute or imply its endorsement or recommendation. The views and opinions of authors expressed herein do not necessarily state or reflect those of Rowman & Littlefield Publishing or its agents. The information and/or products mentioned herein do not imply an endorsement, guarantee, or warranty. This book is for entertainment and educational purposes only.

1

Introduction

Conserve to Preserve: What Does This Mean to Me?

You've made the plunge and closed the deal. This is perhaps the first and largest investment and financial commitment you'll ever make—your own home. Perhaps you're renting, about to remodel, making a major home purchase, downsizing, or looking for something new in which to live. For all the above situations, and for all of us, new rules apply when considering conserving energy, resources, and making constructive changes for our environment and our Earth. Analysis from the Energy Information Administration's (EIA) most recent Residential Energy Consumption Survey (RECS) shows that US homes built in 2000 and later consume only 2 percent more energy on average than homes built prior to 2000, despite being on average 30 percent larger.

After location, size, style, and the number of bedrooms and bathrooms have been locked down, most people miss a very important aspect of their home—energy efficiency, and how much it will cost to run a home from room to room, top to bottom, interior to exterior. Although some homebuyers and even homebuilders appreciate energy efficiency, they often aren't willing to seek it out, let alone pay extra for it. Surveys show that buyers appreciate green features, but it becomes a disconnect when house hunting, or when it involves paying extra for green features, and realtors claim it's just icing on the cake when evaluating a home. However, there is a trend emerging that energy-efficiency and sustainability certifications for homes may result in easier sales and higher sales prices of 8 to 10 percent. Plus, a nice byproduct is a warm glow of conservation.

Watching a home improvement channel's programming about buying a home, the first-time buyer's wish list always includes things such as crown molding, hardwood floors, granite countertops, an updated kitchen, modernized bathrooms, and charm. Rarely do the new homeowners ask about the type and age of the furnace, condition of ductworks, double-pane windows, the type and condition of insulation, energy-efficient appliances, home ventilation and cooling, whether the yard is water-wise, what it will to cost to run the house during each season, and if the house has ever had an energy audit. Moreover, most homebuyers have never heard of, let alone used, what is called an Energy-Efficient Mortgage (EEM).

EEMs provide the borrower with special benefits when purchasing a home that is energy efficient, or one that can be made efficient through the installation of energy-saving improvements. Research and advocacy groups like the National Home Performance Council and CNT Energy (Center for Neighborhood Technology) in Chicago have done research on how energy-efficiency transparency can encourage homeowners to invest in such improvements. When you are buying, selling, refinancing, or remodeling your home, you can also increase your comfort and actually save money by using an EEM. It is easy to use, federally recognized, and can be applied to most home mortgages.

The federal SAVE Act (Sensible Accounting to Value Energy) allows homebuyers to qualify for larger mortgages when purchasing energy-efficient homes. At the same time, the real estate industry is working to standardize and improve how it reports and evaluates energy improvements for existing homes.

Not only is type and overall energy use important to homeowners, but it can have positive or negative consequences for the planet. There has been much sound and fury in recent years about what is called a change in weather patterns, global warming, or lately, climate change, and what each of us can do about it. Simply put, climate change is any alteration of the condition of the Earth and atmosphere over a large number of years. Weather, which is affected by climate change, is what you see when you look out the window. Now let's look at some energy concerns.

Most of the electricity produced in the United States comes from fossil fuels. Worldwide humans put 100 million metric tons of carbon dioxide (CO_2) a day into the atmosphere, and the United States makes the second largest contribution to that figure. China is now the dubious champ. One of the problems of burning fossil fuels is a byproduct called greenhouse gas (GHG), made primarily of CO_2. There are 40 percent more GHGs in the atmosphere than there were at the time of the industrial revolution, roughly 150 years ago, and the world emits 48 percent more carbon dioxide from the consumption of energy now than it did in 1992. Ironically, when in balance CO_2 keeps the Earth's temperature stabilized, but too much can either heat or cool the planet so life as we know it is no longer possible.

Growth Rates of Greenhouse Gas

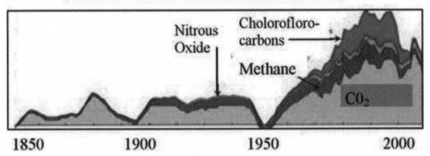

1850   1900   1950   2000

Figure 1.1.   Growth rates of greenhouse gas.
Source: NASA.

The combustion of fossil fuels to generate electricity is the largest single source of CO_2 emissions in the United States, accounting for about 38 percent of all emissions and 32 percent of total US greenhouse gas emissions. Consequently, how much energy homeowners use is vital. Each consumer has choices about the type of power to use. The truth is that there is no perfect energy source, but the fact remains that the demand for electricity will likely triple in the next two decades; hopefully it will come from a renewable and sustainable resources.

And whether or not you believe in climate change, one of the clean, sustainable remedies to this condition is conservation—which is a good thing whether you are liberal or conservative. Conservation is what some scientists call the "low-hanging fruit" of energy resource management. It is the easiest, cheapest, and foremost task in which every person can participate. In fact, conservation can save about 1.7 cents per kilowatt-hour (kWh), while finding new sources of energy costs about ten cents per kWh.

Despite doomsday headlines, there are many bright spots in the combat against climate change and the resolve to conserve energy and resources:

James Hansen, a well-known astrophysicist and climatologist, says, "The real key to preventing climate change is reducing home energy use."

FACTS AND FIGURES

Very encouraging trends include an ongoing improvement in global energy management leading to far fewer emissions, price-induced conservation of energy, and a dramatic increase in solar and wind power over the last decade is causing a rapid transformation in how we produce energy. Global wind power has grown about 25 percent per year in the last decade, and global solar power has grown an average of 68 percent each year over the last five years, according to Bloomberg New Energy Finance. At these rates of growth some scientists optimistically claim that alternative power sources could provide the entire global demand by 2030—if everyone used them, and the fossil fuel industry unplugged from petro chemicals.

Emissions in the United States have declined 8 percent in the last five years. Various states have been employing alternative sources of power—70 percent of Vermont's power is nuclear; California uses water, solar, and wind power; Georgia is regularly ranked among the top ten states for solar resources; and Oregon's legislation has called for decreasing use of fossil fuels, to name a few.

The EPA (Environmental Protection Agency) is moving forward with the regulations required by the Clean Air Act to regulate new power plant emissions of CO_2, the primary greenhouse gas causing global warming. The United States has committed to cut carbon emissions by 26 percent to 28 percent of 2005 levels by 2025. This represents an acceleration of its existing goal to reduce emissions by 17 percent.

There is no single magic bullet that is going to forestall the change in environment and resource management—it's going to take a shotgun approach. Conservation is only one weapon in an arsenal of change that takes planning, work, and energy. Remember when recycling was a pain? Now people do it by habit and scold those who don't.

The treasury of information in this book will offer hard facts and figures about resource and energy use, along with practical suggestions about how to monitor and make decisions that could save you a lot of money and the planet a lot of nasty gases.

This book will take the big picture in small steps: room to room, floor to ceiling, by appliances, fixtures, indoors and outdoors, and more without making you feel hopeless, helpless, or generally overwhelmed.

We'll finish with a do-it-yourself Home Energy Audit to help you get an appraisal of your energy use and efficiency, and to find areas you can easily improve. By using only a fraction of what's inside this book, this investment will pay for itself very quickly—and keep giving over the years if you follow its advice. This home energy and resource guide will get into that and lots more about recycling, resources, and the way we use and misuse our resources.

One last thought about the apocalyptic environmental "end of times" predictors and their "chicken little" acolytes. There have always been prophets of doom and naysayers about population explosions in the past and lately about a topic called climate change. Scientists who are specialists in this field have compiled a lot of compelling information concerning this forecast brought on by man's contamination of the atmosphere and Earth. True, we are witnessing some inconvenient and ominous transformations and perhaps we're in the beginning of a perfect storm of environmental change brought on by our own doing. And because the sky is not falling today doesn't mean it won't fall in the next several decades. Remember the gas shortages in the 1970s that had people fighting over petrol? It only took a year or two before people forgot about it and used more gas in bigger cars.

So it makes a lot of sense to pay attention—both for the investment in the present and for the savings return in the future and to make sure to conserve our precious planet. Making your energy and resource use lean will give a nice green glow to you, your wallet, and our Earth.

2

Your Home

And Its Appetites

When people receive the inevitable and somewhat bothersome monthly visitors—their water and power bills—many wonder what does this mean and where does all that money go? These days people have a lot more things that cost a lot to run and maintain. Think of the house as a very large and complex machine that should run efficiently and be maintained properly when it comes to energy. Our aim is to tune up that machine and ease the burden of climate change while shrinking the size of your monthlies, and to live a little more lightly and slightly.

The good news is that the big energy suckers in your home—air conditioner, refrigerator, clothes washer, and even light bulbs—have become far more efficient. Compared with 1980 models, clothes washers now use 70 percent less electricity. New LED light bulbs use 80 percent less, and refrigerators use 60 percent less power.

Compared to newer homes, those built before 1980 tend to be poorly insulated and leak a lot of energy like poorly constructed cottages and drafty castles. The comfort and condition of the family home and wallet can be improved by remembering energy conservation, checking water systems, insulation, keeping a watch on the kitchen and bathroom appliances, creating more efficient lighting, heating, and cooling, improving ventilation, eliminating drafts and moisture levels in winter, and reducing attic temperatures in summer.

Despite the advances in energy-saving technologies and improvements which have helped cut the energy consumption of appliances by as much as 50 percent in recent years, as a nation, the United States consumes far more energy than it did over forty years ago because of our unquenchable thirst for power to run larger homes and the stuff in them. In fact, our consumption of electricity is due to rise as much as 30 percent or more in the next two decades, which will have far-reaching consequences regarding pollution, power, and water resources.

Our homes cause more air pollution than our cars and Americans spend 90 percent of their time indoors where the air quality is poorer than it is than outdoors. When speaking of power and pollution, most of the energy we use in the home comes from power plants, which burn fossil fuels. So the by-product of turning on the stove, the water, or the heater is air pollution, acid rain, and greenhouse gases that ultimately cause climate change. Hopefully, new technologies of wind, sun, and other alternative and sustainable power sources will close the energy and pollution sinkhole, but in reality many other countries are still planning scores of new fossil fuel–fired plants. Although US carbon emissions have been receding, we are not the best example for energy conservation or reduction of ground, air, and water pollution. But for the most part we are trying to improve and change our wasteful ways. The habit of being a fossil fuel junkie is hard to kick.

President Obama has set a new goal of cutting US carbon pollution by 26 to 28 percent of 2005 levels by 2025 and China has committed to peak CO_2 emissions, and then boost the use of non-fossil energy by 20 percent by 2030. Although President Obama believes we have a moral obligation to take action on climate change, and China seems to be getting on board the non-fossil fuel bandwagon, there is no guarantee that these changes will be abided by the next administration.

In California there are state-mandated standards for homebuilding efficiency known as Title 24, which prescribes methods for calculating the sizes of home windows, the capacities of air conditioners and heaters, and various thicknesses of insulation. A small cottage industry has sprung up to perform the engineering calculations required for any new commercial or residential construction, or for major changes to existing structures. Check your area for this kind of building code.

Efficiency is the swiftest, most inexpensive way to conserve energy, slow down the CO_2 overdose in the atmosphere, and cut your utility bill by 30 percent. Poor insulation, inefficient appliances, drafty homes, and other fixable faults cost US consumers over $300 billion per year—about one-third of our military budget!

FACTS AND FIGURES

Energy use in America is doubling every twenty years. In 2014, the United States used approximately 412 billion kWh of electricity (or a quadrillion

Btus) costing more than $241 billion on home energy use in the United States. According to the Organization of American States (OAS) Department of Sustainable Development (DSD), the average American household uses 12,000 to 18,000 kilowatt-hours (kWh) yearly, which averages $1,500 to $3,000 per year; and unfortunately a lot of that is wasted. Compare that usage with yours.

About 20 percent of the nation's energy dollars are spent in homes. Energy efficiency improvements could cut this number by well over 30 percent. American homes produce 21 percent of US emissions, a greater percentage of CO_2 emissions than the combined emissions from autos and light trucks. That's 1.2 billion tons of greenhouse gas emissions emitted annually (as carbon dioxide) into the atmosphere. According to the US Department of Energy, if US consumers were just 5 percent more efficient in their homes, it would be equal to removing the emissions from 53 million cars.

The American Council for an Energy-Efficient Economy (ACEEE) estimates that if we increase the energy efficiency in just our major appliances by 10 to 30 percent, it would be the equivalent of shutting down twenty-five large power plants.

Homes built between 2000 and 2005 use 14 percent less energy per square foot than homes built in the 1980s, and 40 percent less energy per square foot than homes built before 1950. Thirty years ago the average American home had three to four electronic devices in it. Today the average is more like two dozen which creates about six times the need for energy in the nation, even if those devices are "energy savers."

One study at the Lawrence Berkeley National Laboratory (Berkeley Lab) showed that electricity consumption in American homes is growing faster in the category of small appliances than in any other group. The average American family creates fourteen to fifty tons of carbon dioxide per year. Multiply that by 100 million households and it is evident that consumers are responsible for more than 70 percent of the five to seven billion tons of CO_2 our nation emits each year—an 8 percent increase from 1990.

HOME TROUBLE SPOTS

The following are places where homes lose a lot of energy through improper insulation, air leakage, and poor ventilation.

- Roofs: up to 80 percent of their energy consumption
- Ceilings: 10 percent
- Walls: 12 to 14 percent

- Floors and below-grade space: 15 to 18 percent
- Windows and doors: 18 to 20 percent
- Infiltration and air leakage: 35 percent
- Garden and water conservation: some experts estimate that more than 50 percent of landscape water use goes to waste due to evaporation or runoff caused by overwatering

PRACTICAL SUGGESTIONS

Following a few simple steps could cut your waste amounts and CO_2 discharge by 60 percent. Between 1960 and 1990 trash production doubled and remains at about 4.5 pounds per person per day. Bottom line: Use and buy with care. Borrow, lend, share. This goes for books, magazines, DVDs, CDs, even tools. One study showed that the average power tool bought by a homeowner is used from six minutes to an hour in its lifetime. Buy for the long run and durability, not for throwaway. Think locally concerning transportation costs and related pollution.

Don't buy overpackaged products or products packaged in individual serving sizes. For example, ask your butcher or restaurants to wrap your purchases in paper, not in Styrofoam trays. Be sure to look at whether a package is recyclable before you buy it. If you cannot avoid getting a plastic bag from the store, reuse it for wrapping leftovers or as a trash bag for the bathroom

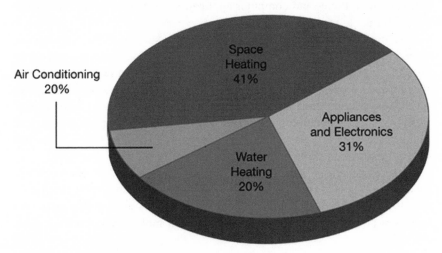

Figure 2.1. Largest users of electricity in the home.
Source: U.S. Energy Information Administration.

or bedroom. Ask that store clerks not bag items that have their own handles, are easily carried, or when the items are going straight from cart to car to kitchen. You can reuse containers instead of plastic bags for wrapping and storage. Buy fresh, unpackaged fruits and vegetables and grains, pasta, and dried fruit in bulk.

Go paperless! Use bags (preferably canvas) when you go shopping. Paper constitutes about 30 percent of average American garbage. Use fabric instead of paper napkins, especially if you can use them for more than one meal. Avoid using nonrecyclable paper plates and plastic tableware. Reduce the paper overload by using the Internet for paying bills, etc. Avoid brochures and flyers by calling and asking to be removed from mailing lists. The energy used to produce, deliver, and dispose of junk mail in the United States produces more greenhouse gas emissions than 2.8 million cars.

Give away or sell what is not used or needed. Look for sites such as freecycle.net, trashnothing.com, recycletheworld.org, ilovefreegle.org, simplegive.com, or donate to local churches or charities. Purchase used products and choose to reuse or repair instead of replacing them.

PRACTICAL SUGGESTIONS: EFFICIENT ELECTRONICS

Many local utility companies offer free or low-cost energy-efficiency home evaluations and rebates for using energy-efficient products. These days, you can use smartphones and computer applications to help monitor energy use in real time.

Do a nightly sweep through the house to make sure all electric devices are turned off before going to bed, and use nonelectric tools and manual appliances such as a can opener. Find alternatives to watching television, playing video games, renting video tapes, and surfing the Internet—like talking, reading books, playing card and board games, doing puzzles and word games, playing charades, and doing crafts and family projects. Camping or being out of doors where there is no electrical power, Internet, or Wi-Fi can do wonders for communication skills between friends, family, and even strangers.

Up to 75 percent of all the energy you pay for is wasted by electronic appliances and devices using phantom or standby electricity. (See chapter on Standby Power.) You could save more than $150 per year by using surge protectors or power strips that can turn off single or multiple electronic devices.

AROUND THE HOUSE AND NEIGHBORHOOD

Buy organic foods as much as possible. Organic soils capture and store carbon dioxide at much higher levels than soils from conventional farms and use fertilizers made from fossil fuels. If we grew all of our corn and soybeans organically, we'd remove 580 billion pounds of carbon dioxide from the atmosphere. Seek out and support local farmers markets; they reduce the amount of energy required to grow and transport the food by one-fifth. Look for a farmers market in your area and at the USDA Web site: http://search. ams.usda.gov/farmersmarkets/.

Start neighborhood potlucks or barbecues featuring utility-free or utility-reduced meals. Put on neighborhood yard sales emphasizing recycling. The proceeds can go toward emergency supplies for yourself, for your town, or for community funds to help needy neighbors with utility bills or home weatherization. Make a neighborhood commitment to saving energy. Choose projects or set goals. Examples: skipping television one night a week, agreeing to forego decorative holiday lighting, or having friends and neighbors over.

Promote sleepovers for neighborhood kids to save energy and get to know your neighbors. Teach the neighborhood kids to look for air leaks, drafts, and places that need to be weatherized—at the expense of making them environmental cops.

Take turns shopping for and with neighbors, especially those who need a little assistance. Distribute lists of energy conservation tips and choose a neighborhood project or set neighborhood goals.

Table 2.1. Life Expectancy of Household Items

Appliances	Life in Years
Compactors	10
Dishwashers	10
Dryers	14
Disposal	10
Freezers, compact	12
Freezers, standard	16
Microwave ovens	11
Electric ranges	17
Gas ranges	19
Gas ovens	14
Refrigerators, compact	14
Refrigerators, standard	17
Washers, automatic, and compact	13
Exhaust fans	20

Source: Appliance Statistical Review, April 1990

REBATES AND INCENTIVES

Check out state and local governments and utility companies that may offer financial incentives for homeowners to upgrade their appliances to newer, more energy-efficient models, especially those identified by the EnergyStar label. The partnership between the Environmental Protection agency (EPA) and the US Department of Energy identifies energy-efficient products and appliances. Check local utilities, state agencies, and Web sites such as Advanced Home Energy for assistance in tax incentives and even cash rebates. Find incentives offered by checking your online state database, or the Database of State Incentives for Renewables and Efficiency (DSIRE).

GREEN-RATED CHECKLISTS AND BUILDING GUIDELINES

Look for your state's adoption of Green Building Standards Codes for residential homes, and download the free GreenPoint Rated checklists. Also, check your county listing for the Green Building Guidelines, a comprehensive resource of voluntary best practices for green building. These guidelines offer recommended practices for improving indoor air quality, increasing energy and water efficiency, conserving natural resources, and planning for healthy and vibrant communities.

SOMETHING TO THINK ABOUT: JAPAN'S TOP RUNNER PROGRAM

In 1998, Japan introduced an innovative addition to its existing Energy Conservation Law. The Top Runner Program is designed to promote ongoing efficiency improvements in appliances, machinery, and equipment used in the residential, commercial, and transportation sectors.

Committees composed of representatives from industry, academia, trade unions, and consumer groups identify the most efficient model currently on the market in a particular product category. The energy performance of this "Top Runner" model is used to set a target for all manufacturers to achieve within the next four to eight years.

As a result, Japan not only has one of the most energy-efficient economies in the world, it plans to be 30 percent more efficient than it is now (measured by energy use compared to economic growth) by 2030.

To begin conserving and saving money, let's take a trip throughout your house from the ground up.

3

How to Read Your Utility Bill

Understanding the Why and the What

Be warned that the following chapter can be as bewildering as your tax return, but it is just as important. So for those who don't care, don't want to learn, and are happy with ignorant bliss, go ahead and move on to the next chapter. All others, ready? Okay.

UTILITY BILL BASICS

Many electric and gas customers open their bill, look at the amount, and simply pay it, because to most of us it looks perplexing. If your utility bill, with its kWh, therms, and tier rates, has you dazed, the California Public Utilities Commission offers this brief primer on how to read a utility bill so you know how much energy you have used and how much it cost.

The Public Utilities Code (PUC) establishes baseline quantities for average residential gas and electricity use within an area. The PUC specifically requires that baseline quantities fall between 50 percent and 60 percent of average use for basic electric customers in both the summer and winter, and for all electric and gas customers in the summer. The PU code also requires that baseline quantities fall between 60 percent to 70 percent of average use for all electric and gas customers in the winter. For example in northern California, Pacific Gas and Electric (PG&E) sets its baseline summer season as April 1 to October 31 for gas and May 1 to October 31 for electric. PG&E's winter baseline season is November 1 to March 31 for gas and November 1 to April 30 for electric.

Your electric bill is based on how much electricity you used during the billing period. Usage is measured in kilowatt-hours (kWh) and is determined by the information on your electric meter. The utility company records the current reading and compares it with the last month's reading. The difference between the two readings is the total usage for the month and is recorded as a total number of kilowatt-hours. Remember that meter readers and even smart meters make mistakes, so watch your bill.

GAS

Gas usage remains at a two-tier structure. Rates for tier 1—the baseline tier— will continue to be billed at the baseline rate; tier 2 rates—over baseline— apply to gas use beyond set baseline quantities. Customers are billed at the baseline rate for gas use up to the baseline limit. Beyond this level consumers are charged at the "over baseline" rate, priced at a higher level.

WHAT TO LOOK FOR IN YOUR ELECTRICITY BILL

Make a note of your utility account number. It will get you faster service if you need it. The rate schedule identifies the type of utility service received and the plan used to bill you. Service dates mark the beginning and the end of the billing period.

"Baseline quantity" is an allocation of electricity that is billed at a lower rate for residential customers. This is predicated on approximately 50 percent of average use for residential customers in a geographic area during summer and 60 to 70 percent during winter.

Baselines are determined by the California Public Utilities Commission established by the number of days in the billing period, season, climatic region, and whether your primary heating source is gas or electricity.

All electricity usage over baseline is charged at a higher rate. Pacific Gas & Electric, for example, bills by tiers 2 through 5. PG&E baseline costs start at $.12 per kWh, and go up to $.40 per kWh for tiers 4 and 5. Baselines will vary by state and location.

A Pacific Gas & Electric bill (in northern California) is calculated by multiplying the number of kWh (hours) used by the kWh rate (cost). The calculation is made according to the "tiers" of usage. For specific information about a bill, contact your utility.

SOME DEFINITIONS

A watt is a measure of power equal to about 1/740 of one horsepower, or calculated by multiplying amperage by voltage. Wattage, measured in watts, is an amount of power produced or electricity consumed.

One kilowatt-hour (kWh) equals 1,000 watts of electricity used for an hour. To understand how kilowatts are calculated, picture a 100-watt light bulb burning for one hour. The bulb uses 100 watts of electricity. If it burns for ten hours, that equals one kilowatt (100 watts × 10 hours = 1,000 watts, or one kilowatt). Burning that one bulb for those ten hours costs about ten cents (depending on your power provider's rates, location, demand for power, type of power used to produce electricity, etc.).

For reference, a medium-sized electric car that consumes 100,000 watts (one horsepower is equivalent to 740 watts) would produce 286 horsepower.

The volt is a unit of electric potential and electromotive force. Just like water needs pressure to force it through a hose, electrical current needs some force to make it flow. A volt is the measure of electrical pressure. The United States uses a 120-volt system, with 220 used for some appliances, like clothes dryers. In Europe a 220-volt system is used.

The rate or amount of electric current is measured in amperes (amps). A typical household circuit carries 15 to 50 amps. The information concerning the amount of amps needed to power a device is found on its label.

A British thermal unit (Btu) is the amount of heat energy needed to raise the temperature of one pound of water by one degree Fahrenheit (°F). A therm is a unit of heat equivalent to 100,000 Btus.

This is the standard measurement used to state the amount of energy that a fuel contains, also the amount of output of any heat-generating device.

PUBLIC UTILITY TERMS

Public Purpose Programs are state-mandated programs such as low-income discount and energy efficiency programs.

Transmission charges are associated with transporting electricity over long distances, from generating facilities to distribution substations in your neighborhood.

Distribution charges cover the costs of providing local service. This in-cludes delivering power to your home or business, wires, poles, repair crews, and emergency and other customer services.

Energy charges calculate the actual cost of the electricity you use by multi-plying the applicable rate by the number of kilowatt-hours consumed.

The usage comparison section shows your usage in the current billing period this year versus the same billing period last year in both total kWh and kWh per day. This information can help gauge your conservation efforts. Under the California 20/20 Rebate Program, customers who reduce their electricity use during summer will receive a 20 percent discount on their bills. Check your utility company for rebates.

Rotating outage block, expressed as a number, is your place in the utility's planned outage schedule. Outage announcements will specify which outage block was or will be affected and may help you plan for scheduled outages in your area.

COSTS OF FOSSIL FUEL ENERGY FOR THE HOME

- Propane (95,000 Btu/gal) @ $1.55 per gal = $16.25 per million Btu.
- Oil (140,000 Btu/gal) @ $2.00 per gal = $14.30 per million Btu.
- Electricity (3410 Btu/KWh) @ $.10 per KWh = $29.00 per million Btu.
- Gas sells at about $9.00 per million Btu.

(Prices are quoted as of 2013 and may change due to location and market fluctuations.)

GAS APPLIANCES

- Cost of operation = Btus × rate of therm × hours used. For example: A gas clothes dryer uses 20,000 Btus per hour.
- Estimate that it runs one hour per load.
- Cost of operation = 20,000 × $1.25/therm × 1 = $.25.

ELECTRIC APPLIANCES

To find the wattage of an appliance, divide the wattage by 1,000 to get the kilowatts used per hour. Multiply this by rate per kilowatt-hour and by the number of hours the appliance is used: Cost of operation = Wattage × rate/ kWh × hours used.

Some appliances cycle on and off automatically, using energy only when they are on. To figure their energy use, estimate the amount of time they're being used. For example, a medium-sized window air conditioner uses 500 watts per hour. Estimate that it runs 10 hours a day. If a utility company charges ten cents per kWh, then multiply it by 1.47 Btus (that would be your consumption for 1 hour of use of your 5,000-Btu window unit air conditioner). That comes to 14.7 cents per hour.

Now multiply that by 24 hours and you see it will cost about $3.52 per day, or $105.60 per month. Actually, it will be much less because the compressor in the unit (the main draw of power) is turning on and off constantly as the room needs it.

If the previous examples were too complicated, simply use this Web site calculator: http://energyusecalculator.com.

THE WATER METER

The water meter may be located outside the house near the front sidewalk in a direct line with the outside main faucet or valve (where you turn the water off to your home or business). It is usually housed in a concrete box below the sidewalk marked with your utility's initials or simply "water." If you have trouble locating your meter, call your water company.

Keep your meter clean by clearing out any vegetation or debris. Insert a screwdriver or a small crowbar in the hole on the cover to pry open the lid. The concrete lid is heavy, so be careful of fingers and toes when handling it. Set the lid aside and check carefully inside the meter box to look for anything that may bite you. To read the meter, lift the metal cover on the instrument. The water meter is read in cubic feet. Always close the cover on your water meter after you are finished.

In addition to providing you with information about how much water you are using, reading your meter can help you detect leaks in your household plumbing. To check for a leak you must first turn off all faucets inside and outside your home. Be certain the toilet is not flushed and the automatic ice cube maker is not operating when performing this task. Mark the position of the meter's sweep hand lightly with a pencil. When the water is turned off, the indicator should not move. A circular motion by the indicator suggests a leak. Wait approximately 30 minutes before rechecking the sweep hand. If it has moved, you have a leak.

Of course, you want to ensure you can easily and correctly read your meter. Do not plant trees or shrubs close to the meter box; their roots may damage the meter or service pipe. Do not ground electrical wires to any water service pipe, which is illegal and potentially dangerous. Make certain that garbage cans, parked cars, or other objects are not covering or in the way of it.

HOW TO READ A WATER METER

Pay attention to your meter; it not only measures the amount of water used, but it can tell if you are paying for more than you are using. A water bill is either based on a flat rate, a tiered rate, or both. You are billed at a base rate prorated on your yearly use, and then further calculated by a tier rate.

Rates increase with usage of water. For billing purposes water consumption is measured in Ccfs, or hundred cubic feet. But you can easily calculate your usage in gallons for tracking your consumption on a daily or weekly basis. One revolution of the water meter sweep hand equals one cubic foot or 7.48 gallons.

HOW TO READ YOUR STATEMENT

The account number is on the bill close to your name. The account details section shows your previous balance, payments, adjustments, and current charges. The headings indicate whether water charges are based on member or nonmember rates and which municipality sets the rates.

Deduct the previous reading from the current reading to determine water consumption, which is measured in hundreds of cubic feet. For example: 1 hundred cubic feet = 748 gallons of water. Most bills should have a thirteen-month consumption summary. This feature compares current water and waste-water consumption to the previous twelve months. It also shows how many days are included in the billing period. If there are more days in the period, consumption may be higher. Fewer days may cause consumption to be lower.

Other reasons for higher consumption may be an addition to your house-hold, a seasonal change (watering lawns), or a plumbing leak that needs to be repaired. To calculate your water use, subtract the previous meter reading from the current meter reading. Example: 563.04 - 561.83 = 1.21 Ccf (1 Ccf = 100 cubic feet or 748 gallons).

There are two sets of charges on the water/sewer bill. The charges show water base fee, how much water was used, and what rates were charged for the water. They also show a sewer base fee, a sewer charge, and the storm drain fee. When totaled, this gives you a total amount due. If under the code heading you find the letter E, it means your bill for this month has been estimated.

The water fees reflect the city or county's cost to treat and deliver water throughout the area, for running daily operations, and paying for the work that has to be done to be in compliance with state and federal government regulations such as the Safe Drinking Water Act.

Conservation information: This box tracks water usage compared to the previous year. New homeowners will have it compared to a citywide average.

Base fee/water: This is a nonvariable amount collected to offset fixed costs of running the Public Utilities Department. Such costs include rent, running the Customer Services Section, and paying for a portion of the fixed operating costs of the water system including routine maintenance and replacement of facilities.

Water used: This is a variable fee based upon the amount of water used. Money collected through this fee pays for buying, treating, and delivering water, as well as for the maintenance, repair, and replacement of the water system.

Base fee/sewer: This is a nonvariable amount collected to offset the fixed costs of running a metropolitan wastewater department. Fixed costs include routine maintenance and replacement of the sewer system.

Sewer: Single-family domestic customers have an individualized sewer rate based upon the amount of water used and costs to run, repair, and replace the sewage system.

Storm drain fee: This fee pays for the cleaning, repair, and maintenance of the city's storm drain system.

IF YOU ARE BILLED SEPARATELY FOR GAS

Most residential gas meters read like an odometer. Gas meters measure the amount of cubic feet of natural gas used in a given month. Though meters vary in size and shape, they all record gas consumption in basically the same way. Well-maintained gas meters have proved to be over 99 percent accurate.

Gas companies bill by hundreds of cubic feet of gas (Ccf) or by therms—approximately the energy equivalent of burning 100 cubic feet (often referred to as 1 Ccf) of natural gas.

Some residential meters are dial meters represented by five or six dials. Some dials run clockwise, but others run counterclockwise. Gas consumption is determined by the top four dials. If the pointer is between two numbers, record the smaller number. Subtract the previous reading from the current reading to find out how many cubic feet were used.

Remember that the above is an example of what and how California utility consumers are billed. Contact your utility provider for more specific information about your area.

4

Smart Meters

Electronic Mentors or Monsters?

Soon, almost every aspect of modern life at home will be "smart," meaning that our homes are going to be run by computers which if not smarter than humans, are better at keeping score. A smart meter is a digital device that records the consumption of electricity and natural gas, and communicates that information to the consumer and to a utility company for monitoring and billing purposes. Even our country's energy grid will be smart one day (see chapter 27, "The Grid").

However, this modern technology hasn't been without controversy. Many consumers from coast to coast have complained that their smart meters logged a 30 percent to 70 percent jump in electricity consumption in just one year, or that the quality of service from their utilities company has nosedived. Further debate concerns the health effects of electromagnetic radiation and radio waves, accuracy, safety, personal privacy, and governmental issues.

FACTS AND FIGURES

A recent tragedy in San Bruno, California, heightened the debate over the safety of PG&E's SmartMeters. On September 9, 2010, a major natural gas leak and subsequent explosion of a gas pipeline killed eight people, injured thirty-eight, and destroyed thirty-eight homes, damaging seventy others. There was speculation that a SmartMeter may have contributed to the explosion by creating minute sparks, much the same as a cell phone could, which may have ignited a gas leak in the pipeline.

In northern California the small town of Fairfax, waggishly nicknamed "Mayberry on marijuana" because of its reputation as a sort of suburban

Berkeley, tried to stop or at least put a leash on PG&E's SmartMeter installation project. The town council raised concerns over the meters producing unhealthy electromagnetic radiation. In northern California, PG&E's main customer region, several citizens' committees asked for a halt to SmartMeter installation pending a full investigation. One point that especially rankles some free-thinking citizens is that smart meters are an example of having a device technocratically forced upon the population without any degree of democratic input. Simply stated: bad vibes, man.

Paul Moreno, spokesperson for PG&E, has said repeatedly that their meters do not pose a health risk as the emitted radio signals are well within limits established by the Federal Communications Commission: "The meters emit a 45-second signal every 24 hours, the strength of which is about .001 watts of energy or about 1/1000 of a cell phone call, far below the levels in many common household appliances, including computers, microwaves, and cell phones. PG&E complies with Federal Communications Commission regulations, by a very wide margin."

The World Health Organization has reviewed the issue and determined there is no connection between low-level electromagnetic emissions and negative health effects. However, PG&E has since instituted an opt-out alternative. (For more info check out: http://www.smartmeterdangers.org/).

Some critics claim that smart meters might actually cause increased customer energy consumption and energy consumption behavior to become worse since electricity is cheap, lessening consumer resolve to conserve. In addition, consumers might be tempted to let the machines make energy decisions that should be their responsibility.

According to Katherine Hamilton, the president of GridWise Alliance, a coalition of technology companies and utilities, there's evidence to suggest that smart meters are far more accurate than older meters. "Analog meters degrade and slow down over time," she says. "Immediately, when you put in a digital meter, the reading will become more accurate." That should translate into consumer savings.

By the way, want a remedy for bad vibes? Those still concerned about the radiation effect from smart meters can attach sheets of tinfoil to the wall behind a meter and attach a grounding wire to a pipe or other ground source. This should absorb any wayward electromagnetic signals.

Despite these concerns, smart systems for homes and buildings are the wave of the future. The worldwide base of smart meters is going to grow rapidly. The estimated annual growth rate will be 31 percent in the next several years reaching 302.5 million devices installed by 2016, and by 2020 it is projected to increase to reach between 75 percent and 100 percent of homes in California. In the next few years the majority of all electricity meters shipped to the world's leading economies are expected to have advanced functions and networking capabilities.

PRACTICAL APPLICATIONS

According to PG&E, this technology is designed to not only allow you more energy management decisions, but also offers options to set personal preferences in financially and environmentally responsible ways, making life easier while lowering your energy bill.

Some utility companies charge more for power during peak hours—typically between 2 p.m. and 7 p.m.—but generally most offer a set price for power, supposedly better regulated by smart meters. Smart technology will help utility companies to detect and manage outages, pinpoint problems on the power grid, and allow utilities to determine which customers are without power. At present many communities rely on customers to report power failures. Smart technology (smart meters, energy panels, and smart appliances) also enables consumer access to accurate information about where energy is being consumed, how much energy is used during peak times, and about how their electricity is priced.

Smart meters will point out certain irregular peaks, which may mean that an appliance, whether a toaster or a furnace, is out of whack and needs to be repaired or replaced. Smart meters, in tandem with smart appliances, work to avoid peak-hour energy prices and demands. For example, a clothes dryer will automatically switch from high to a lower setting if electricity hits a certain rate, or a refrigerator can delay an automatic defrost cycle. Consequently, employing a smart meter allows the consumer to compare prices when deciding when and how much power to buy.

Smart meters can communicate information via smart home energy panels (kind of like a home energy Internet). This detailed information presented online reports how power is distributed and consumed, enabling the meter to make smarter energy choices throughout the day. Smart meters, coupled with advanced metering infrastructure (AMI), will also enable consumers to pre-pay their electricity bill if they wish. The new meter also allows the utility company to read energy usage remotely, eliminating the need for meter readers. Of course the meter readers don't like this.

Reading a smart electric meter is easy. The meter automatically scrolls through several different displays. Each display remains on screen for three to five seconds. These displays will show your kilowatt-hour usage, date and time, and other useful network and diagnostic information. Consumers are responsible for the cost of installing home displays to control appliances and other equipment. According to a study by the US Department of Energy, real-time pricing information provided by the SmartMeter helped consumers reduce their electricity costs by 10 percent on average and 15 percent for off-peak consumption. It is estimated by PG&E that SmartMeters will result in billions of dollars in energy savings to consumers.

ADVANCED METERING INFRASTRUCTURE FOR NATURAL GAS

AMI has been referred to as "the other grid" for gas. The smart gas grid is becoming an area of increasing focus for utilities, especially utilities that supply both electricity and gas. Natural gas information is available via a smart system on a daily basis, and the meters are read the same way as electricity meters.

In the next couple of decades, it is inevitable that smart meters for gas will be installed in most homes and businesses. This will result in:

- Reduction in meter reading labor costs.
- Increase in meter reading frequency and accuracy.
- Power quality monitoring and load planning, protection analysis, troubleshooting, and outage detection which are very important due to the volatility of natural gas.
- Remote disconnect capability, also critical to diminish or stop pipeline leaks.
- Prevention of gas theft.

SMART WATER MEASURE

Droughts, water scarcity, and the need for more food will increase the need for water by about 50 percent by 2050. This is putting pressure on water utilities around the country to manage and modernize water infrastructure (see "Water Watch," chapter 15). That means that smart meters will be coming to your neighborhood soon—or to more than 153 million homes in the next decade. That will enhance badly needed leak detection and water pressure, quality, and quantity management for water operations and distribution. That means that the water company is going to have its nozzle pointed at your consumption and what to do about it.

Switching to smart technology delivers benefits for both the utility and their customers. The ability to analyze and identify patterns in the data is an important piece of overall oversight. Utilities companies say this information will be used to manage many operating mechanisms and to identify performance issues, improve customer service, and better prioritize future investments in infrastructure. Water conservation also positively affects the bottom line of water utilities by reducing their energy consumption. This factor is significant for utilities, since around one-third of their total costs are for energy to treat and pump the water. Less wasted water equates to less wasted energy.

Utilities claim it will reduce the labor necessary to read traditional water meters, as well as streamlining billing origination. It will reveal problem areas within the system and better manage the production, storage, and distribution of water. It can also help utilities substantially decrease nonrevenue water by detecting water loss both in the distribution network and at customer endpoints, a big problem.

It also gives consumers the information they need to conserve water, thereby lowering their water bills, increases accuracy of billing, and reduces water losses and improves maintenance. All of these benefits lead to one bottom line: better water resource management for the utilities, lower costs for the customers, and less stress on water sources.

5

The Smart Home

An Intelligent Choice

Our fantasies of commuter jetpacks, driverless cars, drones delivering packages, computer applications and robots running our homes and being able to distinguish between family members and guests, biometric teddy bears monitoring our children's health, using virtual reality to help run the house, remotely babysitting and tracking the whereabouts of our families, even toothbrush and stool analyzing appliances and far more are just sci-fi fantasies, or a time warp to the future, but they're here now at a house near you.

The ability to run your entire home is no further than the palm of your hand with an application which gives a completely secure 3G/4G connection. The G stands for the generation of the speed. It's kind of like "Wi-Fi everywhere," meaning it provides Internet access via the same radio towers that provide voice service to your mobile phone. Via an "app" it can connect you to your home's lighting, security, energy, comfort, appliances, and entertainment systems as you move from room to room via your Android, iPhone, iPad, or computer connection. Some systems can even shut down consoles and electronic devices when your kid is playing video games instead of doing homework while you're out of the house. Groceries can be ordered by the pantry and refrigerators, the wear and tear of clothes can be monitored by a washer/dryer, utensils can check eating habits, and some systems will automatically put a home in "away mode" when a person is out of town—all the while saving gobs of money on resources and energy bills. And everything will happen automatically and seamlessly because the smart house will understand exactly who you are, where you are, and what you want—robotically.

US homes have become considerably more energy-efficient over the past four decades, despite the growing use of devices. According to figures from the Department of Energy's Office of Energy Efficiency and Renewable Energy, the average US home used 31 percent less energy than in 1970, and will use less in the future when American houses become "smart."

The "smart home" may be defined as an ingenious system with access to assets, communication, various controls, data, and information technologies for enhancing the occupants' quality of life through comfort, convenience, reduced costs, and increased connectivity. It also functions as a switchboard for data flow among appliances and utility companies, employing automated home energy management (AHEM), a network that manages systems based on information from the occupants' smart meters. This idea has been widely acknowledged for decades, but few people have ever seen a smart home, and fewer still have occupied one. Yet.

In the recent past, the term "smart home" conjured up images of expensive home improvements and high-tech gadgets that were only found in the homes of the rich and famous. Since hardware prices and the Internet of Things (IoT) have decreased dramatically over the last few years, home control goods are far more affordable. And US-based retailers have expanded their smart home offerings by forming partnerships with technology providers and ramping up their in-store marketing.

According to a report from the publication *Business Insider*, there are now 1.9 billion connected-home devices, including smart appliances, safety and security systems, and energy-related equipment. This figure will go ballistic to nine billion by 2018—equivalent to the current number of smartphones, smart TVs, tablets, wearable computers, and PCs in the United States combined. Revenue, meanwhile, is predicted to climb from $61 billion in 2014 to $490 billion in 2019. In other words, "smart" is about to happen in a bodacious way.

The publication *Business Insider* Business Intelligence Report figures the connected-home market will make up roughly 27 percent of the broader emerging technology market or the IoT by 2019. While market trends have suggested that although the smart home of the future is close, consumer acceptance may not happen as quickly as technologists, marketers, and businesses have hyped.

Many retailers intend to expand the number of stores where consumers can view a display of home automation products designed to work together, including remote-controlled thermostats, door locks, blinds, lights, and security cameras. Each connects to a wireless hub in the home, allowing people to use a smartphone app to control each device.

Smart systems are now more affordable than ever. After years of hoopla, home control and automation products are gaining speed. The idea of being able to see and control your house via a smartphone makes sense because people are already connected via their phones to everything else in their lives.

Whether people are doing it for status, energy conservation, or simply to save money, the more people get information about their usage patterns, the more they are inclined to take action.

BECOMING MORE ENERGY EFFICIENT

Energy-efficient homes are garnering more attention in the face of a wave of higher utility costs as residential electricity prices are expected to rise nearly 4 percent this year, according to data from the Energy Information Administration. Obviously, poor household energy use has a direct impact on energy bills. Fortunately, with a few smart upgrades, it's possible to make a home more efficient and cost-effective through information and automation.

Home automation is a simple way to shave your energy bill since it eliminates human error that can inflate costs, like leaving the lights on, or running the air conditioning when you're not home, or forgetting to turn off other appliances. The average household could cut a third of its current energy bill by switching to energy-efficient appliances, equipment, and lighting, and a home with a comprehensive, centralized automation system has the potential to increase energy savings from 17 to 40 percent, according to a 2011 study by the Fraunhofer Institute of Building Physics that used a European Smart Home.

Another effortless way to green your home is to take control of your energy consumption by finding out exactly how much you're using. Armed with tools like the Kill-A-Watt meter and the PowerCost Monitor, you can measure how much electricity an item uses or find out how much electricity your whole household uses. These devices can be programmed to reflect two rates—one for off-peak periods and one for peak periods—so you know how much money you're spending on electricity at any given time. Once you determine these facts, you can reduce usage or replace energy hogs with more efficient items. These real-time energy usage meters will help you understand your habits and can get you to become more efficient with your energy consumption.

The next steps toward automating and greening your home are to check out whole-house smart systems that connect the home electronics into an integrated wireless network, allowing control of these items with a remote control, with a PC via the Internet, or with a cell phone. These systems are plug-and-play and wireless so you don't have to deal with any timely or costly installations. They're modular, too, so you can add or remove components as your needs change. Conveniently, they do not require any major renovations to your home and you will immediately save money on utilities costs. In fact, the savings realized in just a few years may pay for your whole smart home system.

This technology allows people to be good to both the environment and the wallet through energy conservation and by reducing the carbon footprint a home or business creates. Cloud-based services can also lower energy bills further. Utilities, for example, can reduce power usage during peak times through smart thermostats or analyze heating and cooling equipment to recommend ways to optimize efficiency.

It's a combination that excites consumers in that, while there might be significant cost savings, nearly half also list helping the environment as what they believe to be a key feature of the smart home. Eighty-five percent of consumers who use connected devices not only find they are more helpful than annoying, but also 83 percent are excited about the possibilities of the smart home. Additionally, these consumers indicated a higher likelihood that they would purchase a connected-home monitoring camera (70 percent), connected thermostat (69 percent), connected door locks (66 percent), smart home hub (64 percent), connected lighting system (65 percent), and smart home services (61 percent) in the next twelve months.

Recently there has been a rise in the level of excitement about smart home technology with 76 percent of millennials, 70 percent of their parents, and 50 percent of the overall population. Millennials are estimated to spend more than $200 billion annually starting in 2017, and $10 trillion in their lifetimes, and these numbers will increase as this younger generation grows older and newer generations embrace this technology with 54 percent of people saying they plan to buy at least one smart home product in the next year.

There are 114 million people who plan at some time to purchase smart products. Adults aged forty-five years and younger accept the inevitably of the future of the smart home and will be the foundation of the next generation of "connected" consumers.

Although in the next decade the typical family home will contain more than 500 smart devices, at present most consumers look at smart homes as a notion without a clear idea as to use and significance. So, although people are checking out the advantages of smart devices, there is a bridge to cross before the mainstream adopts totally smart systems.

And for those consumers who may not be ready to receive a text from their refrigerator, data shows they are ripe to adopt the first wave of home automation—connected thermostats, cameras, lights, door locks, and camera monitoring—90 percent of consumers claim security is one of the top reasons to purchase a smart home system. It makes sense that home monitoring cameras and connected door locks are among the most popular devices when you consider that a burglary takes place every 14.1 seconds in the United States. And 56 percent of break-ins are through the front or back doors. With heating and cooling accounting for up to 48 percent of energy use in a typical home, it is also easy to understand why connected thermostats topped the list of the most popular products this year.

It may look as if we are heading into a world where one can't function without an app to help manage anything and everything. While it's true that virtual assistant apps can be very useful, consumers need to be cautious about what information they are giving up; use of apps that have access to personal information can mean that hackers now only have to find a way to exploit a single app to gain access to all of your data—what you use and how you pay for it.

PEOPLE AND APPS

- Consumers are most excited about connecting their entertainment room to their smart home, followed next by their kitchen and their bedroom.
- 18 to 26 percent say it makes it easier to enjoy music, movies, and Web surfing anywhere in the house.
- 18 to 24 percent claim it helps anticipate needs with shopping lists and minor repairs.
- US consumers aged 55 and older exhibit a higher level of excitement around the cost savings benefit of the smart home.
- US consumers aged 25 to 34 express a higher level of excitement around the benefits of home and family of the smart home and want greater use and ability to manage work-life balance.

ELDER CARE

Smart home technology has the potential to help senior citizens live happier, easier lives, and can be a great resource for family members to keep an eye on their aging parents. In fact, 72 percent of consumers aged 25 to 34 and 74 percent of parents say they would sleep better at night if their parents or grandparents had smart home technology.

SECURITY

Indeed, energy savings isn't actually the prime reason for owning smart homes, according to 62 percent of the 2,000 adults surveyed in 2014 by Lowe's Home Improvement Center. The main reasons were increased security and the ability to remotely monitor homes.

MAKE THE COMPLEX SIMPLE

While the technology to enable the smart home might be complex, more than half of the homeowners want the experience to be easy, intuitive, and friendly. Manufacturers will undoubtedly optimize ease-of-use throughout the entire ownership experience, including purchase, installation, configuration, operation, and management of smart home solutions making smart home technology accessible for everyone.

PRIVACY AND DATA CONCERNS

Seventy-one percent of consumers say their number one concern about the smart home, more than the cost of the technology, is the possibility of a data breach or that their personal information may get stolen and sold.

DEVICES THAT TALK TO EACH OTHER

Overall, 60 percent of consumers say they wished their devices did a better job of talking to each other and 49 percent agree that devices that don't work together cause more stress in their lives. It has been forecast that the number of households with household energy management systems (HEMS) will grow to more than 40 million in 2020. (Companies such as Sony and Hitachi are in the research and development phase with HEMS devices, while Nest and Check-It already have some on the market.) And if HEMS can be combined with services we already use—such as utilities, security, cell, and Internet—then more consumers will buy in.

BOTTOM $$ LINE

The Baby Boomers' concerns are largely about cost savings, while the 25 to 34 set is more likely to factor in lifestyle issues, such enhanced productivity, media access, and interactivity. According to an International Data Corporation (IDC) survey commissioned by the Internet of Things Consortium (IoTC), 61 percent of people have concerns about privacy, while 51 percent thought the costs might outweigh the advantages.

Although many voiced concerns over privacy, surprisingly, a full third of respondents said they wouldn't oppose commercial advertising on connected devices if it meant trimmed costs, while a significant portion insisted on smartphone controllability as a prerequisite to purchasing.

POPULARITY

One reason why more people aren't using home energy management systems is that technological advances in our electrical grid have tended to benefit the utilities more than the consumer. For example, by the end of 2015, approximately 45 percent of all US households will be served by smart meters. *Intelligent Utility* reports as few as 10 percent of those meters will be enabled for two-way communications via HEMS.

Lacking that interactive connection with the energy grid, consumers won't fully benefit from HEMS' capabilities, such as real-time information on energy costs and usage, which would let them save money by using power when its costs are lowest, potentially even earning money by selling unused, locally generated power (from solar panels, for example) back to the utilities.

We've reached the point where we have the technical ability to create a truly interactive smart grid that benefits consumers and utilities and the environment. But we haven't yet put in place the state-by-state rules and regulations that will allow all that futuristic technology to take full effect.

The current Home Energy Management Systems market was valued at $1.5 billion in 2013, and includes utility residential demand response (DR), connected-home subscriptions, software services, and associated hardware. The top two leading home automation companies combined already have over two million customers, demonstrating the HEMS market's remarkable potential. New companies have entered the arena, hungry for the next set of opportunities revolving around software and bundled service solutions, and the market has expanded in its scope of offerings.

GADGETRY

Topping the list of most-desired smart gadgets are those for entertainment systems.

- According to the Coldwell Banker survey, some 44 percent of home-owners use some sort of smart entertainment technology, the most popular being smart TVs and speaker systems.
- Home security systems are next, which may include video monitors inside and outside the house viewed on a smartphone, and 71 percent desired doors which can be remotely locked and unlocked.
- Self-adjusting thermostats interested 72 percent. According to the Coldwell Banker survey, 30 percent of consumers polled already have devices like smart thermostats that can be programmed remotely via computer or

mobile device. Many of these devices quickly "learn" consumer habits so they are able to turn themselves up or down at the right time and by the right amount, based on what has been done in the past. Some related products on the market now include water and humidity monitors that alert you to any leaks in the house while you're away.

- A master remote from which to control all household preferences interested 68 percent.
- Adjustable, automatic, outdoor lighting—65 percent.
- Cost savings from energy efficiency and monitoring—70 percent.
- Greater productivity and enhanced work-life balance—23 percent.
- The ability to anticipate homeowner needs—18 percent.
- Interactive, connective features—13 percent.

ELIMINATE PHANTOM ENERGY

Phantom energy—also known as idle currents, standby power, etc.—occurs when electronics, like microwaves or digital video recorders, are turned off but continue to draw power by being plugged into an outlet.

According to Berkeley Lab (Lawrence Berkeley National Laboratory), standby power accounts for 10 percent of household electrical use that's paid for but not really used. This may seem trivial, but when the average home uses approximately $2,100 worth of energy each year, that small amount adds up.

Certain electronics use more power than others, including computers, printers, and gaming consoles, but there are ways to reduce the output. Smart systems shut down major electronics that drain significant power. Little changes can make a big difference in a home's energy consumption. And with modern technology, it's easy to automate energy use so you don't even have to think about it.

FROM HEAT AND AIR CONDITIONING AND TOILET TO YOUR WALLET

The front line of smart home technology is in the heat and air conditioning, the most energy-intensive, operation-expensive system in the home eating up 40 to 60 percent of its energy consumption. We all want to stay cool in the summer and warm in the winter, but the associated costs can pack quite a punch.

Studies estimate that roughly 70 percent of American homes' heating, ventilation, and air-conditioning (HVAC) systems are either running inefficiently or headed for a breakdown, leading to costly repairs and higher energy bills.

Home automation has potential benefits as it's been estimated that home-owners can save on average $180 per year simply by using programmable or zone-based thermostats.

The number of smart thermostats in North American and European homes increased by 105 percent in 2014 to a total of 3.2 million units. The US Environmental Protection Agency found consumers could reduce energy usage by 10 to 30 percent, or 1.4 billion kilowatt-hours, enough electricity to power more than 135,000 US homes for a year. The problem has been that consumers often struggle to effectively program thermostats and achieve those benefits.

Getting consumers to adopt highly efficient appliances, where the future energy savings outweigh the higher up-front equipment costs, is challenging for three main reasons. There may be nonmonetary costs such as searching for a contractor. Next, there may be uncertainty about the resulting energy savings that keeps homeowners from acting. Third, energy costs may just not be as salient to energy users as other features of the appliances that they are considering and consumers may focus more on the present cost than on the future savings.

With zone-based smart thermostats, your house can be divided into zones so that unoccupied rooms and areas are not being cooled or heated unnecessarily. Additionally, motion sensors in the room can start and stop your heating and cooling system to decrease the amount of wasted energy.

LIGHTING

Reduce your energy usage with automatic timers, motion detectors, and dimmers that can cut lighting costs by as much as 50 percent. And the International Energy Agency (IEA) reports that switching to efficient lighting systems would reduce the world's electricity bill by one-tenth.

OCCUPANCY SENSORS

Motion sensors can control some appliances in your home, lowering utility costs by ensuring that lights, televisions, sound systems, and even small appliances, like coffee-cup warmers or curling irons, are turned off when no one is in the room to use them. With some systems, you can also control lights and appliances remotely from your personal digital devices. This way you aren't paying for the energy that is normally consumed when lights and appliances are mistakenly left on while you are not home.

Using infrared or ultrasonic technology, occupancy sensors can automatically turn lights on and off based on the motion in a room, which conserves power and increases convenience.

Sensor-based technology, as seen with ConnectSense, is another way to control light use. Light sensors can be used to perform "daylight harvesting," which is the concept of using sensors to monitor direct sunlight to ensure that you are only utilizing overhead lighting in an office or home when it's absolutely needed.

MONITOR ENERGY USE

Being aware of the optimal times to run your electrical appliances can save you a bundle. There are several monitoring devices that can give you real-time feedback on how much energy your home is using, as well as the times when your energy costs are lowest. Based on this feedback, you can set power timers to run large appliances like hot tubs, spas, and attic and exhaust fans at optimal times, and have them automatically turned off at set times to avoid wasted energy.

SMART GARDENING

Smart homes extend to the garden, too. Installing a smart irrigation system will save you time and money, giving you the ability to literally enjoy the fruits of your labor. Automated watering controlled through Wi-Fi can control your watering schedule, sprinklers, and outdoor lighting through a couple of buttons. It can actively respond to changing weather conditions in your local area over a period of time, monitoring the nearest weather station and responding accordingly. Using an intelligent hub to monitor your watering habits can help to save up to 50 percent on your gardening water bill, while keeping your outdoor space looking pristine.

In addition to energy savings, you can save on your water bill by using an automatic irrigation system like Cyber-Rain, a sprinkler system that runs depending upon local weather conditions or not at all if rain is expected. You can even monitor water usage, program schedules, and more directly from a computer.

THE FUTURE

The Coldwell Banker Smart Home Marketplace Survey, which polled more than 4,000 Americans, found that 45 percent of all Americans either own smart home technology or plan to invest in it in 2016, while eight out of ten consumers using smart home products said they would be more likely to buy a home if smart technology was already installed. According to the Consumer Technology Association, smart home technology represents a $1.2 billion market this year, up 20 percent from a year ago. One recent report by the research firm MarketsandMarkets found that the industry, which was worth $5.77 billion in 2013, could more than double by 2020.

6

Insulation and Weatherization

To Help Weather the Seasons

No matter where you live you're going to need insulation, whether you're trying to keep cool in Palms Springs, California, or stay warm in Steamboat Springs, Colorado. Good insulation is like having gloves on while making snowballs. Trying to remain comfy during the change of seasons is the job for insulation, the buffer for a comfort zone. "Insulation" refers to materials that deflect and resist heat, and chill or trap small air pockets that work as barriers between warm and cold zones inside and outside your house.

One overlooked benefit of improved insulation is that it makes heating and cooling equipment cheaper and more efficient to operate in your home. If your home doesn't have proper insulation at present and has no sidewall insulation, there are some tricks that will help block or keep cold air out and eliminate condensation on walls, ceilings, and your body.

Heat can transfer itself in three ways. Convection is the transmission of heat by movement of air. As heated air comes in contact with cold surfaces such as windows, it loses heat. Conduction is passage of heat through a material, such as the hot handle of a pan. Some materials, such as glass and metal, conduct heat (and lose it) easily. Thermal radiation is the passage of energy through open space, such as sunlight radiating heat to the Earth.

Cold can also move in three ways: by wind, fans, and the stack effect. Wind is somewhat predictable—at least in terms of average speed and direction. Fans include kitchen and bath exhaust fans, HVAC equipment fans, and clothes dryers. The stack effect is the movement of air into and out of buildings, through chimneys, flue gas stacks, or by other means, resulting from air buoyancy. This occurs due to a difference in indoor-to-outdoor air density resulting from temperature and moisture differences.

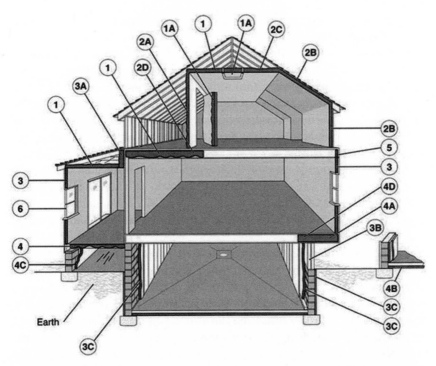

1. In unfinished attic spaces, insulate between and over the floor joists to seal off living spaces below. If the air distribution is in the attic space, then consider insulating the rafters to move the distribution into the conditioned space. (1A) attic access door 2. In finished attic rooms with or without dormer, insulate (2A) between the studs of "knee" walls, (2B) between the studs and rafters of exterior walls and roof, (2C) and ceilings with cold spaces above. (2D) Extend insulation into joist space to reduce air flows. 3. All exterior walls, including (3A) walls between living spaces and unheated garages, shed roofs, or storage areas; (3B) foundation walls above ground level; (3C) foundation walls in heated basements, full wall either interior or exterior. 4. Floors above cold spaces, such as vented crawl spaces and unheated garages. Also insulate (4A) any portion of the floor in a room that is cantilevered beyond the exterior wall below; (4B) slab floors built directly on the ground; (4C) as an alternative to floor insulation, foundation walls of unvented crawl spaces. (4D) Extend insulation into joist space to reduce air flows. 5. Band joists. 6. Replacement or storm windows and caulk and seal around all windows and doors. Source: Oak Ridge National Laboratory

Figure 6.1. Good places to insulate.
Source: Oak Ridge National Laboratory

FACTS AND FIGURES

A healthy home needs fresh air. However, it's important to be able to control when, where, and how outdoor air enters and indoor air leaves.

R-value measures the amount of thermal resistance. The higher the R-value, the better the insulation. Different types of insulation will have different R ratings, ranging from R-11 to R-45. Always check the R-value printed on the foil side of the insulation.

Insulation slows down the rate of heat transfer and retains heat within the house as long as possible. Ten-and-a-half inches of loft insulation can save up to 15 percent of a home's heating costs. Good insulation also improves the value of your home. It reduces high energy costs for low-income families providing an economic boost in low-income communities.

In the United States alone more than 46 million homes are underinsulated according to the North American Insulation Manufacturers Association (NAIMA). The Department of Energy (DOE) estimates that the average cost to fully weatherize a home is around $6,500. This investment will keep giving back year after year, at approximately $437 per annum. Nationwide, every $1 invested in a weatherization program returns $2.51 to the household and society.

Homeowners may be able to reduce their energy bills by 10 percent to 50 percent by decreasing air loss (drafts) and increasing thermal insulation in their homes, or by purchasing additional insulation. Adding insulation to ceilings, walls, and attics can save from 30 percent to 45 percent on heating and cooling costs. Proper insulation can also reduce carbon dioxide emissions by 140 to 2,100 pounds per home per year. If you live in a very cold climate, consider superinsulating. That can save 5.5 tons of carbon dioxide per year for gas-heated homes, 8.8 tons per year for oil-heated homes, or 23 tons per year for electric heat. (If you use electric heat, you might also consider switching to more efficient gas or oil.) For every 10,000 owners who properly insulate their homes, 50 million fewer tons of carbon dioxide are released into the atmosphere each year, which strongly correlates to climate change.

Table 6.1.   Insulation R-Value and Cost

New Insulation R-Value	Existing Insulation R-Value		
	8	15	19
19	$5.90	$1.40	
30	$7.80	$3.30	$1.90
38	$8.50	$4.00	$2.60
45	$8.95	$4.40	$3.00

Source: US Department of Energy

MORE "R" AND "U" INSULATION VALUES

The most important measures of all insulation are its R and U values. R-value is a laboratory measurement of conduction, but it does not effectively measure the other two methods of heat transfer: convection and radiation. It measures the resistance to heat transfer. The bigger the number, the better the building insulation effectiveness against drafts and heat loss. When insulating your walls, you will need an R-value of at least R-11. However, R-values do depend upon the state in which you live, so be sure to check local building codes. Recommended insulation levels for ceilings/attics recently rose from R-19 to R-30.

U-value measures the transfer of heat through a material, or "thermal transmittance" of a building element, as in windows and skylights. U-values are the direct opposite of R-values, representing the amount of heat that escapes through a material. The lower the U-value, the slower the rate of heat flow and the better the insulating quality.

VAPOR RETARDERS AND BARRIERS

Vapor retarders are necessary to protect against moisture development when installing insulation. Condensation can create moisture on many surfaces, which can affect the performance of insulation, and can cause wood rot and rust. A vapor barrier is simply a plastic sheet, usually six millimeters thick, that covers insulation. In cool climates, a vapor barrier is installed on the heated side of a surface; in humid climates, the vapor barrier is installed against unheated surfaces.

Any material with a therm rating of less than 1 is considered a vapor retarder. A rating of 1 or more qualifies as a vapor barrier. This includes:

- Asphalt-coated paper backing on insulation 0.40.
- Polyethylene plastic (6 mil) 0.06.
- Plywood with exterior glue 0.70.
- Plastic-coated insulated foam sheathing 0.4 to 1.2.
- Aluminum foil (.35 mil) 0.05.
- Vapor barrier paint or primer 0.45.
- Drywall (unpainted) 5.0.
- Drywall (painted—latex paint) 2.0.

INSULATION'S SURPRISINGLY VARIED FORMS

Materials for insulation have included old newspapers, clothes, nylon stockings, mud, and many other improvised materials. Although some of the older materials are still used, such as shredded denim jeans, there are many newer, tech-savvy forms.

Basically, there are two types of insulation: absorptive and reflective. The ubiquitous bales of pink and yellow fiberglass insulation (absorptive) are in more than 90 percent of the new homes built in the United States. However, if you have wondered why your home can be so hot on summer evenings, it's because the insulation is releasing some absorbed heat that hasn't dispersed.

Reflective insulation is a new twist on an old technology. You've seen windows facing the sun covered with aluminum foil. Reflection technology uses that same basic idea, but it took the National Aeronautics and Space Administration to harness it fully. Space-age foil insulation was designed for use in outer space where temperatures range from -250° to +460°F, yet it keeps the astronauts' capsule at a comfy 78°F, as reflective insulation reflects 96 percent of all radiant heat.

Insulation alone is not the complete answer to conserving and maintaining air temperature at home. In the North Pole if you wear an Arctic-rated thermal jacket (your insulation) and open it to below-zero wind (drafts), you're going to freeze, so focus on buttoning up your home to air infiltration and leakage via gaps and cracks. Then focus on investing in more insulation (see chapter 7, "Defeating Drafts").

INSULATION OPTIONS

Slag wool is a man-made material that comes from blast furnace slag (waste material) that collects on molten metal—it's good for insulation for material that is typically dumped. It can be fluffy and its R-value is similar to that of fiberglass.

Rock wool is a man-made material that includes natural minerals. Denser types of mineral wool have a higher R-value per inch than fluffy types; if the rock wool is dense enough (8 pounds or more per cubic foot), it can be formed into rectangular panels and installed like rigid foam.

Fiberglass is made from molten sand or recycled glass and other inorganic materials, and is produced in batts, blankets, and loose-fill forms. Batt insulation comes in rolls, blankets, or strips that are pre-cut and laid in between joists. They are available in a variety of lengths, widths, and R-values. Fiberglass is actually spun glass and can irritate exposed skin. So wear a mouth mask rated for fiberglass, as well as a hat, gloves, long-sleeve shirt, and goggles to keep fibers out of your eyes.

Installing batt insulation is a relatively easy project. Choose the new "no-itch" or poly-wrapped batt insulation products (insulation that is wrapped in plastic for a more comfortable installation with less itch and dust, making it safer to handle). You don't have to use the same type of insulation everywhere—for example, it's fine to use batts or blankets over loose-fill, or vice versa. When using loose-fill (that looks like small chunks of gray papery material), be sure to distribute the insulation evenly. Any inconsistencies can reduce the insulating value. "IC" stands for insulation contact and means that it can touch a light fixture without danger.

BATT INSULATION

Fiberglass batts are the cheapest, easiest way to insulate new walls. However, they're often installed poorly—even small gaps can reduce efficiency as much as 25 percent. You'll need a utility razor with a supply of blades and/or large scissors, a tape measure, a straightedge, and a medium putty knife for stuffing insulation around doors and windows.

Measure and cut carefully to pack spaces properly. Cut the batts to length by setting the top of the batt into the space and cutting against the bottom plate. Leave an extra one-half-inch length and width for a tight fit. Fill all voids. Push batts all the way to the back of each stud or joist space and then pull out the front edges until they're flush with the face of the studs. Always point the paper or foil outward toward you.

Fit batts tightly around electrical cables and boxes. Be sure to fill gaps around windows and doors. Stuff skinny strips of batting into spaces around windows and doors with a putty knife. The insulation should fit snugly, but don't overpack it.

When selecting a floor insulation system, it helps to think about the thicknesses of typical fiberglass batts. Here is a list of batt thicknesses to help get you started. Individual brands can vary by as much as one inch. It's a good idea to check with your supplier for the thickness of the brand they use.

- R-19 = 6¼ inches
- R-22 HD = 5½ inches
- R-22 = 7½ inches
- R-25 = 8½ inches
- R-30 = 10 inches
- R-30 HD = 8½ inches
- R-38 = 12 inches
- R-38 = HD 10 inches

BLOWN-IN INSULATION

Blown-in insulation is a product composed of loose-fill fibers or fiber pellets that are blown into building cavities or attics using special pneumatic equipment. This can be tricky, and usually calls for professional equipment and contractors. However, if you're ambitious, equipment for the job can be rented. Cellulose fibers are a popular blown-in insulation material because the small particles fill in the nooks, crannies, and irregular areas of wall space quite well. It is also considered by many to be a "green" material, as it is composed of up to 75 percent recycled newsprint and does not contain formaldehyde, which can release harmful vapors into the air.

To blow it in yourself, first locate studs in the wall with a stud finder. With a hole-saw, cut a small area (about the size of the blower hose) between two studs and near the top of the wall. Save the cutout and reattach it later with spackle or sheetrock "mud." Thread the blower hose into the first hole, and point the nozzle down deep into the wall cavity. Wrap a rag around the hose where it meets the wall to stop blowback into the room. Turn on the blower and pull the hose back as the cavity fills. Stop the machine when you feel resistance and can no longer insert insulation.

Checking a wall's insulation level is more difficult. Select an exterior wall and turn off the circuit breaker or unscrew the fuse for any outlets in the wall. Be sure to test the outlets to make certain that they are not "hot." Once you are sure your outlets are not getting any electricity, remove the cover plate from one of the outlets and gently probe into the wall with a thin, long stick or screwdriver. If you encounter a slight resistance, that's insulation.

You could also make a small hole in a closet, behind a couch, or in some other unobtrusive place to see if a wall cavity is insulated. Only infrared scanning can verify if the whole wall is totally insulated.

CELLULOSE

Cellulose insulation is plant fiber used in wall and roof cavities to insulate and reduce noise. It is considered "green" because it's made from wood fiber (newsprint in many cases) that is naturally more resistant to the conduction of heat. The fiber is chemically treated with nontoxic borate compounds (20 percent by weight). It comes in several forms, from blown or sprayed to loose-fill and low-dust form.

Installations have shown that even several months of water saturation and improper installation did not result in mold. The borate treatment also gives cellulose the highest (Class 1 or A) fire safety rating. Many cellulose companies use a blend of ammonium sulfate and borate.

Cellulose provides an R-value of approximately R-35 per inch of thickness. Cellulose is a superb air-blocker; when packed, it provides a thermally efficient, cost-effective, and comfortable solution to drafts. In a Massachusetts survey a cellulose-insulated building consumed 32 percent less energy for heating than buildings insulated with fiberglass, even after extensive air sealing of all the buildings was done.

The Cellulose Insulation Manufacturers Association (CIMA) claims that insulating a 1,500-square-foot house with cellulose will recycle as much newspaper as an individual would read in forty years. Cellulose also earns "green" points because it requires less energy than fiberglass to manufacture, yet fewer than 10 percent of the homes built today use cellulose.

Cellulose is also hygroscopic, able to soak and hold liquid water, whereas water leaks can compress a blanket of fiberglass and, in extreme cases, can create a void space, degrading its thermal value. However, chemicals used to protect cellulose from fire make it potentially corrosive in wet environments. Tests conducted by the Oak Ridge National Laboratory show that metal fasteners, plumbing pipes, and electrical wires can corrode if left in contact with wet, treated cellulose insulation for extended periods of time.

In addition, loose-fill cellulose can be made from rock wool fibers, fiberglass, cellulose fiber, vermiculite, and perlite minerals. Loose fill tends to slump after application, which, in some situations, can leave areas of wall uninsulated. Loose fill can be applied by pouring directly from the bag or with a blower. Be careful, any inconsistencies can reduce insulating value. For a given R-value, loose fill cellulose weighs roughly three times as much per square foot as loose fiberglass.

FOAM BOARDS

Rigid foam board insulation is used primarily in new construction and major renovations. It consists of either fiberglass or mineral wool material and is primarily used for insulating air ducts, especially where there are high temperatures. While other types of insulation are installed in wall or ceiling cavities between the studs, rafters, or joists, rigid foam board insulation is used on exterior walls beneath the siding and on exposed interior basement walls where studs are not used. Rigid foam board insulation is also an excellent moisture deterrent. Green building experts say that rigid foam board insulation offers benefits including higher R-values per inch than other types of insulation and rigid foam, from 1 inch to 2.5 inches, typically has an R-value between 5 and 8. Building codes may require a covering such as gypsum wall board as a fire barrier for foam board insulation products.

REFLECTIVE INSULATION

Reflective insulation, usually composed of aluminum, is also known as a radiant barrier. It resembles metallic foil and has a reflective surface.

This type of insulation is versatile and fairly simple to install in new or existing homes, usually in attics to reduce summer heat. Some studies show that radiant barriers (especially on ducts) can lower cooling costs by 5 to 10 percent. In cold climates, this form of reflective insulation in attics/roofs might not work well. It's usually more cost effective to install higher levels of common insulation (fiberglass, sprayed foam, cellulose, mineral wool materials) than to apply a radiant barrier in an attic.

The simplest way to install reflective insulation is to lay the radiant barrier directly on top of existing attic insulation, with the reflective side up. But be mindful of problems due to moisture (even if products are perforated) and dust accumulation, which will strongly reduce the performance of the material. A much more efficient alternative is to apply the reflective material between the roof sheathing and the attic floor insulation. Many radiant barriers are placed at the top of trusses or draped over them.

LIQUID FOAM

Liquid foam is an organic material developed by the petrochemical industry. Icynene insulation is a water-based formula that contains no formaldehyde, CFCs or HCFCs (chlorofluorocarbon and hydrochlorofluorocarbon compounds that are harmful to the Earth's ozone layer).

The insulation has the texture and look of angel food cake and is made up of millions of tiny cells. These cells are filled with air and provide permanent control of air and airborne moisture movement. There are no VOCs (volatile organic compound) detected in Icynene after thirty days.

Spray foam insulation can be categorized into two different types: open cell and closed cell. Open cell is a type of foam that is sponge-like in appearance. Open cell is less expensive because it uses fewer chemicals. It is a very good air barrier but does not provide any type of water vapor barrier. It is often used for interior walls because it provides sound reduction by damping the movement of existing insulation. The product is environmentally safe, has been tested, and shows no corrosive qualities that would damage electrical wiring or metals. In the event of fire it will not sustain a flame upon removal of the flame source, however, like fiberglass, it will be consumed by flame.

Closed cell foam insulation is a much denser type of foam than open cell. It has a smaller, more compact cell structure. It is often used in roofing projects or other outdoor applications, but can be used anywhere in the home. It repels water well. If placed in water it will float, and on removal it will dry rapidly, losing none of its insulating properties. This material can be sprayed, foamed in place, injected, or poured.

Some foam insulations have twice the R-value per inch of other traditional insulations in that they effectively fill the smallest cavities. But be careful when using foam, it can be easily underestimated and blow out part of a wall.

STRUCTURAL INSULATED PANELS

Structural insulated panels (SIPs) are a composite building material. They consist of an insulating layer of rigid polymer foam sandwiched between two layers of structural board. The board can be sheet metal, plywood, cement, or oriented strand board (OSB). The foam can be either expanded polystyrene foam (EPS), extruded polystyrene foam (XPS), polyisocyanurate foam, or polyurethane foam.

SIPs have high R-values and also high strength-to-weight ratios. The pre-fabricated and insulated elements are used for building walls, ceilings, and floors. They provide superior and uniform insulation compared to the more traditional methods. They can offer energy savings of 12 to14 percent when installed properly. SIPs also result in a more airtight home, making a structure quieter and more comfortable.

BE SELECTIVE WHEN YOU CHOOSE

All insulation materials reduce greenhouse gas emissions (by saving energy). However, some thick layers of material made with "blowing agents" of HCFCs or XPS, such as Dow Styrofoam or Owens Corning Foamular, are made from materials considered environmentally unfriendly, and may result in out-gassing, the release of a gas that was dissolved, trapped, frozen, or absorbed in some material.

Standard closed-cell spray polyurethane foam (SPF) results in very long "payback periods" due to the toxic emissions in the production of the insulation. This can thwart attempts to create carbon-neutral structures.

The bottom line is that if you are aiming to minimize the impacts of climate change you should choose fiber insulation made from cellulose, fiberglass, mineral wool, or non-hydroflurocarbon foam insulation, and consult a professional just to be safe.

THE CURE FOR HOLES IN YOUR HOUSE, CAULKING, AND WEATHER STRIPPING

Caulk is a chemical-based sealant made from silicone, polyurethane, polysulfide, silyl-terminated-polyurethane or polyether, and acrylic sealant. It usually comes in tubes, which is then squeezed into seams.

Table 6.2.   Common Types of Weather Stripping

Weather Stripping	Best Uses	Cost	Advantages	Disadvantages
Tension Seal: Self-stick plastic (vinyl) folded along length in a V-shape or a springy bronze strip (also copper, aluminum, and stainless steel) shaped to bridge a gap. The shape of the material creates a seal by pressing against the sides of a crack to block drafts.	Inside the track of a double-hung or sliding window, top and sides of door.	Moderate; varies with material used.	Durable. Invisible when in place. Very effective. Vinyl is fairly easy to install. Look of bronze works well for older homes.	Surfaces must be flat and smooth for vinyl. Can be difficult to install, as corners must be snug. Bronze must be nailed in place (every three inches or so) so as not to bend or wrinkle. Can increase resistance in opening/closing doors or windows. Self-adhesive vinyl available. Some manufacturers include extra strip for door striker plate.

Source: US Department of Energy

Weather stripping is adhesive-backed foam or metal strip used around the perimeters of doors and windows. Spray foam out of a can may also be used to fill holes.

Select the right caulk—100 percent silicone, not acrylic, is used more for painted surfaces. Silicone it is permanently waterproof, flexible, and shrink- and crack-proof. Acrylic caulk can shrink and crack over time, leaving gaps for air and water to seep through. When shopping, look for low- or no-pollution materials.

Gaps in between walls and windows should be caulked. Closing the gaps in your home can reduce your utility bills by up to 20 percent. Check windows for loose panes and seal them. Be aware that some caulks will blacken after a period of time, especially when exposed to moisture. Caulking costs less than $1 per window, and weather stripping is under $10 per door. These steps can save up to 1,100 pounds of carbon dioxide in the atmosphere per year for a typical home. It's estimated more than half the homes in America need weather stripping and/or caulking. That's more than 100 million homes, that's a lot of caulk and weather stripping!

INSTALLING CAULK

Buy an inexpensive caulk gun for around five to ten dollars. Clean the surface to be caulked with a household cleaner, and wipe with a dry cloth. Where you cut the caulk tub nozzle determines the thickness of the caulk bead. Oh yes, be sure to break the seal through the tube nozzle.

Steady, don't press too hard. Hold the caulk gun at a 45-degree angle and squeeze gently. This will supply a smooth, even bead. Avoid "globs" by maintaining an even hand from start to finish.

Next comes tooling, or smoothing, the caulk. Don't overlook this important step. Your finger is often the best tool (although you can also buy a cheap smoothing tool that fits on your finger if you're fussy). Run your finger along the bead to ensure that it's neat, even, and most importantly, fills the gap to form a tight seal.

Clean it up with water, but be careful to maintain a tight bead. Some caulk requires up to 24 hours or longer before it can be exposed to water.

HOW TO INSTALL WEATHER STRIPPING

Most forms of weather stripping are fairly user-friendly. Ask at your home improvement store which application is going to work best for your needs and uses. You'll need a few instructions and common sense, along with the proper materials and the tools. Be patient and by the time you tackle the first project, the rest will be easy.

TOOLS TO HAVE HANDY

Here are the tools you'll want to have on hand to apply pressure-sensitive types of weather stripping:

- Tape measure.
- Pencil.
- Hammer.
- Screwdriver.
- Razor knife or scissors.
- Dishwashing detergent.
- Clean rags or paper towels.
- Petroleum jelly.
- Tin snips or heavy scissors for metal weather stripping.

- Proper size nails or tacks for metal weather stripping.
- Nail set or pilot holes drill bit for metal weather stripping.

Pressure-sensitive adhesive-backed foam is the easiest weather stripping to apply, and is quite inexpensive. Available in both rubber and plastic, adhesive-backed foam comes in rolls of varying lengths and thicknesses. Pressure-sensitive types of weather stripping can be used only on the friction-free parts of a wooden window, such as the bottom or top of a sash (window) frame. If the strips were installed snugly against the gap between sides, the movement of the window would pull it loose.

To install, clean the entire surface to which weather stripping will be attached. Use dishwashing detergent and water to clean the area, making certain no dirt or grease remains. If pressure-sensitive weather stripping has been installed previously, use petroleum jelly, cleanser, or light solvent to remove any old adhesive. Clean and dry the surface. Cut the strip to fit, but do not remove backing paper yet. To peel, start at one end, slowly pulling paper backing off as you push the sticky foam strip into place. If backing proves stubborn at the beginning, stretch the foam until the seal between backing and the foam breaks.

Nailed spring-metal weather stripping is another option. Spring-metal strips (V-shape or single) are available in bronze, copper, stainless steel, and aluminum finishes. Most spring-metal weather stripping comes in rolls and installing this kind of weather stripping requires some patience. Spring-metal weather stripping fits into the window tracks closest to the outside. Each strip should be about two inches longer than the sash so the top end of the strip is exposed when the windows are closed. Here's how to install it:

Position vertical strips so the flared flange faces outside. The center strip should be mounted to the upper sash with flare aimed down, while the other horizontal strips are mounted to the top of the upper sash and bottom of the lower sash with flared flange facing out. Cut the spring-metal weather stripping to size. Be sure to allow for window pulley mechanisms. Attach strips to the window frame. Position the strip properly and note any hinges, locks, or other hardware that might interfere. Trim away metal where needed; also trim the ends of strips at an angle where vertical and horizontal strips meet. Tap in one nail at the top and one nail at the bottom of the strip. Do not put in more nails and do not drive top and bottom nails all the way in. Since some vertical strips do not come with nail holes, you may have to make pilot holes with a punch, ice pick, drill bit, awl, or larger nail.

Check to make sure strips are straight and properly positioned. Then drive a nail into center of strip—but, again, only partway. Add more nails between the starter nails. To avoid damaging the strip, never drive any of the nails all the way in with the hammer. Instead, drive nails flush with a nail set (or a larger nail). To get a snug fit use a flat-edged screwdriver or chisel.

Self-sticking spring metal has a peel-and-stick backing. These are like standard spring-metal strips, but they are far easier to install. This type of weather stripping works best on wood-framed windows.

To install, measure and cut strips to fit the window, then clean the surface where the strips will be placed. Put the strips in place without removing backing paper, and mark spots for trimming. Indicate points where the vertical and horizontal strips meet. Peel off the backing at one end, and press the strip in place, peeling and pressing as you work toward the other end. Trim the excess.

Felt weather stripping is one of the old standbys and is very economical. It comes in a variety of widths, thicknesses, qualities, and colors. Felt strips are somewhat unsightly for sealing gaps on wooden-frame windows. There are places where felt can be used to good advantage, however. Attach felt strips to the bottom, top, or interior side of a sash or double-hung window. The strips will then function as horizontal gaskets.

To install, measure and cut the felt strips to fit the window. Keep in mind that the strips can go around corners. Push the material snugly against gap. If the weather stripping is not self-adhesive, apply adhesive (there are many types, ask your hardware adviser). The adhesive forms a better bond if applied when the temperature is at least 60°F. Start at one end and drive a tack in every two to three inches of felt, pulling it tightly as you go. If you find slack when you reach other end, remove the tack, pull to tighten, and trim off any excess.

Tubular gasket weather stripping is made of extremely flexible vinyl. It is usually applied outside where it easily conforms to uneven places. Foam-filled tubular gasket weather stripping includes a foam core in the tube of the gasket. The foam provides extra insulating qualities and strength. Neither should be painted.

To install, measure the strips and cut them to size with scissors. Cutting all strips for a window at one time will save you trips up and down a ladder. Position each strip carefully and drive a nail into one end. Space nails every two to three inches, pulling weather stripping tight before you drive each nail.

Metal windows are grooved around the edges so the metal flanges will interlock and preclude the need for weather stripping. However, sometimes gaps do exist and you must apply weather stripping in such instances. Generally, the only kind of weather stripping that can be applied to metal windows is the pressure-sensitive type, as screws or nails would obstruct movement of the window.

The average door has more gaps than a loose-fitting window, and doors don't run in grooves as windows do. Before you start weather stripping, inspect the door to be sure it fits properly in the frame opening. Close the door and observe it from the inside and outside. Look to see if the distance between the door and the frame is uniform all along both sides and at the top. You may want to do this first in the dark and have someone use a flashlight on the opposite side to locate gaps. The distance does not have to be precisely the same all the way around, but if the door rests crooked in the frame weather stripping may make it impossible to open or close.

The cause of most door problems is the hinges. Therefore, the first thing to do is open the door and tighten all the hinge screws. You may want to remove them and use an adhesive sealer on the screws when reinstalling them. If the screw holes have been reamed out and are now too big to hold the screws, you can use larger screws as long as they fit. Sometimes the door must be planed or sanded to prevent binding.

Spring metal is quite popular for door weather stripping. It works effectively when installed properly and is not visible with the door closed.

CAVEAT EMPTOR—LET THE BUYER BEWARE

Be sure to find out what insulation contractors must tell their customers. Check out Title 16, Section 460 of the Federal Trade Commission's Code of Federal Regulations, as the purpose of this regulation is to ensure that consumers are provided essential pre-purchase information about R-values.

It's always best to hire professional help when installing insulation. Look for contractors who are members of the Insulation Contractors Association of America (ICAA), the nonprofit trade association of insulation contractors and suppliers. Be certain that the job specification includes cost, method of payment, and warranty information provided by the insulation material manufacturer. Make sure that the contract lists the type of insulation to be used and where it will be used; make sure that each type of insulation is listed by R-value. Avoid contracts with vague language, such as R-values with the terms "plus or minus," "+ or –," "average," or "normal."

Beware of quoting the job in terms of thickness only ("14 inches of insulation"). Remember, it is the R-value—not the thickness—that tells how well a material insulates. When buying insulation, don't be sidetracked by the thickness of the material.

HOMEOWNER'S BILL OF RIGHTS

For any type of home repair, be safe and hire only licensed contractors or those vetted by a referral company (check them and any subcontractors out with your state Department of Consumer Affairs for proper licensing and complaints).

Also record the names and addresses of all people working on the job. From the contractor, require a list of exactly what needs to be done and the materials needed. Read estimates closely; the cheapest bid may have overlooked work that other bids factored in. Tell the contractor the contract must include a timetable that stipulates the job will be "continuously processed" (no stopping to work on another project). Get at least three bids.

Control the money. Tell potential contractors you won't pay more than 10 percent up-front and you'll withhold 15 percent for thirty days after the job is done to make sure all is well. A reputable person won't balk. Do not pay in cash. If you have to, get a detailed receipt of what the payment is for and the deadlines it entails. Never consolidate existing loans through a home improvement contractor. Make payments as work is completed and never let payments get ahead of work.

Require that the work has one project price, including work and material. Demand an agreement to provide lien releases at job's end showing subcontractors and suppliers have been paid, or demand a release of liability. Negotiate and clearly understand a contract with clear payment and completion schedules of specific projects and the project as a whole.

Create a job file with started and completed individual job deadline dates. Contractually arrange to withhold 10 percent of each payment until completion. This ensures that the contractor finishes the renovation right down to the last item. Before signing a certificate of completion, get an itemized breakdown of final details and deadlines to be completed.

Require that the contactor receive a building permit for your project and require a one-year warranty on all work. Put everything, including any changes, in writing with signatures or initials. If you need to cancel a contract, do it within three business days.

Call your state Contractors State Licensing Board if you have any unanswered questions. Also you might want to check your issues with the National Association of the Remodeling Industry (NARI) at 1-800-966-7601 (http://www.nari.org).

CAVEAT VENDITOR—LET THE SELLER BEWARE

Homeowners must put specific information about insulation in every home sales contract (Federal Rule 460.16). Local and state governments may have additional rules and regulations governing consumer contracts.

7

Defeating Drafts

Infiltration and Exfiltration

We all know what a draft is, that warm or chilly breath of a breeze that causes a quiver or a shiver. But the technical terms are either infiltration (coming in) or exfiltration (going out). A draft can be one of the biggest energy vampires in your house, even if the offending area is well-insulated. A draft is like wearing an untied robe outside in the winter. No matter how warm that robe is, you're going to feel the weather. Besides the annoyance of chilly or overheated air currents, leaks are also expensive.

Sealing the exterior envelope of a house, or what builders call a "shell," against unwanted air getting in or getting out helps increase comfort and reduces the energy bill. Unless you live in a rustic log cabin or the ruin of a castle, there is no need to put up with drafts.

FACTS AND FIGURES

Infiltration and exfiltration are two of the leading causes of home energy losses (right next to inefficient insulation). Air leakage accounts for 5 percent to 30 percent of the costs to heat and cool buildings. They can cost you $500 or more a year in lost energy, so there is a big incentive to track them down and eradicate them. The majority of air leakage originates from spaces like basements, crawl spaces, attics, and garages. These are also spaces that generally contain large amounts of pollutants: dust, insulation particles, fumes from paints, gasoline smells, carbon monoxide from cars, mold, insecticides, etc.

"Wind washing" (air leaking into and through insulation) can reduce effectiveness of insulation by 15 to 50 percent. Making use of the highest-rated insulation will be of little benefit if your building is leaking warm or cold air. A one-inch square hole in a wall, roof, etc., will let in thirty quarts of water vapor over the course of a season, creating a cascade of problems. Moisture rots wood, creates mold, lets dust mites thrive, and can attract other pests. Most homes have enough gaps and voids equaling a one-foot-square hole in an exterior wall—not something you want to live with during a chilly winter, or a hot or humid summer.

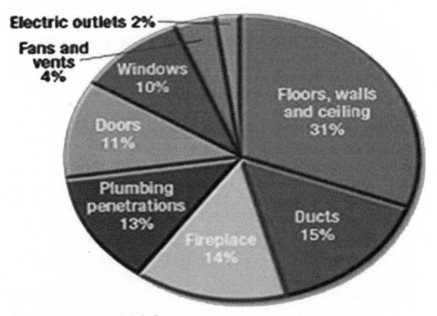

Figure 7.1. Sources of air leaks.
Source: International Association of Certified Home Inspectors, https://www.nachi.org.

WHERE TO LOOK FOR LEAKS

There are areas where infiltration/exfiltration shows up repeatedly in energy containment efficiency tests. Check these places out:

- Look for dirty spots on your ceiling, paint, and carpet, which may indicate air leaks needing caulk.
- Dropped ceilings.
- Recessed light fixtures.
- Attic entrances.
- Sill plates, the seam between the top of the foundation wall and the wood framing.
- Door and window frames.

- Water and furnace flues, laundry chutes, pipe and wire entry and exits in the walls.
- All ducts, including exhaust fans.
- Chimney flashing.
- Electrical outlets, switch plates, and along baseboards.
- Plumbing and utility access, both inside and out.

FIXING YOUR HOME'S LEAKS

Be sure to caulk and seal air leaks where plumbing, ducting, or electrical wiring comes through walls, floors, ceilings, and soffits (beams or arches) over cabinets (see chapter 8, "Roofs, Attics, and Ceilings"). It's also a good idea to install foam gaskets behind outlet and switch plates on walls.

Cover single-pane windows with storm windows or replace them with more efficient double-pane low-emission windows (see chapter 9, "Windows and Doors"). Use a foam sealant on larger gaps around windows, baseboards, and other places where air may leak out. Be careful with foam sealant as it expands and can pop sheetrock out.

Seal any air leaks around fireplace chimneys, furnaces, and gas-fired water heater vents with fire-resistant materials such as sheet metal or sheetrock and

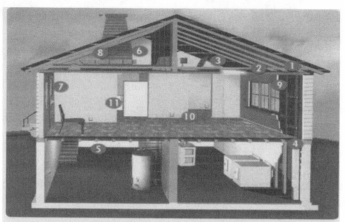

1. Dropped ceiling 2. Recessed light 3. Attic entrance 4. Sill plates 5. Water & furnace flues 6. All ducts 7. Door frames 8. Chimney flashing 9. Window frames 10. Electrical outlets, switch plates, baseboards 11. Plumbing and utility access
US EIA

Figure 7.2.   Common areas of leaks.
Source: https://www.energystar.gov.

furnace cement caulk. Keep the fireplace flue damper tightly closed when not in use. Also, cover your kitchen exhaust fan to stop air leaks when you're not using it. Check your dryer vent to be sure it is not blocked, which will save energy and may prevent a fire. Replace door bottoms and thresholds with ones that have pliable sealing gaskets.

A PRACTICAL TEST

Technicians use a "blower-door test" to accurately measure air leakage in houses. The test involves sealing a portable, frame-mounted fan in an exterior doorway to the house.

First, seal any known openings to the outside, such as the fireplace flue, bathroom vent fans, and the flues to the water heater, furnace, or boiler. After the sealing and setup is complete, and the blower fan is switched on, devices called smoke pencils (or anything that safely creates smoke) can identify areas where air is entering the house. Professionals use infrared meters that will paint a picture (literally in reds and blues) where the house is losing energy.

Another approach is to shine a flashlight at night over all potential gaps while a partner observes the house from outside. Large cracks will show up as rays of light, though this is not a good way to detect small cracks. For those, shut a door or window on a dollar bill. If you can pull the dollar bill out easily (without it dragging through the sill), you're losing energy.

8

Roofs, Attics, and Ceilings
Don't Let Your Top Down

It can ruin your day and your utility bill when your roof lets you down, figuratively if not literally. No one needs raindrops falling on their head, and the ceiling can be a headache when it is too hot or not cool enough. Below are some sustainable suggestions to help keep your home toasty in the winter and chilled during the summer.

In the world of sustainable building, roofs and ceilings do more than put a structure over your head. They can help put bucks back in your pocket while conserving enormous amounts of energy when cared for and properly constructed. Roofs can also be modified to be innovatively green, even when they are a reflective white.

Insulation is very often overlooked in attics, especially in older homes and in awkward hard-to-get-to areas. The more complex the architecture, the more challenging it is to insulate. Taking care of the space in between your ceiling and roof is an effective way to reduce your heating bills and produce less carbon dioxide, as you will be using less energy. You can do it yourself.

FACTS AND FIGURES

Poorly insulated attics and roofs can lose up to 40 percent of a house's heated and cooled air. Adding insulation to ceilings, walls, and attics can save up to 30 percent on heating and cooling costs. The recommended minimum insulation for roofs is R-30 to R-40, depending on your geographic location. In addition, a white roof (light or bright white in color) typically saves 10 to 20 percent on cooling costs. Metal roofs reflect heat better than conventional roofs, and most US homeowners can get a 30 percent tax credit by installing a metal roof.

The attic floor should be covered with the recommended amount of insulation (approximately R-38). Upgrading insulation from three inches to twelve inches in your attic can cut heating costs by 20 to 40 percent, and cooling costs by 10 to 20 percent. It can cost from $500 to $1,000 to bring a typical attic up to best weatherized standards. Keep in mind that insulation is effective for at least 40 years, and when properly utilized, pays for itself in about five years. However, if attic insulation is already more than six inches deep, other energy improvements are usually a better investment. Think about using Earth-friendly chopped cellulose, which is chemically treated to resist fire and insects, and holds up well.

Any uninsulated patch in your attic will reduce its total R-value insulation. Be sure to check that the following areas are well-insulated:

• Between, over, and into floor joists.
• Attic door.
• Finished attic room.
• Between the studs of knee walls (a short wall, typically under three feet in height, used to support the rafters in timber roof construction) and rafters of exterior walls and roof.
• All exterior walls and walls between living spaces, unheated garages, and other spaces.
• Foundation walls above ground level and in basements.
• Floors above cold spaces.
• Any portion of a floor that is cantilevered.
• Slab floors built directly on the ground.

ROOFING MATERIALS PROS AND CONS

Composition Pros: Asphalt or fiberglass shingles offer a durable option, may be available with recycled content, are easy to install, and in some applications can be nailed in place over an existing roof. They are also low maintenance and can be walked on without damaging the material. Most brands offer Class A fire protection. They last from ten to twenty years.

Composition Cons: They can blow off in high winds and are easily scarred when hot. They also do not have the dimensional look of tile or shake.

Metal Pros: These roofs can be made to resemble wood shakes, clay tiles, shingles, and Victorian metal tiles. They are durable, fire retardant, almost maintenance-free, and are also energy efficient. Metal reflects heat and blocks its transfer into the attic. Research by the Florida Solar Energy Center showed that metal absorbed 34 percent less heat than asphalt shingles, causing homeowners to save up to 20 percent on their energy bills. They are made of 60 to 65 percent recyclable material. Because it weighs very little, metal roofing can be installed over existing roofs, eliminating the need to dispose of excess material in a landfill.

Metal Cons: Installing some metal roofing can be an intricate and expensive process best done by a professional, and the initial cost of a premium metal roof is higher than most other roofing materials.

Tile Pros: Tiles last a long time. They won't rot or burn and insects can't harm them, so they require little maintenance.

Tile Cons: The biggest drawback to tiles can be their weight. Tiles are fragile and may break during roof maintenance, and they can also be very expensive.

Slate Pros: Slate has a very long lifespan, good fire protection, low maintenance, and an invulnerability to rot and insects. It comes in a good selection of sizes and colors.

Slate Cons: It can be very heavy and can break during roof maintenance.

Concrete Tile Pros: These have a long life and are the most economical of roofing materials. They can be the most cost-effective solution for durability, aesthetics, and environmental friendliness and the material can be reused. They are fiberglass reinforced, require low maintenance, offer good fire protection, and are resistant to rot and insects.

Concrete Tile Cons: They can be heavy and can break.

Wood Pros: Wood offers a natural look with a lot of character and it allows a house to breathe, circulating air through the small openings under the felt rows on which wooden shingles are laid.

Wood Cons: A wood roof demands proper maintenance and repair or it will not last as long as other products. Mold, rot, and insects can be a problem. Installing wood shakes is also more complicated than roofing with composite shingles. The cost of wood shingle and shake roofs may be high, and, unfortunately, the old wood can't be recycled. Many use wipe or spray-on fire retardants, which offer less protection and are only effective for a few years, although pressure-treated materials are available. Some communities are rejecting wood roofs for various reasons.

Asphalt Pros: Also called hot mopping, asphalt's main advantage is that it is less expensive than other roofing materials and holds up fairly well when properly applied. Most of the time patching is easily done.

Asphalt Cons: This technique results in a roof that's not very pretty, although it is often covered with a layer of decorative gravel to improve the appearance. In addition to being unpleasant, the hot asphalt poses a health risk to installers. It should be professionally installed, and small leaks can be a hassle and hard to find and fix. Because its fumes contribute to smog (outgas), hot mopped asphalt may be restricted in some urban areas. Check your city's building department.

ATTIC ENERGY-SAVING SUGGESTIONS

Never cover attic vents or recessed light fixtures with insulation (without using the proper material), and allow a three-inch clearance around chimneys and flue pipes to prevent overheating and avoid the risk of fire. Check if openings for pipes, ductwork, and chimneys are sealed. If not, seal gaps with expanding foam or a permanent foam sealant.

Verify whether there is a vapor barrier (plastic sheet, roofing felt, tar/felt paper) under the attic insulation. Never use more than one vapor barrier as this can trap water and cause rot. If there is no vapor barrier, paint the interior ceilings with vapor barrier paint to reduce the water vapor that passes through the ceiling.

Attic stairs create a big hole in your ceiling. An easy and inexpensive solution is an attic stair cover which with weather stripping, provides a good seal for air leaks. See if you observe any gaps and light coming through your attic door. This can represent huge air leakage—both in and out. Be sure to seal exhaust fans to the outside and use an airtight box to cover the case. Also, caulk any electrical boxes in the ceiling.

Most new homes have metal chimneys. Repair and seal around any gaps between the brick chimney and the wood framing the chimney with high-temperature exterior sealant. Where walls meet the ceiling, use caulk for the smaller holes and strips of wood in conjunction with expanding foam for the larger gaps.

Fill gaps around plumbing vent stacks and pipe holes with an expanding foam. Expanding foam can be tricky, so follow instructions carefully. Venting in attics and basements (the little screen openings) allows air flow and is important for preventing moisture from becoming trapped in the insulation.

A layer of aluminum foil-type material across the underside of the roof in your attic blocks heat radiated and reduces energy use by 3 to 8 percent. Use a mask to prevent inhalation of insulation fibers. Vermiculite insulation may contain asbestos, a carcinogen.

SAFETY TIPS FOR INSULATION

Follow the manufacturer's directions for all products. Before insulating, ensure that electrical connections and wires are in good condition. Consult with an electrician if old knob-and-tube wiring is present. Treat electrical wiring with care. Do not try to pull or bend it.

Check for nails protruding through the roof. Keep cellulose three inches away from chimneys, even if it is fire retardant, and keep all insulation at least three inches away from other heat sources for fire protection. Do not cover or pack insulation around bare stovepipes, electrical fixtures, motors, or any heat-producing equipment. Make sure the insulation meets either federal or American Society for Testing and Materials (ASTM) standards and specifications.

CEILINGS

According to the US Department of Energy, energy losses from a roof can account for 40 to 50 percent of the total thermal losses of a ceiling. In some homes these concealed air leakage areas can add up to 20 square feet of leakage. It's like leaving an outside door wide open. One of the simplest ways to reduce this loss is by checking out the value and amount of insulation you have in your attic. Batt insulation is an easy fix, and can be easily placed in between the joists of your ceiling.

High ceilings can result in significant stratification where much warmer air becomes trapped close to the ceiling. This is heat you pay for, which you don't use. Even for a standard seven- to eight-foot ceiling, several degrees difference in temperature between floor and ceiling is not unusual. A cathedral ceiling can range up to 15 degrees warmer at the top. A heat harvester, simply consisting of a fan placed so that it creates a flow of air up to and across a high place, will reclaim the heat by circulating it down to the living space. It will save far more in heating costs than the electricity required to operate it.

ICE DAMS

An ice dam is a ridge of ice that forms at the edge of a roof and prevents melted water from draining off the roof. Heat and warm air leaking from the living space below melts the snow, which trickles down to the colder edge of the roof (above the eaves) and refreezes.

Ice dams cause millions of dollars of structural damage to houses every year. There are many ways to treat the symptoms, but proper air sealing, insulation, and attic venting are the best ways to eliminate the problem. Another way is to remove snow from the roof with a "roof rake" and push broom, being careful not to damage roofing materials. In an emergency where water may be running into the house, create channels through the ice dam, allowing the water behind the dam to drain off the roof. Block melted water running into the house by installing a rubber membrane on the roof under the roof shingles.

Another temporary solution is to hose the roof with tap water, working upward from the lower edge of the dam. Make sure the ceiling is watertight. Block all air leaks leading to the attic from the house so warm, moist air can't flow from the house into the attic space and potentially melt the ice. Increase the amount and/or thickness of insulation on the attic floor. Be sure the air and insulation barrier are continuous.

NATURAL ATTIC VENTILATION

Proper insulation and air sealing keeps attics cold in winter by blocking the entry of heat and moist air from below, ensuring against ice dams on the roof. In the summer, natural airflow in a well-vented attic moves super-heated air out of the attic, protecting roof shingles and removing moisture. Attic fans are intended to cool hot attics by drawing in cooler outside air from attic vents and pushing hot air to the outside.

If your attic has blocked vents and is not well sealed from the rest of the house, attic fans will suck cool air up out of the house and into the attic. This will use more energy and make your air conditioner work harder, which will increase your summer utility bill. To prevent this, follow the air sealing and insulation strategies in this book and make sure the attic is well-ventilated, using passive vents and natural air flow.

COOL AND GREEN ROOFS

They can be called green roofs, cool roofs, living roofs, eco-roofs, or roof-top gardens and are largely an untapped conservation resource. Truly green roofs embrace several technologies. It can be a living roof of a building that is partially or completely covered with vegetation—a growing medium, planted over a waterproofing membrane. It may also include additional layers such as a root barrier and drainage and irrigation systems. On hot summer days, the surface temperature of a green roof can be cooler than the air temperature, whereas the surface of a conventional rooftop can be up to 90°F (50°C) warmer.

On a wider scale green or cool roofs last longer than conventional roofs, reduce energy costs, are naturally insulated, make for peaceful retreats for people and animals, and absorb storm water, lessening the need for complex and expensive drainage systems, and they filter impurities out of the air (which helps lower disease rates and respiratory conditions such as asthma). Cool roofs also absorb carbon dioxide, provide insulation, and reduce heat loss and energy consumption. They improve air quality and help reduce the urban heat island (UHI) effect, which causes buildings to absorb and trap heat. Anyone who has walked across a scalding parking lot on a hot summer day has felt an effect of an urban heat island.

Cool roofs come in a variety of colors, most commonly white, and today's "cool roof" pigments allow metal roofing products to be EnergyStar-rated in dark colors—even black. They aren't as reflective as whites or light colors, but can still save energy over other paints.

Heat-absorbing buildings, especially those with dark roofs and nonreflective surfaces, release heat absorbed from sunlight that can increase outdoor air temperature from 2° to 8°F and a concentration of green roofs in an urban area can reduce a city's average temperatures by up to 2° to 4°F during the summer.

Green roofs can insulate buildings for sound and, if installed correctly, many can contribute to LEED (Leadership in Energy and Environmental Development) points. Getting LEED certification can mean good things for your home's resale value and potential tax incentives, not to mention bragging rights to your eco-savvy friends. The system, created by the US Green Building Council, was developed to promote guidelines for achieving conservation and protection of resources, reduction in greenhouse gas emissions, reduction in waste sent to landfills, and improved air quality. LEED guidelines can help you do this by making sure every part of your home is properly insulated, ensuring you'll be using less energy to operate your home.

Green roofs also add beauty and landscape design to commonly unused space, or can be used as outdoor recreational areas for urban structures. An extensive green roof may cost $10 to $25 per square foot, although less expensive alternatives are available. Green roofs play an important role in reducing urban temperatures and air pollution, and they have a cooling effect on your town and neighborhood.

9

Windows and Doors

Openings You Want to Keep Closed

Windows and doors provide our homes with portals to the outside for light, warmth, and ventilation, but unless they are efficient they can also be energy robbers. Windows and doors are some of the most common places for air to leak, after all, they are big holes in the wall. According to California's Pacific Gas and Electric Company, the gaps in windows and doors of the average house represent about a foot-sized square hole in the wall.

According to the National Resources Defense Council, approximately 30 percent of a home's total heat loss usually occurs through windows and doors. This is why windows and doors should be inspected each season. An investment of under $50 in weatherizing supplies can save two to three times that much in heating costs each year.

FACTS AND FIGURES

Replacing the windows in an old house is one of the most expensive energy upgrades you can make. To improve performance of existing windows, consider storm windows, window films, exterior roller shades, and simple fixes like caulking and weather stripping before buying replacement windows.

Windows alone lose 5 percent of all US energy produced yearly, at a cost of $35 billion. The Department of Energy states that the amount of energy escaping through windows in the United States equals the energy produced by all the oil flowing through the Alaskan pipeline in one year.

Windows, the prime energy bandits offering only R-1 to R-3 in insulation value, are responsible for 25 to 50 percent of energy loss in buildings. Windows, through heat loss, can account for 10 to 25 percent of your home's heating bill. If all windows were as efficient as possible, the average household would save $150 a year and reduce its carbon dioxide emissions by about 4,300 pounds per year. Double-glazed windows save 2.4 tons of carbon dioxide emissions per year for homes heated by natural gas, 3.9 tons for those heated by oil, and 9.8 tons for electric heat.

The initial cost of an efficient window is going to be 2 to10 percent higher than a nonefficient window, however, you'll start seeing the payback in energy savings around two years after installation. Then it's the gift that will keep on giving for fifteen to thirty years, depending on the (double-pane) type you choose—aluminum lasts approximately fifteen to twenty years, sustainable wood up to thirty years, and vinyl twenty to thirty years.

Low-emittance (low-E) coatings are microscopically thin, virtually invisible metal or metallic oxide layers deposited on a window or skylight surface, primarily used to reduce radiative heat flow. High-performance windows have at least two panes of glass and a low-E coating. They can also be filled with argon gas. Argon gas is an inert form of gas that window makers seal between panes of glass to act as an insulator, slowing the heat transfer through the window. These windows are designed to reduce heat loss, but admit solar light.

Recently, some reflective insulation manufacturers have switched to a metalized polyethylene facing. The long-term efficiency and durability of such facings are still undetermined. There are nine different technologies in material science and manufacturing windows to get insulation values from R-5 to R-20.

TERMS TO GET WIND OF

When shopping for windows the following are some key words you should know.

A casement window opens with a crank or a lever. They are efficient because they seal tightly.

Double-hung windows open by sliding up and down, and both window sashes (frames) are moveable. Single-hung windows have only one moveable sash.

Low-E is a measurement of how much heat a window radiates. Many windows are coated with invisible, metal oxide e-coatings that reduce the amount of heat radiating from the glass. When there is a temperature difference between inside and outside, heat is lost or gained through the window frame and glazing by the combined effects of conduction, convection, and radiation.

The U-factor of a window assembly represents its insulating value. The lower the U-value, the more efficient the window.

Solar heat gain coefficient (SHGC), regardless of temperature, is the ability of the window to control heat gain though direct or indirect solar radiation.

PRACTICAL SUGGESTIONS FOR WINDOWS

It might not be necessary to replace windows unless they are actually falling apart, unsafe, or if they no longer work properly. Replace any cracked or broken panes promptly and keep all exterior surfaces painted; it protects wood. Pay particular attention to horizontal surfaces such as windowsills, where water collects.

Check windowpanes to see if they need new glazing. If the glass is loose, remove and replace the putty. Some types of window glazing require painting for a proper seal.

Some energy-saving devices are very low tech. A simple drape can stop a 33 percent heat loss through a window. An insulated drape can increase that to 50 percent, a savings of 10 percent of your annual energy bill. Drapes will save energy only if they fit snugly against the window and the floor. This means weighted bottoms, side guides, and a valance at the top. You could also secure them together or to a wall with Velcro or self-sealing strips. In winter, keep drapes and shades on south-facing windows, which receive the most sunlight, open during the day. Close them at night to reduce the chill. In winter cover older windows (on the exterior) with a plastic sheet.

Pay special attention to south-facing (during the summer) and north-facing (during the winter) windows. Keep all south-facing window glass clean to maximize the amount of sunlight coming through the windows during the winter. Remember that condensation can cause rot. Check the condensation resistance factor (CRF) with the manufacturer.

Don't count on Venetian-type blinds or louvered windows to be efficient window insulation. They have too many gaps between the blades. To keep the heat out, the most effective window treatment option is to keep the sun out. Retractable awnings and even fixed awnings tend to be expensive, but economical exterior roller shades are available for as little as $25 per window.

WINDOW FILM

Use reflective window coverings (on the outside) to mitigate heat through sunlight. Reflective film blocks 40 to 60 percent of solar heat, but doesn't block sunlight. Installing window film can save up to 70 percent of warm and cool air loss. Using reflective window film will also keep furniture and carpets from fading.

Film improves shatter resistance, blocks up to 99 percent of ultraviolet radiation, and reduces glare. There are two primary types of window films: permanent surface-applied films, and the stretch-plastic that you install temporarily to interior windows. Surface-applied films are now rated by the National Fenestration Rating Council and have a wide range of performance properties. Standard sun control window films run about $80 installed while spectrally selective films are about $125 per typical window. Spectrally selective window films reduce solar heat gain effectively while transmitting more of the sun's visible light than do standard films.

The DIY stretch-plastic film kits you tack onto window trim can be installed relatively airtight for better thermal comfort and reduced heating in cold climates. They typically run about $1 to $2 per square foot, with a payback period of 3 to 5 years, available at any building supply or hardware store. Use aluminum foil on the sunniest windows, reflective insulation can stop 97 percent of radiant heat transfer.

STORM WINDOWS

If everyone in the Frost Belt installed storm windows, the nation would save as much oil as it now gets from Alaska. Thirty-five million cubic feet of natural gas would be saved and four million pounds of carbon dioxide would be removed from the atmosphere.

In cold weather, exterior storm windows can reduce heat loss by 25 to 50 percent and can reduce air leakage by 45 to 75 percent. Interior storm windows can reduce air leakage by 80 to 95 percent. Storm windows preserve interior windows from wear and tear.

Super-insulated windows let in more heat than they let out, even on the north side of the house. These windows outperform the best-insulated wall, because they conserve furnace heat and gather solar energy.

Newer, airtight storm windows with low-E coatings can rival the performance of just about any window replacement. Interior units are easy to install, although exterior units do a much better job of protecting your existing windows.

Storm windows also add value to your house, are less expensive than replacement windows, and are relatively low maintenance. Most door manufacturers sell pre-hung storm doors in kits so installation is easy and can be a DIY project. The kits, including those for temporary storm windows, include all the hardware you need to install the door and window, such as hinges, pneumatic closers, and latches.

READY TO REPLACE A WINDOW?

When selecting windows, look for low U-factors and low solar heat gain coefficient (SHGC) ratings to maximize energy savings. Ask the retailer or manufacturer for product literature to determine whether windows and doors meet building code requirements, and look for whole unit U-factors and SHGCs rather than center of glass (COG) U-factors. Use ASTM rating (American Society for Testing and Materials) E283, "Standard Test Method for Determining Rate of Air Leakage through Exterior Windows, Curtain Walls, and Doors." For state codes check out: http://www.efficientwindows. org/standards_codestate.php.

Install double-pane windows filled with argon gas. They are twice as efficient as single panes. If you live in the Sun Belt look into low-E windows, which can cut the cooling load by 10 to 15 percent.

Use or ask for a computer simulation program, such as RESFEN (a program for calculating the heating and cooling energy use of windows in residential buildings). This lets you compare window performance options by calculating performance based on utility rates for your climate, house design options, and window design options.

Make sure design and window workmanship results in a good and durable choice for your specific application. Check out frames and sashes, insulating glass seals, weather stripping, and local requirements for structural integrity. Window warranties can be an indicator of the reliability of the window and its manufacturer.

For metal frames, install rubber gaskets between inner and outer pieces to lessen heat loss. Proper installation is necessary for optimal window performance, to ensure an airtight fit, and to avoid water leakage. Always follow manufacturer's installation guidelines and use trained professionals for window installation.

Before you make the final decision on your replacement windows, be sure to investigate rebates and other tax incentives from your utility companies.

PRACTICAL SUGGESTIONS FOR DOORS

Never add a glass storm door if the door gets more than a few hours of direct sun each day. The glass will trap too much heat against the entry door and possibly damage it. When a storm door is properly sealed and adjusted, it should make the house door a little difficult to close. When opening the house door, the storm door should suck in slightly as air is pulled out of the area between the doors. If large amounts of moisture condense on the inside of windows and freeze on cold days, the storm windows are not working properly.

The R-values of most steel- and fiberglass-clad entry doors range from R-5 to R-6 (not including the effects of a window). Look for glass doors manufactured with several layers of glazing, low-E coatings, and low conductivity gases between the glass panes. These options are a good investment especially in extreme climates. Over the long run the additional cost is paid back many times over in energy savings.

Consider an insulated metal or fiberglass door when replacing exterior doors, as they are more durable, have lower maintenance needs, seal and insulate better. They also have the added advantage of offering a strong deterrent to intruders. When replacing patio doors, hinged doors offer a much tighter seal than sliding types. Look for glass doors with metal frames that have a "thermal break," a plastic insulator between inner and outer parts of the frame.

Because doors open and close constantly, door jams, sweeps, sills, and weather stripping are under constant use and can increase energy loss around the door. Be certain that the vinyl strips that seal the storm doors from the thresholds are clean and not worn out. Check them yearly. Doors also shrink and expand, causing gaps in the door jams and at the bottom where they meet the door sill.

Door sweeps come in strips that you can measure and cut to the size of your door. They are then screwed (you might want to drill "pilot" holes to make the job easier) into the bottom of the door. Make sure the bottom of the sweep fits snugly, but not too tightly, and fits the bottom door sill. Adjustable door threshold bottoms are made from wood or metal and covered with a removable, replaceable strip of vinyl or rubber. Under the strip are several screw heads. By adjusting the screws, you can cause the threshold to rise or fall, creating a close fit.

Adhesive-backed foam insulation strips for door jambs come in various widths and lengths. Make sure all surfaces are clean. Measure the length of the sides and top of door jamb, cut, remove adhesive backing, and press into place. Metal- or wood-backed rubber strips work essentially the same as the foam strips, except that the metal-backed rubber strips are sturdier and last longer. The strips contain a vinyl bulb or padded strip set into the edge of a wood or metal strip. This is nailed or screwed to the side door jamb and is flexible enough to conform to even a badly warped wooden door. Thin bronze or brass strips can be attached inside the jamb. When the door closes, it contacts the metal strip, bending it a bit and ensuring tight contact with the door edge.

With any weather stripping, use a thickness so that when the door closes, the stripping tightly presses between the door and the doorjamb without making the door too hard to close. Clean glass with a general household cleaner or a mixture of warm water and mild detergent using a soft cloth or paper towel. Do not use abrasive cleaners, thinners, or strippers.

For a cheap fix when drafts sneak in, simply block them with a rolled-up towel, blanket, or "snake" (a manufactured "plug-like sausage") that fits under or against door bottoms. If you do it yourself, it's probably not a good idea to use grain or rice or any filler that could attract rodents. Fish bowl gravel is dense, won't rot, attract vermin, or degrade. Unused doors and windows should be sealed with rope caulk (soft, malleable material primarily used to seal around doors and windows). Don't seal them shut permanently—you might need quick ventilation or an escape route during an emergency.

SIMPLE LOOK AND SEE

Thermal imaging or infrared instruments can detect heat loss. Some can be purchased at hardware and home improvement stores, they can also be rented, or you can hire a professional service.

10

Floors and Basements

Protecting Your Bottom

Anyone who has a home with an uninsulated cement slab foundation will never be caught walking around barefoot in winter. The basement ceiling can affect the floor of your living space, so when you think about one, think about the other. The basement walls and floor are the perimeter to the "outside" of your home and can be the cause of a lot of lost heat. Foundation and basement leaks account for 20 percent of heat loss in a poorly insulated home.

In the past, floors were not very well insulated because heat rises, so homeowners concentrated on preventing heat loss through ceilings and walls. However, heat loss through flooring can still occur when the area under the floor is neither insulated nor climate-controlled. Neglecting to insulate a floor can contribute to higher energy bills because heating systems will need to work harder to keep that space warm.

FACTS AND FIGURES

The process of hot air rising is called convection. It's one way that heat can escape a building. Two others are conduction and radiation. Floor insulation limits all three modes of heat loss. A warmer floor reduces the temperature difference that drives convection. Floor insulation also directly impedes conduction and radiation to the colder air below the floor.

Floors lose up to 10 percent of a home's heating, but some of that can be retained with floor coverings (carpets and throw rugs, etc.) and can result in an estimated energy savings of up to one month's worth of heating per year. Carpets additionally trap and immobilize harmful allergy producing particles, making vacuuming more effective and improving overall household air quality.

The initial cost to upgrade floor insulation from R-19 to R-30 or even R-38 can save several times its cost over the life of the house. While homes in colder climates will benefit most, even upgrading in moderate climates makes sense economically. According to the Department of Energy, $50 or more can be saved in heating costs each year by increasing the insulation in, on, or under the floor.

The best way to insulate floors is to place batt insulation between floor joists, using (at least) R-19-rated insulation. Proceed the same way you would insulate the attic. Insulation must contact the subfloor and both joists/walls, and floor cavities should be completely filled with insulation, without gaps or voids.

PRACTICAL SUGGESTIONS FOR BASEMENT PROBLEMS

Problems of cold air, heat leakage, moisture, and vermin control arise where the house meets the foundation. Always check first for dry rot (use a screwdriver to poke holes into dry or moldy looking wood) and signs of termites or carpenter ants (look for small piles of sawdust-looking matter or weak, brittle, or eaten-away wood) in the floor joists or subflooring. These problems must be remedied before you begin to install under-floor or perimeter insulation. You'll need to have crawl space in your basement area to access the joists.

Do not insulate floors over heated basements. If your basement is unheated, determine whether there is any insulation under the living area flooring. The sill plate (which sits on top of the foundation) should be caulked if gaps are present. During new construction, an insulating gasket should be installed under the sill plate. If you have a floor over an unheated space, such as a basement or garage, insulate the space between the floor and the garage with R-20 or greater. A big heat loss culprit is the rim joist (the final joist that caps the end of the row of joists) that supports a floor. Leaks at the top around the floor joists and leaks at the sill plate are common in older houses. To remedy, cut a batt of fiberglass insulation and fit it into the cavity.

Using (at least) R-19-rated insulation, proceed the same way you would insulate the attic (as seen previously in chapter 6, "Batt Insulation"). An R-value of 25 is the recommended minimum level of insulation. Plastic mesh, metal or wood strips, or specifically designed wire hangers can help secure the batt between the joists. Hanging the mesh can create "sagging bellies," and they should be taut against the bottom of the floor framing. To avoid gaps in this situation, the batt must be pushed up into the cavity and supported properly. A polyethylene vapor barrier should be installed on the unfinished (sometimes dirt) floor after insulation to prevent the collection of moisture. Check local building codes for proper insulation R-value.

Chapter 10

A WORD ABOUT SUMP PUMPS

If you are in a flood zone, below sea level, or near a levee, sump pumps can protect basements and houses from flooding. Check your homeowners insurance for flooding; it usually doesn't cover damages from sump-pump failure or overflow. Things to know:

- Sump pumps often vibrate while running, which can cause the float mechanism that regulates water flow to get stuck.
- Fouled ground water and sediment can clog intake screens, discharge pipes, and float switches. Check running pumps regularly.
- Battery backups offer a measure of protection if the primary pump fails, or in case of a power outage.
- Once a year, pour a gallon of distilled white vinegar into the sump pump basin to break down calcium deposits.
- Listen for grinding noises that might mean the pump may be on its last leg.

11

Walls

If They Could Talk, They Might Criticize

It's good that walls don't have mouths, because they would complain about how we neglect to properly insulate them, or fix the little holes and gaps that eat up energy.

An energy-efficient wall is built to minimize energy transfer in the form of warm or cold air moving through the chinks and cracks of your home. The exterior walls of the building envelope are the dividing line between the warm, cozy interior and the chilly exterior. Because walls are exposed to the outside, they also are special target areas for energy loss. Plus, insulating walls offers a noise barrier between the outside world, inside walls dividing rooms, or "party walls" dividing apartments or condos.

FACTS AND FIGURES

The loss of air temperature through the walls of a building depends upon the condition of the walls, their thickness, layers of insulation, and the difference between the inside and outside temperatures. One of the most important parts of insulating a home is making sure that it is insulated with the correct material and R-value.

Up to 40 percent of heat is lost through uninsulated walls and good quality wall insulation is a way of preventing energy waste and cutting up to 25 percent of your fuel bills. Efficient wall insulation can mean saving $50 to $350 per year.

Wall insulation is normally made up of protected air barriers, vapor retarders, and thermal bridges—all of which contribute to preventing heating and cooling from escaping through the walls of homes. Cavity wall insulation, between-wall framing, is one of the most cost-effective energy efficiency measures in the home.

PRACTICAL SUGGESTIONS

Feel the walls for warmth or chill. If the wall lacks sidewall insulation, place heavy furniture like bookshelves, armoires, cabinets, and sofas along exterior walls, and use decorative quilts and wall hangings. These will help block cold air. Make sure where walls meet floors and roofs there are no cracks or drafts.

Insulation is placed between the two-by-four wall framing and stapled to the inside or the face of the studs. If you are using unfaced batts, place the insulation into the cavity, making sure that it is the correct size and fits snugly at the sides and ends and does not protrude in the back.

Add pieces of batt insulation to the rim joists—the area along the top of the foundation where it meets the exterior walls. When using batt insulation with a reflective aluminum facing, allow one inch between the facing and the wallboard. To achieve this gap, staple the insulation to the inside of the stud instead of the edge. This air gap will significantly increase the amount of thermal energy reflected back to the home.

If construction is airtight, all air leaks should be sealed during construction and prior to the installation of insulation. It is sometimes feasible to install rigid insulation on the outdoor side of masonry sidewalls, such as concrete block or poured concrete. However, if that is not an option, use batts to insulate the interior of masonry walls that can be attached via tacking strips of wood to the masonry first with construction adhesive or cement nails.

For basement walls, a vapor barrier should first be installed on the walls. The vapor barrier on insulation is always installed toward the living space. Air leaking into walls and attics carries significant amounts of moisture. Any exterior rain drainage system, continuous air barrier, and vapor barriers (plastic sheathing over insulation) should be located on the appropriate side of the wall.

Foam boards are a good choice for insulation in basement renovations since they do not absorb water. For new construction, reduce exterior leaks by using house wrap, a replacement for the older asphalt-treated paper or asphalt-saturated felt. These materials are all lighter in weight and usually wider than asphalt designs, so contractors can apply the material much faster to a house shell, then caulk and seal.

Table 11.1.　The Look and R-Value of Insulation

What You See		What It Probably Is	Total R-Value
Loose Fibers	Lightweight yellow, pink, or white	Fiberglass	2.5 × depth
	Dense gray or near white, may have black specks	Rockwool	2.8 × depth
	Small gray, flat pieces or fibers (from newsprint)	Cellulose	3.7 × depth
Granules	Small and lightweight	Vermiculite or perlite	2.7 × depth
Batts	Lightweight yellow, pink, or white	Fiberglass	3.2 × depth

Source: www.energystar.gov

TAKE A LOOK

It is difficult to add insulation to existing walls unless you see what you need.

Interior wall insulation contributes to your home's overall energy efficiency and adds significantly to the enjoyment of peace, privacy, and comfort in your home by keeping heat and cool in and by keeping sound out, or at least preventing it from migrating from one room to another.

12

Fireplaces
Old Style Is Romantic, Modern Is Resourceful

A roaring blaze, glass in hand, cuddled up to your special someone, or maybe a favorite book, and kept warm by the rosy glow and mesmerizing flames of the fire on the grate. Sounds wonderful, right? Not so fast. Home is where the hearth used to be. No matter how romantic old-style fireplaces seem to be, they're going the way of coal scuttles. Some cities have strict building codes regulating fireplaces even in remodeled homes where they already exist. Increasingly, fireplace use is forbidden during "clean air" days, and because of fire hazards and insurance hassles, in some cities you can't get a building permit for one. As for producing, distributing, and conserving heat, fireplaces and chimneys are another big hole in your house from which precious heat can escape. But hold on, if you do have a fireplace relax and enjoy. We have some tips to keep it safe and sane while saving some energy.

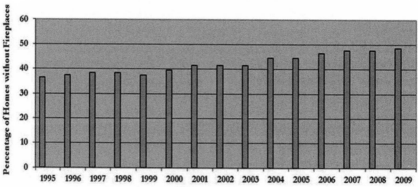

Figure 12.1. Percentage of American homes without fireplaces.
Source: Hearth, Patio and Barbecue Association, www.hpba.org.

FACTS AND FIGURES

As prices for oil and natural gas drive more Americans toward alternative fuels to stay warm in winter, environmental watchdogs are awakening to the unhealthy effects of the pollution from burning wood in the home. Although wood is our most renewable resource, it's not commercially grown for fuel in the United States. A cord of wood (8' × 4' × 4') can cost approximately $200 to $300, is a bother to store, and is not a very efficient way of heating a home.

A single open fireplace damper sends 8 percent of your heating bill up the chimney. In 2011, an estimated 19,500 home structure fires were reported involving fireplaces, chimneys, and chimney connectors that resulted in twenty civilian deaths, seventy civilian fire injuries, and $195 million in direct property damage. According to the US Census Bureau, the number of new homes built without a fireplace in 2009 hit 49 percent, a new low, following a steady upward trend over the past fifteen years.

A wood-burning fireplace can exhaust as much as 24,000 cubic feet of air per hour to the outside. Burning paper products not only increases greenhouse gas pollution, but like other cellulose products, it can cause combustible residue called creosote to collect inside a chimney and invite chimney fires. It is formed when gases from burning wood condense to form a gummy, foul smelling, corrosive, and extremely combustible substance. If it builds up in sufficient quantities and if the flue temperature is high enough, it can combust and cause chimneys to crack, liners to collapse, and may allow flames to reach the wood frames of your house—good reasons to look for a chimney sweep to keep the house safe.

Wood-burning is the primary contributor to particulate pollution during winter months and wood-burning produces particulate matter (particles less than ten micrometers in size) that are far in excess of those produced by agriculture or industry combined. Almost half of our particulate matter pollution comes from wood-burning fireplaces. For folks with asthma, this can be life-threatening. According to federal standards, a fireplace burning for three hours emits over 113 percent of the allowable particulates into the air and an all-day fire emits more than one thousand times the allowable particulates into the atmosphere. During the winter in Southern California, fireplaces produce an average of more than ten tons per day of particulate matter emissions—equal to nearly seven times the amount of daily primary particulate matter emitted from all of the power plants in the area. In Oregon, a very green state, smoke from fireplaces and woodstoves is one of the largest threats to healthy air.

Smoke contains gases and tiny particles known as PM2.5 (particulate matter less than 2.5 microns in diameter). These particles are so small that the

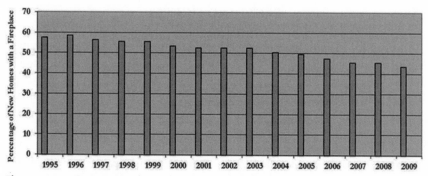

Figure 12.2.   Percentage of American homes with fireplaces.
Source: Hearth, Patio, and Barbecue Association, www.hpba.org.

body's natural defense mechanisms can't keep them from entering deep into the lungs, where they can damage the structure of lung tissue, trigger asthma, and aggravate heart disease as they reduce the blood's ability to supply oxygen to body tissues. Even small amounts that include carbon monoxide (CO) can stress your heart and reduce your ability to exercise. Smoke contains nitrogen oxides (NO_x), which may lower a child's resistance to lung infections. Other contaminates like hydrocarbons (HC) can injure the lungs and make breathing difficult as well.

Old wood stoves that are not Environmental Protection Agency (EPA)–certified waste up to 60 percent of the wood's energy burned in them. Any stove you purchase now must be EPA-certified, which sets limits on emissions.

FIREPLACE EMISSIONS

Following are the hourly and PM10 emissions produced from different sources:

Table 12.1.   Particulate Emissions

Pollution Source	(grams/hour)	(grams/day)
Open Hearth Fireplace (upper range of emissions)	59	1,416
Open Hearth Fireplace (lower range of emissions)	30	720
One New 300-HP Diesel Truck (running full throttle)	18	432
One Non-EPA-Certified Fireplace Insert	15.6	374.4
One EPA-Certified Phase II Fireplace Insert	8.2	196.8
One Chain-Smoker (0.04g/cigarette at 12 cigarettes/hour)	.48	
One Average Smoker (0.04g/cigarette at 1 pack/day)		0.8

IF YOU ARE AN INCURABLE ROMANTIC, REMEMBER THESE PRACTICAL SUGGESTIONS

Check local ordinances for the legality of operating or installing a fireplace. Check with local agencies concerning "Spare the Air Days" before operating your fireplace. Also, be sure your firewood is "seasoned," unpainted, untreated (with chemicals), and bug-free. Moisture level should not be above 20 percent (ask if the seller uses a moisture meter), or be assured that the wood has sat for at least one season. Burning unseasoned (green) or even partially seasoned wood in your stove or fireplace will cause excess creosote build-up in your chimney, which can lead to a chimney fire, a poor quality fire, and a roomful of smoke.

To speed drying, split large logs and stack loosely in a crosswise fashion to get good air circulation. Avoid sappy wood such as pine and oily woods such as eucalyptus, which cause an overkill of creosote. A side note just in case: Planting trees to make up for the wood you're burning decreases your carbon footprint.

Catalytic converters (kind of like those in your car) are devices that channel wood smoke, mixing the gases with air to allow them to reignite at lower temperatures, which reduces emissions and increases efficiency. The converters may need to be changed every few years, which can add a couple hundred dollars per replacement to the cost of your fireplace heat. A baffle, which reflects heat back toward the fire causing a secondary combustion during which unignited gases are burned off, is simpler, less expensive, and lasts longer than a catalytic converter.

Install a fireplace heater system that works by pulling fresh air from the room via a small pump, circulating the heat through the tubular grate, and then blowing the heated air back into the room. These heaters are closed systems, so no smoke from the fireplace will invade the home, and they can be easily installed as an insert. Even during a power failure the system will still passively deliver heated air back into your home.

For the best efficiency, a wood stove should be placed against a wall made of material such as brick or stone, to protect the wall from heat, and radiate it back into the room.

Sealing or blocking a fireplace flue can reduce or eliminate soot and odors that are prone to enter the house during windy or stormy days. Of course, any flue-blocking material must be removed before a fire is started.

When using the fireplace, turn down the furnace to at least 55°F, otherwise much of the warm air from the furnace will go right up the chimney, wasting energy and money.

Add fireproof caulk where the chimney meets the wall, inside and outside. If you never use your fireplace, plug the chimney with fiberglass insulation and seal any doors with silicone caulk.

SAFETY TIPS AND MAINTENANCE

Always have a fire extinguisher on hand. Hundreds of Americans die every year from carbon monoxide poisoning, so remember that a smoldering fire, even though it might not be visible through a layer of ashes, produces carbon monoxide. If you have a wood-burning, open fireplace, install a carbon monoxide detector along with a fire alarm. Be certain a wood-burning fire is completely out and the ashes are cold before you shut the damper or put other seals in place.

Inspect for creosote deposits in the flue. If greater than one-eighth inch in thickness, then the chimney flue should be cleaned. When cleaning your fireplace, simply look up the flue, with a mirror if necessary, and use a flat screwdriver to carefully scratch the interior of the flue and inspect the residue. It's always best to employ a chimney sweep (see below). Check the flue for broken or damaged bricks on the flue liner. Brick, mortar, or metal cracking is a sign that there has been a flue fire (caused by the build-up of unburned combustible materials in the smoke accumulating along the chimney walls) and is a potentially serious problem. Check the damper for operation and a snug fit. Also inspect for cracks, pitting, or rusted-out sections. A chimney sweep will check this out as part of their services.

Chimneys that are used on a regular basis should be inspected or serviced by a chimney sweep every two years, even if you burn only dry, non-sappy, non-oily woods.

MAINTENANCE FOR CERAMIC LOG
AND ALL GAS BURNING FIREPLACES

During the summer months shut off a gas-burning pilot light. Clean and check controls. Inspect, clean, and adjust the pilot light. Always remember to turn off the gas valve before cleaning the fireplace. Before relighting it, make sure to follow manufacturer's instructions, or call the local gas company to relight the pilot. Most will do this at no cost.

Before you use the fireplace, especially the first time at the beginning of the new season, check the venting system to make sure there is nothing clogging it. Look for any areas that show wear or corrosion, which would look like streaks or rust spots that will need to be replaced before using the fireplace. Be sure to remove the vent cap on an exterior wall and use a flashlight to look down the vent to see if any birds or insects have built nests or if any leaves or other debris have accumulated in the chimney. Look for any condensation like water droplets forming in the vents. If condensation continues, the caps will corrode, along with fittings and pipes.

Gas (ceramic) "logs" can be fragile and easily damaged so use a good glass cleaner and a clean, soft paintbrush or cloths to clean them. If you discover any broken logs, turn the gas valve off and let the fireplace cool. Make sure the pilot light is off, and replace with an appropriate log, as not all fireplace logs are the same. Check the position of the logs as well to make sure they are connected firmly and safely. If the logs are not positioned according to the manufacturer's guidelines, carbon build-up can occur and ultimately damage them.

It is important that the (glass) door gasket of your fireplace be the right type to handle high temperatures. Continually inspect and clean glass to note irregularities. Keep burners clean by brushing and vacuuming them once or twice per year. Gold and brass trim should be cleaned with a damp cloth. Do not use abrasive materials, chemical cleaners, or anything else that may damage the finish. Check and clean the blower if applicable. Most gas fireplaces are installed with pilot lights that are on continuously on a 24/7 basis. If you convert these standing pilot lights to on-demand pilot lights that fire up only when necessary, you can save $10 or more every month.

FIREPLACE DAMPERS AND CHIMNEY CAPS

Don't confuse the flue with the damper. The flue is simply the open middle of the chimney that the smoke goes up. Dampers are sometimes miscalled flues, but they are intended to shut off—either fully or partially—the stuff that goes up the chimney.

A chimney cap is a screened or grated cap that covers the top of a chimney. A cap's functions are to keep rain, debris, and "critters" out, especially birds. The screen also serves as a spark arrestor as it will keep most dangerous hot sparks that come up in the smoke from landing somewhere hazardous. These are important functions and no chimney should be uncovered.

After the fire has gone out, most homeowners forget to close the fireplace damper the next day. Remember that the chimney and flue are designed as an exhaust system for expelling air to the outside, which shouldn't come from an expensive furnace or air conditioner on the inside.

An open chimney damper can easily account for the same effect as leaving open two 12" × 12" windows—that can cost you a heating loss of about $500 per year. Even when a fireplace damper is closed, the sealing is often not very effective. In the off-season, placing insulation, a piece of plywood or rigid foam board, tightly under the damper opening will seal the damper. Check the seal on the damper by closing it off and holding a piece of tissue paper or candle inside the firebox. If a draft blows the tissue or flame around, repair or replace the damper.

Top-sealing dampers (about $150 to $200) replace the fireplace throat damper and are installed at the top of the chimney. They have a seal that acts like a storm door, which keeps the expensive heated air inside the house and the cold air outside. A top-sealing damper can be easily installed by a handy person. A chimney cap ($25 to $85) and a top sealing damper are easily installed either with screws, special caulk, or a compression fit, depending on make or model.

HOW TO HIRE A CHIMNEY SWEEP

The Chimney Safety Institute of America (CSIA) suggests annual inspections to ensure against fires and carbon monoxide poisoning and recommends using a CSIA-Certified Chimney Sweep. There are more than 1,900 CSIA Certified Chimney Sweeps located within North America. To ensure that homeowners receive a certified sweep at every job, all chimney sweeping companies promoting the credential are required to have a CSIA Certified Chimney Sweep on every job site.

Ask these questions when interviewing a chimney sweep:

- How long has the chimney sweeping company been in business?
- Does the company offer current references?
- Does the company have unresolved complaints filed within the city or state consumer protection agency or Better Business Bureau? (Check this out yourself.)
- Does the company or individual carry a valid business liability insurance policy to protect your home and furnishings against accidents?
- Does the company ensure that a CSIA Certified Chimney Sweep will be on the job site?

Table 12.2.   Comparable Cost and Efficiency of Fuel Versus Fuel

Fuel	Heating Value	Efficiency	Cost	Cost/ MBtu	Annual Fuel Cost
Wood Pellets	16.4 million Btu/ton	83%	$250/ton	$18.37	$918.50
Firewood	20 million Btu/cord	77%	$250/cord	$16.23	$811.50
Coal (Anthracite)	25 million Btu/ton	80%	$200/ton	$10.00	$500.00
Fuel Oil #2	134,500 Btu/gallon	83%	$2.50/gallon	$22.39	$1,119.50
Natural Gas	1.03 million Btu/Mcf	80%	$2.16/Ccf	$26.21	$1,310.50
Propane	91,200 Btu/gallon	80%	$3.00/gallon	$41.12	$2,056.00
Electricity	3,413 Btu/kWh	100%	$.12 per kWh	$26.10	$1307.52

The average price people in the United States pay for electricity is about twelve cents per kilowatt-hour. (Context: A typical US household uses about 908 kWh per month of electricity.) But there's huge variation from state to state. "The Price of Electricity In Your State," *Planet Money: The Economy Explained*, NPR (podcast). Accessed at http://www.npr.org/sections/money/2011/10/27/141766341/the-price-of-electricity-in-your-state

Source: https://basc.pnnl.gov

NATURAL GAS

Gas fireplaces provide the look, feel, and heat of wood fireplaces without the hassle of firewood. Natural gas and propane are the fuels available for gas fireplaces. Natural gas is the most widely used, while propane is often used where natural gas is not available. Gas fireplaces can range from small to extremely large. Choosing a size is based on the amount of heat it needs to generate, or simply the desired aesthetic appearance of the fire.

A natural gas fireplace is by far more economical, energy-efficient, and nonpolluting than a wood-burning or electric fireplace. Gas stoves are more cost-effective than electric stoves, which cost about twice as much as gas to operate, but electric heaters generally cost less to purchase.

Natural gas heating offers other advantages, because it is 94 percent efficient, and burns more thoroughly and cleanly. Electricity generated from coal or other fossil fuels is only 30 percent efficient. Some natural gas fireplace models have built-in blowers to increase heating effectiveness by circulating heat to a larger area.

The operation of a gas fireplace is generally controlled by use of a wall thermostat. The fireplace is equipped with either an electric ignition or a standing safety pilot light that burns continuously and lights the main burner whenever the gas is turned on. Remember to turn off continuously lit pilot lights in the off-season as they can burn gas that is wasted.

Simulated to look like real wood logs, natural gas logs are made of ceramic material and are mounted on a metal rack similar to those in wood-burning fireplaces. If efficiency and heat are priorities, a firebox insert is a better option than log simulation.

Complete fireplace inserts can be retrofitted into existing wood-burning fireplaces. Usually they require no additions, such as glass doors, screens, or other decorative accessories. They consist of a closed combustion chamber with ceramic logs and a glass front.

FIREPLACE VENTS

Natural vent, direct vent, and vent-free are the basics. Within these categories there are models that are "heater-rated" and those designed solely for decorative purposes.

A natural vent fireplace does not have a sealed combustion chamber and relies on hot air rising to vent effectively. It must be installed either with an existing chimney that meets the local building code standards or it can be installed using a B vent, which is a vent pipe that must be installed according to the same parameters of a masonry chimney but it can be enclosed in combustible material.

A direct-vent gas fireplace has a sealed combustion chamber that prevents any combusted gases from entering the room. It vents horizontally to an outside wall or vertically through the roof.

Vent free fireplaces are fireplaces that do not require any type of vent system. They are designed to burn clean, but stringent requirements are required for installation. A highly sensitive sensor is employed to turn off the gas to the fireplace should the level of oxygen within the area begin to deplete. No heat is lost through this system, making the fireplace virtually 100 percent efficient. Currently, these types of gas fireplaces can only be installed in some areas of the United States. They are not approved for use in Canada.

SYMPTOMS OF A VENTING SYSTEM PROBLEM

- Damp patches on interior walls or exterior walls may be the sign of a leak.
- Peeling wallpaper.
- Blistered paint.
- Stains on the ceiling around the chimney.
- White stains (efflorescence) on the outside of the masonry chimney.
- Eroded mortar joints.
- Crumbling bricks.

WOOD-BURNING PELLET STOVES AND FIREPLACE INSERTS

Insert or pellet stoves may look like old wood-burning stoves, but instead of burning wood they burn pellets with electrically controlled combustion, providing reliable heating that is far more efficient and produces less pollution than traditional fireplaces.

These are a good combination of fairly clean and innovative, nonpolluting and safe wood-burning "stoves." A pellet stove or fireplace burns compressed wood or biomass (renewable organic material) pellets. Many city planners are stressing the use of a "pellet" or "insert" fireplace instead of traditional ones.

When choosing a wood- or pellet-burning appliance, it's important to select one that's properly sized for the space to be heated. When an appliance is too big, residents tend to burn fires at a low smolder to avoid overheating, which wastes fuel and is one of the biggest causes of air pollution. An undersized unit will not provide sufficient heat.

A good rule-of-thumb is that a stove rated at 42,000 Btus can heat a 1,300-square-foot space and one rated at 60,000 Btus can heat a 2,000-square-foot home. The two main styles for pellet stoves are freestanding and fireplace-insert models. Freestanding units are like conventional fireplaces and can heat a single room well. For more heating requirements, you'll need a fan to force the warm air into other spaces. Several companies now make pellet-fired furnace inserts as replacements for or to supplement gas- or oil-fired furnaces and boilers in residential heating systems.

Pellet-fuel appliances burn small, ⅜ to 1 inch-long pellets that look like rabbit food. They are made from compacted sawdust, wood chips, bark, agricultural crop waste, waste paper, and other organic materials. Some models can also burn nutshells, corn kernels, and small wood chips. Pellets are slightly more expensive than cord wood, but wood takes up more space, is bulky to deal with, and discharges more pollutants. By slowly feeding fuel from a storage container (hopper) into a burn-pot area, it creates a constant flame that requires little to no physical adjustments. Most pellet stoves produce a small, concentrated fire that burns very hot.

Their combustion efficiencies are 78 percent to 85 percent, making them exempt from United States EPA smoke-emission testing requirements. They are easy to operate, have much higher combustion and heating efficiencies than ordinary wood stoves or fireplaces, and they produce little air pollution making them the cleanest of solid fuel-burning residential heating appliances.

Pellet stoves have a variety of moving parts and motors that require maintenance. It's a good idea to select a model that offers easy access to parts. The motors of a pellet stove require electricity (some models have battery backup units), so it should be positioned near a 110-volt outlet.

BOTTOM- AND TOP-FED PELLET STOVES

Pellet stoves use two types of automatic pellet-feeding systems: top-fed and bottom-fed. When choosing between these two, consider the benefits and drawbacks of each.

Bottom-fed designs feed the fuel horizontally into the fire chamber, and incoming pellets shove aside ashes and clinkers (partially burned pellets), which fall into the ash pan. It's not necessary to use higher quality low-ash pellets in this system.

A top-fed stove has a lesser chance of fire burning back into the pellet hopper because the feeder is inclined at an angle to its pellet delivery system. But the combustion chamber is more likely to become clogged by the deposits caused by reheating ash and pellet debris. As a result, many manufacturers of top-fed models recommend burning high-grade, low-ash pellets.

COMBUSTION AIR CONTROLS

To get the maximum heat and clean burn from each pellet, the appliances use a draft-inducing fan to supply combustible air and vent combusted gases. The fan either draws air out of the firebox or blows air into it. Because these fireboxes use an electric fan, manufacturers advise against opening the firebox door while the appliance is operating.

Most pellet stoves are self-igniting and cycle themselves on and off, controlled by a thermostat, or by remote controls. Recent innovations have created computer systems within pellet stoves that monitor various safety conditions and can run diagnostic tests if a problem arises.

PELLET FUEL PRICE, QUALITY, STANDARDS, AND AVAILABILITY

Most pellet fuels have a 5 to 10 percent moisture content (well-seasoned firewood usually has around a 20 percent moisture content). Some pellets contain either petroleum or nonpetroleum lubricant (lignin) to increase heating value in the pellet-production process, though most contain no additives. Pellets made from agricultural waste contain more ash, but may produce more heat than pellets made from wood. Pellet stoves designed for low-ash (typically top-fed stoves) tend to operate poorly when used with pellets of higher ash content. Many pellet appliance manufacturers are redesigning their products to burn pellets with varying ash contents. Standard is less than 3 percent inorganic ash content.

Pellet fuel is normally sold in 40-pound (18-kilogram) bags at about $3 to $4 each or about $180 to $250 a ton. Most homeowners who use a pellet appliance as a main source of heat use two to three tons of pellet fuel per year. Pellet-fuel appliances are almost always less expensive to operate than electric heating, oil, and propane-fueled appliances.

The availability of stove pellets is increasing. They usually are available at local nurseries, at home and garden supply stores, or where pellet stoves are sold. Check pellet fuel quality by inspecting the bag for excessive dirt and dust. There should be less than one-half cup of dust at the bottom of a 40-pound bag. Store away from moisture and from the house in case termites discover it. If possible, store the wood a foot off the ground (on concrete blocks) for air circulation and to avoid insects.

Pellet Stove Pros: Most pellet appliance exteriors (except glass doors) stay relatively cool while operating, reducing the risk of accidental burns. Since pellet stoves burn fuel so completely, very little creosote builds up in the flue. Because of this, pellet appliances pose less of a fire hazard and do not require cleaning as frequently as conventional wood-burning appliances.

Pellet stoves come in sizes adequate to heat small homes all the way up to multi-family living environments such as apartments, townhomes, or condominiums. They consume about 100 kWh or about $9 worth of electricity per month to run. You can start the fire simply by pushing a button or adjusting a thermostat. Pellets require less storage space and are easier to handle than wood. Pellet stove heat is easily regulated by using a thermostat or changing the heat output directly on the stove itself. No trees are cut down, no gas reserves are used, and no large amounts of electricity are necessary for the fuel that runs pellet stoves, and they effectively combust fuel so they are rated the very cleanest of all residential heating appliances that burn solid fuel.

Pellet Stove Cons: Most residential models are expensive, ranging in price anywhere from $1,700 to $3,000. The annual fuel costs for pellet stoves run, on average, from $300 to $600, not including the cost of electricity. (See table below for comparative costs of operation). Because they require electricity, loss of power is lost of heat, and loss of power can cause smoke to enter the house, which can be inconvenient and even dangerous.

Pellet stoves are mechanical and therefore more prone to failure than a wood or gas stove, particularly if they are not properly maintained. They may also make a noise—a constant, dull, mechanical rumble. Pellet stove fires are not as pleasing to look at as those of a wood stove or even a gas stove. You should have the stove cleaned by a professional yearly, as well as cleaning the burn debris regularly. Most families go through two or three tons of pellets each winter. This comes out to about 50 bags of pellets per ton (2,000 pounds) times two or three each year, which can be more expensive than alternative forms of energy. Pellet stoves can also be expensive to repair.

PELLET STOVE MAINTENANCE

- During the summer months, shut off the gas-burning pilot.
- Inspect door gasket.
- Clean glass, interior, and exterior of firebox.
- Inspect, clean, and adjust pilot light.
- Inspect and clean burners.
- Inspect all feeder pipes to the fire-producing element.
- Clean and check control compartment.
- Check venting system.
- Check on/off switch or thermostat.
- Check fan and clean blower (if applicable).
- Adjust the primary air shutter for proper regulation of the air feed to the flame.
- Check combustion chamber for any cracks.
- Make sure of proper ignition and combustion.
- Paint firebox if chipped or worn.

FUEL VERSUS FUEL FOR HEATING VALUES AND COSTS

You can estimate how much fuel you will need for a heating season by noting that one ton of pellets is equivalent to approximately 1.5 cords of firewood.

So depending on your location, your level of romanticism, economic condition, and environmental regulations, pick the flame and fuel of your choice.

13

Air Ducts

A Clean and Clear Air Supply

People think of "home" as being a safe shelter where they are protected from the grit, grime, and pollution of the outside world. Don't kid yourself. The Environmental Protection Agency tells us that the build-up of toxins and the degradation of indoor air quality can be up to ten times worse than outdoor air pollution. To make matters worse, we gritty people spend up to 90 percent of our time indoors.

Think of your air ducts as the respiratory system of your home, delivering the heating, cooling, and clean air to your house, critical to the health and well-being of your family. Like lungs, if they are kept clean, clear, and airtight, they will keep your interior atmosphere comfortable and uncontaminated, and will save you energy, while reducing the risks of asthma and other respiratory complaints.

FACTS AND FIGURES

A duct system is a branching network of round or rectangular tubes—generally constructed of sheet metal, fiberglass board, or a flexible plastic and wire composite—located within and around the walls, floors, and ceilings of your home.

If a duct leakage is 20 percent of total airflow, the efficiency of the cooling system can drop as much as 50 percent. Insulation around ducts should be a two-inch thickness of R-6 or greater. However, Residential Energy Efficient Distribution Systems (REEDS) have found that in a typical house about 20 percent to 40 percent of the cooling and heating energy that moves through the duct system is lost due to leaks, holes, and poorly connected ducts. The efficiency to heat and cool can also be compromised by as much as 50 percent to 70 percent when passing through cold or hot spaces such as the attic, crawlspaces, or basements.

Leakage of treated air in our homes is equivalent to the annual energy consumption of 13 million cars. This represents an additional 18 percent use of electricity at an average cost of $233 a year, or about $160 per year in natural gas. For furnaces and ducts, look for high annual fuel utilization efficiency (AFUE) ratings. The national minimum is 78 percent AFUE, but there are EnergyStar models on the market that exceed 90 percent AFUE.

Faulty or leaky ducts can be hazardous as the low pressure can suck flue gases from the furnace back in the house or carbon monoxide in from the garage, distribute radon gas from the soil in the basement (which is a known carcinogen), pull VOC (volatile organic chemicals) contaminants from the house or fumes from the kitchen, and will cool or heat air surrounding the ducts. If your ducts are insulated by asbestos (an off-white, stiff, heavy cloth), also a known carcinogen, you may want to change it.

PRACTICAL SUGGESTIONS

Make sure that your ducts are up to code—you can lose a lot of heat from thin-walled ducts. Be sure a well-sealed vapor barrier exists on the outside of the insulation on cooling ducts to prevent moisture buildup. Warming heating ducts prevent pipes from freezing in cold weather. Sealing ducts well in existing homes reduces cooling costs by about 33 percent.

The EPA recommends that fuel-burning furnaces, stoves, or fireplaces be inspected for proper functioning and serviced before each heating season to protect against carbon monoxide residue poisoning through your ducts (all homes should be equipped with a carbon monoxide and radon detector and fire alarms). Home air quality test kits are available at home improvement centers and check your ducts for the presence of mold, fungus, bacteria, formaldehyde, carbon monoxide, and carbon dioxide. Or you can have professionals do the testing for you.

REMOVING ASBESTOS

Getting rid of asbestos insulation is not particularly challenging, but don't take it lightly—it can make you very uncomfortable when it gets in your eyes or on your skin. If you want to remove some types of asbestos ("popcorn" from your ceiling, for example) think about calling a certified asbestos abatement contractor. But if you want to tackle the project, here are some things to consider. Enquire at your local dump or landfill to determine if they will take hazardous substances like asbestos and the proper way to dispose of the material. Use protective clothing, preferably paper overalls, protective goggles, gloves, paper slippers, and a respirator. A fine particle dust mask will do if the area to be removed is not too large. Use a plastic drop cloth to work on.

To ensure that no asbestos dust is spread, spray the asbestos with water. Pull away asbestos materials and place them in a bag that can be taped shut, or bag the material twice, along with all rags and plastic sheets you have used. Remove and throw away overalls and slippers. Using clean, wet rags, wash off and wipe down your respirator (and change the filter), goggles, and boots used in the removal and place tools in a bucket for a more thorough cleaning. You may want to leave the plastic sheet down for a day to collect any remaining particles. Double-bag all remaining debris, including all cleaning rags, disposable items, and the plastic drop cloth, in properly labeled asbestos waste disposal bags. Take a shower!

CLUES TO POOR AIR DUCT PERFORMANCE

- High summer and winter utility bills.
- Rooms that are difficult to heat and cool.
- Stuffy rooms that never seem to feel comfortable.
- Check ducts that are located in an attic, crawl space, or the garage for cloggage.
- Tangled or kinked flexible ducts in your system.
- Uninsulated ducts.
- Disconnected, torn, or damaged ducts.
- Blind-alley ducts.
- Inadequate return ductwork.
- Ducts that have become unsealed or show holes, rips, or tears.

WHERE AND WHAT TO LOOK FOR LEAKS

- Joints between sections of duct.
- Joints between branches and trunks.
- Seams in ducts and in air handlers (connections to a ductwork ventilation system from an air conditioner or heater).
- Holes in air handlers for pipes and wires.

- Access slots or filters.
- If there is permanent water damage showing.
- If there is slime growth in or around ducts.
- If there is debris that restricts airflow.
- If dust is actually seen emitting from air supply registers.
- If offensive odors originate in the ductwork or HVAC system.
- Look for discolored insulation around duct elbows and connections—these are symptoms of leakage and dust. Moisture can enter the duct system through leaks, or if the system has been improperly installed or serviced.

PRACTICAL SUGGESTIONS TO KEEP YOUR DUCTS CLEAN

It's good to learn about air duct cleaning before you decide to spend the money to have your ducts cleaned. Find out whether your ducts are made of sheet metal, flex duct, fiberglass duct board, are lined with fiberglass, or a combination of materials. This is important to know because cleaning methods will vary. If the ducts in your home are older than ten or fifteen years, they might need to be replaced.

Air ducts should be constructed so that maintenance personnel have easy, direct access to all components and drain pans for proper cleaning and maintenance. Keeping your ducts clean is a good idea, though duct cleaning has not been documented as a preventer of health problems by the EPA, and they do not recommend that the air ducts be cleaned routinely, but only as needed. Change filters regularly. The disposable AC filters that should be changed every three months are around $4 each. Here's an instance where the cost is very reasonable for the safety benefits.

Keep water and dirt out of ducts by keeping joints tight and heating vents clean, and by being careful when using a hose around them. Water and dirt can cause mold due to moisture, rust, and rot, and provide living and breeding space for insects and vermin. Fiberglass, or any other insulation material, that is wet or visibly moldy (or if an unacceptable odor is present) should be removed and replaced. Steam cleaning and other methods involving moisture should not be used on any kind of ductwork. Research suggests that condensation on or near cooling coils of air conditioning units is a major factor in moisture contamination of the system.

Be sure you do not have any missing filters or that air cannot bypass filters through gaps. During any construction, seal off supply and return registers, and do not operate the heating and cooling system until after cleaning up construction dust. Dust and vacuum your home regularly. Change or clean your vacuum filters as vacuuming can increase the amount of dust in the air. When your air ducts are cleaned professionally, ask if they were visibly contaminated with substantial mold growth, pests or vermin, or clogged with substantial deposits of dust and debris.

No chemical biocides are currently registered by the EPA for use in internally insulated air duct systems. The use of chemical biocides and sealants may be appropriate under specific circumstances, but research has not demonstrated their effectiveness in duct cleaning or their potential adverse health effects. Permit the application of biocides in your ducts only if necessary to control mold growth and only after being assured that the product is not toxic and will be applied strictly according to manufacturer's directions. As a precaution, family and pets should leave the premises during application.

Some states require certification for duct cleaning. Go to the National Air Duct Cleaners Association (NADCA) for more information: https://nadca.com. Make sure the serviceperson follows the NADCA standards or the guidelines of the North American Insulation Manufacturers Association (NAIMA). Commit to a preventive maintenance program of yearly inspections for your heating and cooling system, regular filter changes, and steps to prevent moisture contamination.

SEALING MATERIALS

Make sure ducts are properly sealed and insulated in all non-air-conditioned spaces (attics and crawl spaces). Caulk is best used for small cracks and gaps, and is available in different grades (interior, exterior, high temperature) depending on application. Expanding foam can be used for sealing larger cracks and holes. Recommended products to seal ducts include mastic (duct), butyl tape, foil tape, or other heat-approved tapes. Look for tape with the Underwriters Laboratories (UL) logo.

Sealants should never be used on wet duct liner, to cover actively growing mold, to cover debris in the ducts, and should only be applied after cleaning according to NADCA or other appropriate guidelines or standards.

If you choose to use a cleaning service here are some questions to ask:

- Are there observable or known contaminants in the ductwork?
- Are odors or byproducts leaving the duct and entering occupied space?
- Can the contaminants be identified and can the source be controlled, or is this only a temporary measure?
- Will the proposed duct cleaning effectively remove or kill the contaminants?

- Is duct cleaning the only (or the most cost-effective) solution?
- Will the cleaning process protect HVAC equipment and the occupants of the space during cleaning?
- Will they give you a guarantee that the duct will be clean after completion?
- Any "no" answer should delay duct cleaning until adequate answers are obtained.

When hiring a duct cleaner, contact the National Air Duct Cleaners Association. Check references. Insist that the serviceperson give you knowledgeable and complete answers to your questions. Talk to at least three different service providers and get written estimates for their services. Do not hire duct cleaners who make all-encompassing claims about the health benefits of duct cleaning. Ask for any evidence of mold growth or any biological contamination and/or get a laboratory or professional opinion. Do not hire duct cleaners who recommend duct cleaning as a routine part of your heating and cooling system maintenance.

You should also be wary of duct cleaners who claim to be certified by the EPA. The EPA neither establishes duct cleaning standards nor certifies, endorses, or approves duct cleaning companies. Contact your state department of consumer affairs, county or city office of consumer affairs, or the local Better Business Bureau for complaints against any of the companies you are considering, or to lodge a complaint.

Be sure that the people hired are experienced in duct cleaning and have worked on systems like yours—look for a product label on your furnace. Be certain that the contractors will use procedures to protect you and your home from contamination. If the service provider charges by the hour, request an estimate. Make sure they will provide a written agreement outlining the total cost and scope of the job before work begins. Ask for a written guarantee for work performed.

Table 13.1. Duct Cleaning Consumer Checklist

General	Did the service provider obtain access to and clean the entire heating and cooling system, including ductwork and all components (drain pans, humidifiers, coils, and fans)?
	Has the service provider adequately demonstrated that ductwork and plenums are clean? (Plenum is a space in which supply or return air is mixed or moves; can be duct, joist space, attic and crawl spaces, or wall cavity.)
Heating	Is the heat exchanger surface visibly clean?
Cooling	Are both sides of the cooling coil visibly clean?
Components	
	If you point a flashlight into the cooling coil, does light shine through the other side? It should if the coil is clean.
	Are the coil fins straight and evenly spaced (as opposed to being bent over and smashed together)?
	Is the coil drain pan completely clean and draining properly?
Blower	Are the blower blades clean and free of oil and debris?
	Is the blower compartment free of visible dust or debris?
Plenums	Is the return air plenum free of visible dust or debris?
	Do filters fit properly and are they the proper efficiency as recommended by HVAC system manufacturer?
	Is the supply air plenum (directly downstream of the air handling unit) free of moisture stains and contaminants?
Metal Ducts	Are interior ductwork surfaces free of visible debris? (Select several sites at random in both the return and supply sides of the system.)
Fiberglass	Is all fiberglass material in good condition (i.e., free of tears and abrasions; well-adhered to underlying materials)?
Access Doors	Are newly installed access doors in sheet metal ducts attached with more than just duct tape (e.g., screws, rivets, mastic, etc.)?
	With the system running, is air leakage through access doors or covers very slight or nonexistent?
Air Vents	Have all registers, grilles, and diffusers been firmly reattached to the walls, floors, and/or ceilings?
	Are the registers, grilles, and diffusers visibly clean?
System Operation	Does the system function properly in both the heating and cooling modes after cleaning?

Source: National Association Air Duct Cleaning Association and the EPA.

14

The Thermostat
Controlling the Controller

When it's sweat-searing hot or ear-tweaking cold outside, you dread going home to a house that's sweltering or frigid because you can't program the thermostat while away. Fear not. Your comfy cozy dream zone is literally at your fingertips enabling you to manage the temperature of the house—the largest use of energy for your home—from anywhere, anytime. Modern thermostats are automatic and programmable, can be manipulated by a computer (via the Internet) or a smartphone app, and are a great resource for saving money, energy, and bodily comfort.

FACTS AND FIGURES

According to the US DOE, the proper use of a programmable thermostat can cut heating and cooling bills by 5 to 20 percent. That could mean saving $180 a year on your energy bill by automatically reducing your heating or cooling when it is least needed. However, the EPA's assessment differs. In May 2009, the EPA suspended EnergyStar certification for programmable thermostats, writing, "EPA has been unable to confirm any improvement in terms of the savings delivered by programmable thermostats and has no credible basis for continuing to extend the current EnergyStar specification." But play it safe and you may save some money.

An Internet-programmed (IP) thermostat can e-mail you when the temperature in your home drops to a pre-set low or high setting, alerting you when to reset it. Simply turning the thermostat up or down 10° to 15°F for eight hours can save around 5 to 15 percent a year on heating and cooling bills.

Mechanical and nonprogrammable digital thermostats are manual thermostats—each time you want to change the temperature in the house, the thermostat has to be reset by hand. A programmable (setback or clock) thermostat is designed to adjust the temperature according to a series of programmed settings that take effect at different times of the day. According to the DOE, homeowners can save as much as 15 percent on their energy bills by replacing an obsolete thermostat with a setback (programmable, but non-Internet-controlled) thermostat, which will pay for itself in a year.

System zoning involves multiple thermostats that are wired to a control panel, which operates dampers within the ductwork of a forced-air system. The thermostat constantly reads the temperature of their specific zone, then opens or closes the dampers within the ductwork according to the thermostat's settings. On programmable thermostats, multiple heating and cooling levels utilize an internal clock that has the ability to switch between a night and a morning program. According to the DOE, zoning or multistage systems can save homeowners up to 30 percent on typical heating and cooling bills.

The downside is that some digital thermostats can be hard to read and program, which is a constant complaint from consumers. It's a good idea to have a professional help install them, read instructions carefully, or surf the Internet for help.

PRACTICAL SUGGESTIONS

Look for an EnergyStar-qualified programmable thermostat. From $40 to $70 buys a really nice setback thermostat that you can program to meet your specific needs. Several models allow different programs to be set up to fit with daily and weekly schedules with digital touch-pads, voice, or phone programming, along with other high-tech features.

Keep the thermostat in a neutral spot, not by a drafty or excessively sunny area. During winter, turn the thermostat down while asleep or off when at work. According to California's Pacific Gas and Electric Company, as much as 2 to 3 percent of energy can be saved simply by lowering your thermostat only 1°F in winter (when set between 55° to 65°F at night).

Setting the temperature around 78° to 80°F in summer will save 6 percent to 8 percent of cooling costs for each degree above 78, while still remaining comfortable. Keep the house at a toasty 75°F during your active hours in winter; it's easy to program your thermostat to drop to 58° or 60°F during the night. And family night owls can choose alternate settings for separate rooms while others are warm beneath the covers.

IP thermostats are especially useful when you forget to shut off a furnace or air conditioner before leaving home, when you are running late, or if you want the house to be comfortable upon your arrival. The temperature can be monitored in case someone else changes the programming. Do not over or under set temperatures to get cooler or hotter faster—the air conditioning or heating will work at the same rate no matter how low or high it is set.

Avoid using the hold/permanent/vacation feature to manage day-to-day temperature settings. Hold or vacation features are for when you're planning to be away for an extended period. Set this feature at a constant, efficient temperature when going away for the weekend or on vacation. All programmable thermostats temporarily make an area warmer or cooler without erasing the pre-set programming. This override should be cancelled automatically at the next program period.

Keeping your systems well-maintained extends the life of your air conditioner and heater, reduces operation costs, and minimizes environmental impacts. Don't forget to check and change the batteries regularly.

TESTING THE THERMOSTAT

To estimate if a setback will save money, you can run a simple test. To start, record the amount of time your heating system takes to achieve a random temperature. Next, turn the thermostat to a desired (higher or lower) temperature. Give the house time to equalize at the set temperature and then determine the amount of time the system is running to readjust to the setback (original) temperature.

If the heating system runs for 20 minutes at the higher setting and 14 minutes at the lower setting, you will be saving 10 percent on your heating bill each hour the temperature arrives at the prescribed setting.

To calculate the savings, subtract the minutes the heating system runs at the lower setting from the minutes the system is on at the higher setting (20 minus 14) and divide by 60. Units with adaptive, smart, or intelligent recovery features are an exception to this rule. They reach desired temperatures using formulas based on your historical use.

15

Water Watch

H_2O Health and Husbandry

It's odorless, colorless, and tasteless. It's quite common, but extremely precious. It's essential for all forms of life and it takes up more than 70 percent of our planet, and approximately 65 percent of our bodies. It makes up almost 25 percent of the food we eat. We travel on it and enjoy being in it. It's used to manufacture almost everything we use in one way or another. It's necessary for civilization, and political and legal wars are constantly fought over it, yet it is taken for granted in many places. It's easy to come by, often hard to find, and often squandered. In some places it's treasured and incredibly difficult to obtain. Everywhere it is a substance more necessary to our existence than anything save air.

Noted oilman T. Boone Pickens sagely said, "The new oil is water." Ben Franklin wrote, "When the well is dry, we learn the worth of water." And Fats Domino sang, "What'ya gonna do when the well runs dry?" If we keep wasting water in the way we have been, we're in for a nasty lesson in harsh water rationing and conservation. The US Drought Monitor reports that from the Midwest all the way to the West Coast almost every state is in a drought of some form at this writing. In some it's the worst drought since the mega-drought dust bowl years in the 1930s, and the worst in California's recorded rainfall history.

Ironically, the Earth has the same amount of water it has always had, but we have a lot more people using a lot more of it, and more of it is getting polluted. Most states rely on aquifers or rivers, reservoirs, and lakes, which are dependent on the vagaries of weather, and represent large, but limited, nonsustainable reserves.

Americans use 24 gallons of water each day, approximately 5.8 billion gallons, to flush their toilets. Orange County, California, is doing something with their water, having spent $481 million dollars on a so-called toilet to tap system that takes human waste water and turns it into drinkable water. For those who gag at the idea, recycled water has been shown to have fewer contaminants than existing municipally treated water supplies. It's so successful that it's undergoing a $150 million expansion demonstrating that purified wastewater can be safe and clean, and help to ease water shortages. This is the world's largest water purification system for potable reuse and has supplied more than 112 billion gallons of purified water a day.

Desalinization of seawater has been suggested, but is not practical for most of the states that have no access to oceans, and it is an expensive proposition that uses enormous amounts of energy and may propose eco-problems. Conservation is still the main watchword and experts agree that the first and best course of action is to husband and proficiently manage fresh water.

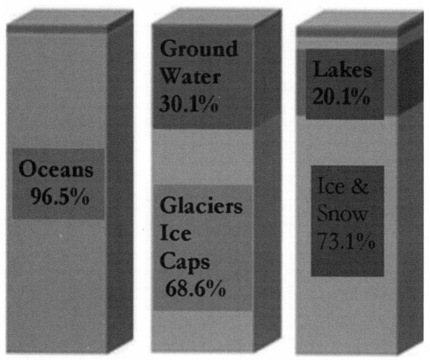

Figure 15.1.   The world's water.
Source: U.S. Geological Survey, https://www2.usgs.gov/water/.

FACTS AND FIGURES

The United States uses more than 410 billion gallons of water per day and wastes more than a trillion gallons a year. Dams provide water for 140,000 farmers in the west; the largest users produce 60 percent of the vegetables in the United States. The population of the country doubled between 1950 and 2000, but the demand for water rose 300 percent.

About 95 percent of the water entering a home goes down the drain. The average American uses 140 to 170 gallons of water per day. If all US households installed water-efficient appliances, the country would save more than three trillion gallons of water and more than $18 billion dollars per year (http://www.waterrights.utah.gov/sustainability/watersustainability.asp).

Twenty years ago, thirty states in the United States reported "water-stress" conditions. In 2000, the number rose to forty. In 2009, the number was forty-five. In another fifteen years it's predicted that all states will be in a water-stressed condition. And water is still inexpensive. The average price of water in the United States is about $1.50 for 1,000 gallons. If drinking water and soda pop were equally costly, your water bill would skyrocket more than 10,000 percent.

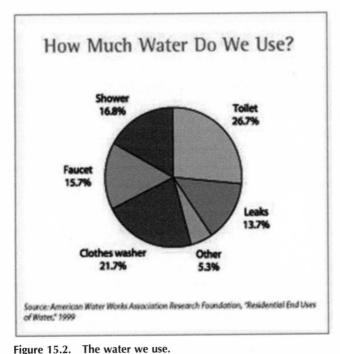

Figure 15.2.   The water we use.
Source: U.S. Geological Survey, https://www2.usgs.gov/water/.

According to the United States Geological Survey, 99 percent of all fresh water is stored in the ground in aquifers, which are being pumped dangerously low. The Ogallala Aquifer, one of the largest in the world, holds up to four quadrillion gallons of water. It yields about 30 percent of the nation's groundwater used for irrigation and five trillion gallons of water is pumped from the Ogallala Aquifer every year. By 2020 it's been estimated that the Ogallala Aquifer will contain only 20 percent of its original content, and if withdrawals continue unabated, some estimates claim that the aquifer could be depleted by 2050, after only 150 years of human exploitation.

The Great Lakes contain 21 percent of the world's freshwater. The Colorado River, which runs into California on its lower southwest border, provides 20 to 25 percent of Southern California's water and is the most litigated river in the world. In one second, the flow of the Colorado River could supply an average American household for one year. In Nevada, the water level of the Hoover Dam has dropped 130 feet in the last ten years. At this rate the dam could be rendered dry within the next decade. The Nevada (underground) Aquifer holds one trillion gallons of water, but it's been contaminated by radioactivity because of underground nuclear testing. Finally, less than 1 percent of the treated water produced by water utilities is actually drunk.

THE BOTTLED WATER BAMBOOZLE

Bottled water is more expensive than gasoline. The Delaware Environmental Institute states the recommended amount humans should drink is eight glasses of water a day. That equals about $49 per year at tap water rates. That same amount of bottled water is about $1,400. Americans now drink more bottled water than milk, coffee, or beer. Coca-Cola's Dasani and PepsiCo's Aquafina, the two top-selling bottled waters on the American market, come from a municipal tap and 44 percent of "purified" bottled water sold in the United States comes from a municipal water source.

BOTTLES, BOTTLES EVERYWHERE

There are 50 billion bottles of water consumed every year, about 30 billion of them in the United States (which means we use roughly 60 percent of the world's water bottles, even though we're about 4.5 percent of the world population). There are 1,500 bottles of water consumed every second in the United States. There are enough plastic bottles thrown away to stretch from San Francisco to New York—every day.

Our national recycle rate for PET (polyethylene terephthalate) plastics is only 23 percent, which means we throw 38 billion water bottles into landfills a year. That's $1 billion worth of plastic that should end up in the recycling stream, where it can be reused as carpeting, synthetic decking, playground equipment, clothing, or new bottles and containers. Most ends up in landfills, where it may take up to 1,000 years to decompose and could potentially leak pollutants into the soil and water. It's estimated that there are also 100 million tons of plastic debris floating around in the oceans, threatening the health and safety of marine life, hence our own.

Three gallons of water is required to produce one gallon of bottled drinking water. It takes 1.85 gallons of water to manufacture the plastic for the average commercial bottle of water alone and, because of the chemical production of plastics, that water is unusable. Seventeen million barrels of crude oil are used to produce a year's worth of water bottles. That's enough oil to keep a million cars going for a year. The energy we waste using bottled water would be enough to power 190,000 homes a year.

At least 90 percent of the price of a bottle of water is for things other than the water itself, like bottling, packaging, shipping, and marketing. It takes about 1,000 to 2,000 times as much energy to produce and transport the average bottle of water to your home as it does to produce the same amount of tap water.

WASTED WATER, WASTED $$

In the United States there are 240,000 water main failures each year, and ten times that from lesser municipal water pipes. Two hundred million people could be served by water lost to leaks, theft, and waste in the United States each year.

New York City uses 1.2 billion gallons a day, of which more than 36 million gallons are leaked. Buffalo, New York loses up to 40 percent of its water due to poor infrastructure. Los Angles consumes 600,000 gallons of water a day, and leaks 7 billion gallons a year. Like most of America, its water pipes are seventy-five years old. Montgomery County, a suburb of Washington, DC, has the dubious honor of being the leakiest place in the country—suffering more than 4,000 water main leaks in four years; 2,129 in 2007 alone.

US homes leak around one trillion gallons per year. That's more than the annual water use of Los Angeles, Chicago, and Miami combined. A leak of one drip per second from only one faucet can mean losing over five gallons of water a day and over 2,000 gallons in a year. A leak of a gallon per minute means that you are losing (and paying for) 1,440 gallons of water per day, or 525,600 gallons per year; which is 43,200 gallons extra, or from $200 to $700, depending on where you live.

Household water leaks rob homeowners, accounting for about 12 percent of their water bill through problems such as worn-out toilet flappers, dripping faucets, and leaking valves.

Estimates vary, but the average American uses from a low of 40 to a high of 180 gallons of water on a daily basis and unknowingly wastes up to 30 gallons of water every day. The average household spends as much as $500 per year on its water bill.

By installing simple water-saving devices, that bill would drop to $330 per household. By using water-saving features, water use in the home can be reduced by 35 percent.

WATER, WATER EVERYWHERE–NOT SO MUCH TO DRINK

Desalinization of seawater has been suggested as 97 percent of the Earth's water is nondrinkable (impotable) but is not practical for the nation, as it is not accessible or inexpensive to produce.

Reverse osmosis desalination is a type of screening, filtering, and sifting of saltwater. The process requires roughly two gallons of water for every gallon of desalinated water produced. Food and Water Watch reports that in the United States, desalinated water costs from two to five times as much to harvest as other sources of fresh water.

San Diego's Poseidon Carlsbad desalination plant, at a cost of around $1 billion, will produce up to 50 million gallons a day, enough water for 300,000 residents or about 10 percent of its population.

Environmentalists fear that desalination is a potential hazard and will discharge chemicals and brine two to three times saltier than seawater back into maritime environments, causing environmental disruption.

WATER AND POWER

If one out of every 100 American homes were retrofitted with water-efficient fixtures, we could save about 100 million kWh of electricity per year—avoiding 80,000 tons of greenhouse gas emissions. That is equivalent to removing nearly 15,000 automobiles from the road for one year. If just 1 percent of households replaced high-flush toilets with products approved by the EPA WaterSense program, the nation would save 38 million kWh of electricity per year, worth approximately $38 billion. It takes about 56 billion kWh per year to deliver and treat the water we use every day in the United States. That's enough electricity to power more than 5 million homes for an entire year, or a cost of more than $62 billion. More than one-third of all water used (and reused) in the United States each year is for cooling power plants. That also accounts for millions of tons of greenhouse gasses.

PRACTICAL SOLUTIONS

If all US households installed water-saving features, water use would decrease by 30 percent, saving an estimated 5.4 billion gallons per day. Stopping water leaks in the home can save more than 10 percent on your water bills. A good method to check for leaks is to examine your water usage. It's likely that a family of four has a serious leak if its water use exceeds 12,000 gallons per month. Monitor your water bill for unusually high use. If every home installed low-flow plumbing fixtures, as much water as the Mississippi empties into the Gulf of Mexico every week could be saved.

Grab a wrench and fix that leaky faucet, especially if it's hot water. It's simple, inexpensive, and one drop per second can add up to approximately 174 gallons a month. Consider installing WaterSense-labeled appliances, which use less water while offering superior performance from older devices. Report broken pipes, open hydrants, and errant sprinklers to the property owner or your water provider.

Use a broom instead of a hose to clean your driveway and sidewalk. When buying new appliances that use water, consider those that offer cycle and load size adjustments for water use. Consider air-cooled appliances for significant water savings as some refrigerators, air conditioners, and icemakers are cooled with a wasted flow of water. Turn off faucets tightly after each use, or when you are doing a task, such as brushing your teeth. Empty soapy water from washing your car, etc., into the kitchen drain or toilet. This way it will be treated properly by your sanitation district. Use a hose nozzle or turn off the water while you wash your car and save up to 100 gallons every wash. Better yet use a car wash that recycles its water.

TO TEST YOUR WATER PRESSURE

Turn off all plumbing fixtures inside and outside your home. Locate the outdoor water spigot closest to where the water enters the house from the municipal water supply on the street (generally it will be in the front of the house). Screw a water pressure gauge into the faucet. A gauge can be purchased inexpensively from most hardware stores. Turn on the spigot. The needle on the gauge will land at the number that indicates your water pressure.

For best results, as the pressure from your water company might vary, test early in the morning, late afternoon, and at night. The optimum range is 55 to 65 pounds per square inch (psi). If your test reveals that your water pressure is higher than 65 psi, install a pressure regulator to even out the flow. This might be a job for a plumber. If you want to do this yourself, it's not that difficult. Check out YouTube for instructions.

WATER SOFTENERS/TREATMENT DEVICES AND FILTERS

There are three organizations accredited by the American National Standards Institute (ANSI) that certify that water filters meet EPA standards and work properly: Underwriters Laboratories, NSF (National Sanitation Foundation) International, and the Water Quality Association.

No single filtration system can protect against all contaminants. Choosing a filtration/purification device will depend on what you want to remove, how much water you use, and how much you want to invest. Depending on your needs, water filters vary from pitcher types that run about $30 to $50 plus $25 for seven replacement filters to large, reverse osmosis systems with under-counter filters ranging around $150. The filters should be changed every 40 gallons or every two months for the average family.

Replacing a large home water filter is a somewhat involved procedure that entails installing pressure intake and outflow gauges to observe changes in pressure denoting deposits in the filter. Some filter systems will have a display that shows its status; others may show a simple readout that changes color when it's time to replace the filter system. Not every unit requires replacement; it may only need a good cleaning. Again, keep a regular monitoring schedule of your unit and, if needed, follow manufacturer's guidelines to clean your home water filter system. If the display shows a problem and you've cleaned the unit, it might be a telltale sign of another problem. Call a professional or the manufacturer. There comes a time when no matter how many times you clean or replace parts, the unit needs replacement. When that time comes, go through the manufacturer's recommended guidelines for replacing the unit.

If your water softener back-flush line is connected to the septic system, recharge your softener as infrequently as possible to reduce water use and avoid overloading the septic system. If you have a point-of-use water treatment device, be sure it has a shut-off valve so the system doesn't run continuously when the reservoir is already full.

IS YOUR TAP WATER SAFE?

In 1972, Congress passed the Clean Water Act, which regulates the nation's public drinking water. The US EPA is charged with enforcing standards for contaminants in public drinking water. Water suppliers are required to issue to their customers an annual water quality report or Consumer Confidence Report (CCR) that indicates what contaminants have been detected and how those levels compare to drinking water standards. They are also required to notify the general public if water isn't fit for human consumption.

Nearly 10 percent of water systems in the United States fail to meet the EPA's standards for tap water quality and there are towns in America that have to boil their water (vigorously for one minute) to make it potable (safe to drink). The EPA has drinking water standards in place to address only approximately 114 out of a possible 82,000 other chemicals that may be in tap water. In setting the drinking water standard for a contaminant, the EPA first estimates what level somebody could drink daily for seventy years without expecting to have their health impacted. Some contamination of water occurs naturally, while other contaminants are knowingly or unintentionally introduced by man (think the Detroit lead situation). Private wells are the owner's responsibility to test for contaminants. The EPA does not regulate household wells (some states or local governments may provide regulation).

If you haven't used your water for some time, run the tap for 60 seconds to flush out any rust or contaminants that may have accumulated in your pipes. Many older homes contain dangerous lead from pipes or lead solder that leaches into tap water, especially hot water, and may also contain lead, arsenic, chloroform, chromium-6, perchlorates (toxic salts), and other cancer-causing chemicals. Most contaminants have no smell, color, or taste so you may not be able to detect a problem if you have one.

If you notice anything out of the ordinary about your water, don't hesitate to call your water company. Here are a few indicators:

- A sudden or gradual change in taste, odor, color, or transparency.
- If family members frequently get upset stomachs, nausea, or diarrhea. If visitors get sick even when family members don't—those who use the water regularly may have become accustomed to it.
- If an oily sheen appears when the water stands for a while (this might also result from dissolved iron, which is not a health risk).
- The build-up of soap scum in bathrooms and on faucets.
- If there is new or unexplained water pooling in your neighborhood.
- If your water is fed by old (lead) pipes.
- There are livestock, agricultural crops, or a toxic dump nearby.

- Stained sinks, tubs, and laundry.
- Indoor radon gas. (Radon detectors are available at hardware or home improvement stores.)
- Poorly lathering soaps, shampoos, and detergents.
- Rapidly corroded water treatment supplies.
- If fracking is taking place around your neighborhood.

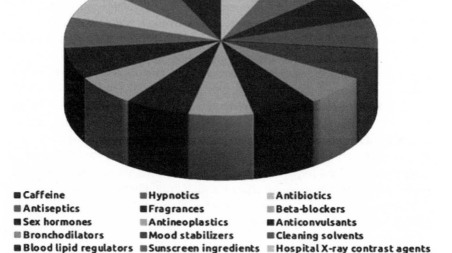

■ Caffeine	■ Hypnotics	▩ Antibiotics
▩ Antiseptics	■ Fragrances	▩ Beta-blockers
■ Sex hormones	▩ Antineoplastics	■ Anticonvulsants
▩ Bronchodilators	■ Mood stabilizers	▩ Cleaning solvents
■ Blood lipid regulators	■ Sunscreen ingredients	▩ Hospital X-ray contrast agents

Figure 15.3.   These might be in your tap water.
Source: U.S. Geological Survey, https://www2.usgs.gov/water/.

WHAT TO DO ABOUT SUSPICIOUS WATER

If you have any questions about your drinking water, call the Consumer Confidence Water Report Safe Drinking Water Hotline at 1-(800)-426-4791, or call your local health department and/or your water company to ask about the safety of your tap water. Have your water tested. Share the tests with your community. Get educated about what contaminants are in water. Get involved with water health and safety.

Activist and author Jerry Yudelson has produced "The Pyramid of New Water Sources," derived from the research for his book, *Dry Run: Preventing the Next Urban Water Crisis*, in which he outlines opportunities for extending our urban water supplies in a pyramid of ten steps. A version of "The Pyramid of New Water Resources" can be found without cost at http://www.prweb.com/releases/2011/3/prweb8230506.htm.

HOME WATER AUDIT

A household water audit is an assessment of how much water is used and how much water can be saved in the home. Conducting a water audit involves calculating water use and identifying simple ways for saving water in the home.

HOW MANY GALLONS A DAY DO YOU USE?

- 80 gallons per day—Excellent. You use water wisely. Please share your conservation techniques with friends and neighbors.
- 80 to 100 gallons per day—Very good. You use less water than the average citizen.
- 101 to 120 gallons per day—Average.
- 120 gallons per day—Water hog! Go over the conservation tips in this book to learn how you can better conserve water.

16

Getting in Hot Water

A Big Energy Eater

Some people take drag-strip or Navy showers—get wet, soap with water off, rinse and out in less than ten minutes. And then some like it hot and long, indulging in scalding, monsoon-like, everlasting showers that exhaust the water heater and skyrocket the water and energy bills. Adding to that the unrelenting surge of laundry, dishes, and various ablutions in and out of the house that drain the hot water tank still more. This chapter offers some information and relief on how to mitigate extravagant water use, and the energy it takes to pump and heat it.

FACTS AND FIGURES

The water heater is one of the largest consumers of energy in your home, second only to heating and cooling the house. According to the California Energy Commission, heating water alone uses up to 33 percent of a home's energy consumption. Water heating typically accounts for about 25 percent of home energy dollars, or 18 percent of your utility bill. Standard tank water heaters have an average life expectancy of eight to thirteen years.

Natural gas water heaters cost about $20 to $40 a month to operate; electric or fuel oil water heaters are about twice as expensive to run. Over the lifespan of a water heater, using natural gas rather than electricity can save a family more than $2,000 according to the Interstate Natural Gas Association of America (INGAA). Electric water heaters eliminate the risk of fuel leaks, NOx fumes (nitrogen oxide, a pollutant), and carbon monoxide. Gas-fired water heaters produce higher flow rates than electric ones, however they waste energy with constantly burning pilot lights, which can offset energy savings.

Another consideration for storage-tank water heaters is recovery rate—the number of gallons of water they can heat in an hour. The greater the demand for hot water, the higher the recovery rate needed. When buying a water heater, look at its cited energy efficiency and yearly operating costs. This information can be found on the EnergyGuide label. Newer models have an intermittent ignition device (IID), which resembles an on-demand piezoelectric igniter on newer gas kitchen ranges and ovens, which saves gas as it ignites only on demand. According to the US DOE, Americans deposit an estimated 7.3 million traditional tank-based water heaters in our landfills annually.

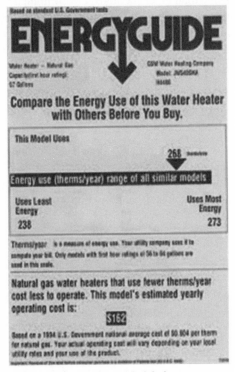

Figure 16.1. Energy guide label.
Source: energystar.gov/index.

TYPES OF WATER HEATERS

Conventional storage water heaters, the most popular type, provide a storage tank of 20 to 80 gallons of hot water, heated by several possible fuels—natural gas or propane, electricity, or even fuel oil.

Tankless or demand-type water heaters heat water directly (via a heated coil) as it is used without relying on a storage tank. They can be fueled by either electricity or gas. Researchers have found energy savings can be up to 30 percent compared with a standard natural gas storage-tank water heater.

Heat pump water heaters move heat from one place to another instead of generating heat directly to provide hot water, which makes them two to three times more energy efficient than conventional electric water heaters. Heat-pump water heaters can be cost effective in some areas, using 50 percent less electricity to heat water than conventional electric water heaters.

Using electricity for water heating can be either for stand-alone systems or combined into a system that heats water while heating and cooling the home. This is more expensive than other methods, but combined systems can be two to three times more energy efficient than conventional electric water heaters.

Solar water heaters use the sun's heat to produce hot water and the power is free. They use a passive system (very little electricity) that is fairly inexpensive in the long run.

GAS HEATERS VERSUS ELECTRICAL

Gas water heaters work more quickly than electric ones, so they produce more hot water in an hour. A gas water heater that holds 40 gallons may turn out as much hot water in an hour as a 65-gallon electric one. Electric heaters are more expensive to buy, install, and operate.

Table 16.1. Water Heating System Comparison

Water Heating System	Monthly Operational Costs (dollars)	Hot Water Delivery (gallons)	Recovery Time (minutes/seconds)
Natural Gas Water Heater	16.20	95.5	21:35
Electric Water Heater	25.05	62.3	61:04
Tankless Water Heater	11.25	Continuous hot water	No recovery required

This is only an approximation. Costs will vary due to location, cost of fuel, and models used.

PRACTICAL SUGGESTIONS

Dos: Consider installing a drain-water, waste-heat recovery system (see the section below on Drain-Water Heat Recovery). A recent DOE study showed energy savings of up to 25 to 30 percent from using such a system. Wrap your water heater in an insulation blanket, but be careful not to cover the water heater's top, bottom, thermostat, or burner compartment.

Place one inch of extruded polystyrene foam insulation under an electric water heater, as most electric water heaters have no insulation on the bottom. Additional water heater insulation can reduce standby heat loss by 25 to 45 percent, saving 4 to 9 percent in water heating costs. Insulate the first six feet of the hot and cold water pipes connected to the water heater with two-inch thick insulation of R-6 value or foam sleeves for more immediate hot water at the faucet; this can save up to 2 percent in energy savings. Set the thermostat on your water heater to 120°F to get comfortable hot water for most uses.

Manufacturers recommend draining and refilling the water heater every 90 days. Also, drain a quart of water from your water tank every three months to remove sediment (at the bottom near the drain faucet); that sediment impedes heat transfer and lowers the efficiency of your heater. Follow the manufacturer's directions. Check your anode a couple of times a year. (It's a rod that mitigates corrosion. Find it at the top of the tank. It looks like a recessed top of a bolt. See instructions below.)

Don'ts: The EPA estimates that a heater set at 140°F or higher can waste $36 to $61 annually in standby heat losses to keep water at that temperature, and more than $400 to bring fresh water up to that high temperature. Operating a water heater at unnecessarily high temperatures increases energy consumption and causes more sediment to accumulate at the bottom of the tank, contributing to shortened tank life. Every 10°F the temperature is lowered represents a savings of approximately 4 to 5 percent of energy used. Water heater dial controls are unreliable. Check the temperature of the water with a hand-held thermometer.

A water heater in the basement will also provide dehumidification in the summer months. However, this technology can pose some installation challenges, so consult an installer. Turn off the heater when away from home for extended periods. Although it takes four hours to reheat the water, this will still save you money.

ON-DEMAND TANKLESS WATER HEATERS (TWHS)

Consider natural gas on-demand or tankless water heaters that deliver a constant supply of hot water on demand directly without using a storage tank.

HOW IT WORKS

The hot water faucet is turned on and water enters the heater unit. A sensor detects water flow in the tank and the burner is ignited by computer command. Water circulates through the heater-coils heat exchanger and the water is heated to the correct temperature. When the faucet is turned off, the system stops.

Pros: TWHs deliver water at a more consistent temperature than standard tank water heaters. They will deliver a constant and endless supply of hot water, providing hot water at a rate of 2 to 5 gallons (7.6 to 15.2 liters) per minute.

Researchers have found energy savings of 30 to 40 percent compared with a standard natural gas storage-tank water heater. A tankless water heater uses 30 to 50 percent less energy than units with tanks, saving a typical family about $100 or more per year, depending on water usage. They take up less space since they are normally wall-mounted, mounted outside, or in the attic. A typical large unit measures only 14 inches wide × 24 inches high × 9 inches deep.

TWH systems have neither an open-flame pilot nor a tank of stored hot water, so they are free of many of the energy and safety issues that accompany tank-based systems. The temperature setting on tankless systems is digital and precise, unlike the inaccurate twist knob settings on most tank-based heaters. The environmental benefits from converting to a TWH system are twofold: a reduction in greenhouse gas emissions due to using less energy and a longer service life (and smaller size) of the tankless units.

An on-demand water heater at each hot water outlet can raise savings by 50 percent over the long run. The initial investment for a tankless system is going to be far more than the cost of a conventional water heater, but when factoring the lower operating cost and longer (twenty-year average) service life, the savings may be substantial. Plus, TWHs may be eligible for up to a $300 tax credit. TWH systems would eventually cut the number of water heaters deposited in landfills to less than half of the number of conventional heaters, and take up less space.

Cons: If you have a large family, plenty of water appliances, and people are multitasking at the same time, a tankless water heater might not be up to the task or suitable for your family's particular needs. A tankless water heater is going to cost twice as much as a gas heater and might require five times the Btus to heat the same amount of water. It also has intricate parts, so reliability might be a problem. Depending where you are in the house, getting hot water could take up to 15 to 20 seconds. Finally, tankless electricity is on all the time.

SOLAR WATER HEATERS (SWHS)

There are two basic types of solar water heaters: passive and active. Active systems utilize a circulating pump and some type of temperature control. This allows greater flexibility than their passive counterparts since the hot water storage tank does not have to be above or near the solar collectors. Generally it takes from three to five hours of sunlight to heat water from 122° to 203°F. Then water can remain hot, and on immediate demand, for up to 80 hours, with a storage capacity of 80 to 120 gallons.

Passive systems do not have any moving parts and rely on the basic principle of physics that hot water rises and cold water falls. The sun heats the thermal collector within which is a system of water pipes. When the collector is hotter than the solar storage tank, the water or antifreeze is then heated as it is pumped through the copper tubes in the collector, and a heat exchanger transfers this heat to the storage tank. Then it can be connected directly to the current water heater during the installation, as sometimes there may be a need to increase the temperature of water.

Homeowners with high electric rates and unshaded, south-facing locations (such as a roof), should consider installing a solar water heater, although solar hot water technologies can be operated efficiently and affordably in any climate. Using a solar water heater may save up to 85 percent of heating water. For a typical family of four at a water temperature of 120°F using 80 gallons a day, it would come to about $650 a year. A $5,000 solar water heating system can reduce annual water heating bills by

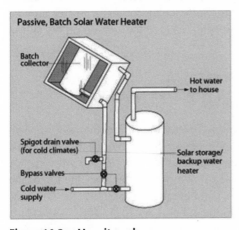

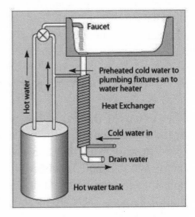

Figure 16.2. How it works.
Source: www.mnenergysmart.com.

65 percent. Costs vary widely and depend on the type of system installed. Typical costs range from $3,000 to $5,000 for a standard home installation, with a life expectancy of fifteen to thirty years. When calculating a payback period, lots of issues have to be considered, such as factors like location, family needs, future energy increases, inflation, savings in boiler servicing or replacing. In general, most thermal solar systems offer a payback of between six and fifteen years, or more. However, factoring in the federal tax credit of 30 percent, this cuts the cost to $3,150. This will reduce your payback to approximately ten-and-a-half years.

By using innovative solar water heating systems, 50 to 100 percent of a typical household or business's needs can be met, even in winter, as there is radiant heat even on overcast days. Generous government incentives include cash rebates (up to $10,000), federal tax incentives, and grants.

Consider installing an EnergyStar-qualified solar water heater certified by the Solar Rating and Certification Corporation. More than 1.5 million homes and businesses in the United States have invested in solar water heating systems. Surveys indicate that more than 94 percent of these customers consider the systems a good investment.

Solar systems can be installed by relatively experienced home handypersons. Solar water heating systems are also beneficial for the environment because the power is free and has none of the greenhouse gas emissions associated with electricity production. During a twenty-year period, one solar water heater can eliminate more than fifty tons of carbon dioxide emissions.

Solar systems can also blend with the architecture of the home and increase its value. There is no worry about future increases in power costs, or loss of hot water due to blackouts. Some solar companies offer no-cost installation partnerships, and other incentives (see the section on the sun in chapter 26, "The Renewables").

DO YOU NEED A NEW WATER HEATER?

It's obvious if the old heater is leaking, corroding, or costing a fortune in heating. Age alone is not the deciding factor. Some older tanks are often more sturdily built than newer ones, but tanks do deteriorate with time. A tank's age is usually encoded in its serial number located near the top of the unit, by year numbers and/or a letter. If it begins A-96 or 0196, the tank was built in January 1996. B-96 and 0296 mean February (02) 1996; C-96 stands for March 1996, etc. If the number reads 9601, the tank was built in the first week of 1996, and so on.

READ THE LABEL

The Federal Trade Commission requires EnergyGuide labels on all new conventional storage water heaters (but not on heat pump water heaters). It compares the average yearly operating costs of different water heaters, using the same criteria for all models tested. It lets you see which one would probably cost you less to run. EnergyGuide labels feature the first hour rating as "Capacity" on the upper left corner of the yellow label.

The big number in the center of the EnergyGuide is the estimated cost of energy needed to operate a water heater for one year. On the bar immediately below the yearly cost, the label displays the range of yearly costs of comparably sized water heaters, from the least expensive to most expensive. That's why an EnergyGuide label is such a valuable tool—it makes comparison shopping easy. Water heaters are sometimes crammed into tight spaces—check the manufacturer's specifications on any model you buy to make sure it will fit.

Another label on new water heaters lists the "Energy Factor." The best indicator of the water heater's efficiency, it provides a number with a decimal point, usually listed on a separate tag beside the EnergyGuide. The higher the Energy Factor number, the more efficient the water heater. In California, electric resistance water heaters have a minimum Energy Factor of 0.97; gas-fired storage, 0.67; oil-fired storage, 0.59; gas-fired instantaneous, 0.62; and electric instantaneous, 0.93.

WHAT CONDITIONS TO WATCH FOR WEAR

Inspect the tank and fittings for rusting, leakage, or corrosion. See if it delivers less hot water to the tap, even when the temperature is raised on the water heater dial. Look into the combustion chamber and the flue of fuel-burning units for obvious damage. (A flashlight and an inspection mirror are a big help.)

You can help reduce your family's risk of exposure to potentially harmful air pollutants by inspecting the color of your gas heater's flame at least once every other month. A properly burning gas heater should produce a sharply defined, blue-colored flame with just a little yellow glowing near the tip.

If the pilot light in your gas heater shows a lot of yellow, orange, red, purple, or green color, this indicates inefficient combustion. These condensates might include tar, dust, rust or oil, all of which are potentially hazardous chemicals. Flames showing a lot of color other than blue should be adjusted by a professional service technician to ensure your gas heater burns properly and safely.

A pile of rusty scale on top of the burner suggests that tainted air has damaged the flue. Light condensation of water or rust marking are not a problem, but heavy rust and water streaks are danger signals. Check out the "sacrificial" zinc anode rod. The rod dissolves diverting corrosion and protects the tank. It should be located on top of the appliance and looks like the top of a large bolt. Unscrew it. If it is eroded, remove and replace it with a collapsible rod. Although it can be difficult to remove, the effort is worthwhile because the anode provides the best clue to conditions inside the tank. If six inches of the core wire is exposed, it's time to replace the anode. If it has little or no sacrificial metal left, probably some damage has occurred to the tank. Replace the anode yourself and save up to $200.

If the inspection of fittings, combustion chamber, or anode suggests that the tank has undergone substantial damage, think seriously about replacement.

DIY: REPLACING THE ANODE ROD IN WATER HEATERS

Items and Tools needed:

- Closed end wrench, ratchet socket wrench, adjustable wrench.
- Standard garden hose.
- Teflon sealing tape or plumbing pipe dope compound.
- New anode (think flexible for easier installation).

How to Do It: Turn off the power supply to the heater and shut off water supply. For an electric heater, turn off the circuit breaker for the heater. If the power to the electric water heater is left on and air comes in contact with the heating element, the element can burn out. For a gas heater, turn the gas control valve to the lowest setting or the vacation setting, or simply to off. The anode rod will be located on top of the water heater or on the side. It will look like a hexagonal plug screwed into the heater.

An up/down valve on the side of the heater relieves pressure in the tank by allowing air into the tank to escape and break the vacuum, which in turn drains the water heater—be careful the water is under pressure and can be hot. If the tank is still under pressure when you try to loosen the anode, look out—it may fly out.

Open any faucet on the hot water supply side. Connect a regular garden hose to the drain valve at the bottom of the heater and drain. If the anode rod is on the top of the heater, draining only about one-half gallon of water is needed. If the anode is located on the side, drain the tank until the water is below the anode rod port. The hose must remain lower than the water level in the tank in order for the water to drain. When draining, the water will be hot, so be careful when handling the hose. Save the water to use on your plants (when cool).

Remove the anode with your selected tool. If the water heater is not strapped to prevent moving, have someone hold it. Don't bang the anode or use chemicals to loosen the anode; you could damage the heater or contaminate the water.

Lift the anode out of the heater. If it is hard to remove and cannot be pulled through the inlet hole, then there is still enough of the anode material to be working properly. Simply screw the anode back into the heater and replace it later. If it comes out smoothly, wrap the threads of the new anode rod with the Teflon tape or sealing compound in a clockwise direction with five or six wraps around the threads. Insert the new anode rod and tighten it down.

Open the cold water supply to the heater to refill the tank, keeping the faucet, as mentioned earlier, in the hot position. The tank is full when water comes out of the faucet and should be rid of any air when the water runs freely. The faucet will usually spit some air out with the water until the air is expelled. Check for any leaks. Turn the power on for electric. For gas, set the control back to the original temperature setting, or follow directions to relight the pilot light.

TO INSTALL A NEW WATER HEATER

If you're not handy it's probably best to call a professional. If you wish to do it yourself, first, measure the tank to be certain a new tank will fit in the current space. Turn off the water and power. Release pressure on the tap valve on top of the tank. Drain the water heater (see above).

Disconnect both hot and cold water connection filler pipes above the water heater tank. Disconnect the power source, turn off the gas valve, and shut off the breaker switch if electric.

Remove cap from the flue above the tank. Remove the tank. Replace the new tank and reverse the process. Open all windows and doors. Before connecting the gas line, you can bleed air through the system by running it for 30 seconds, but be very careful! Wait for gas smell to clear before proceeding to anything else. DO NOT switch anything on or off until the smell clears.

Smell for gas again and also use a soapy brush to ensure there is no gas leaking from the connections to the gas main pipe. (You may have to do this more than once to ensure gas flow if the pilot light won't ignite.) Ignite the pilot light and set the temperature to 120°F. Of course as with any project, get complete instructional details online, from any local hardware store, or contact your utility company to relight and/or inspect the heater at no cost.

DRAIN-WATER HEAT RECOVERY

Water heat recycling (also known as drain-water heat recovery or graywater heat recovery) is the use of a heat exchanger to recover energy and reuse heat from drain water from various activities such as dishwashing, clothes washing, and especially showers. Any hot water that goes down the drain carries away energy with it. Standard units save up to 60 percent of the heat energy that is otherwise lost down the drain.

Some storage-type systems have tanks containing a reservoir of clean water that flows through a spiral tube at the bottom of the heat storage tank. This warms the tank water, which rises to the top. Intake water is preheated by circulation through a coil at the top of the tank. Nonstorage systems usually have a copper heat exchanger that replaces a vertical section of a main waste drain. As warm water flows down the waste drain, incoming cold water flows through a spiral copper tube wrapped tightly around the copper section of the waste drain. This preheats the incoming cold water that goes to the water heater or a fixture, such as a shower. By preheating cold water, heat recovery systems help increase water heating capacity. This increased capacity really helps if you have an undersized water heater. You can also lower your water heating temperature without affecting the capacity.

COST AND INSTALLATION

Prices for drain-water heat recovery systems range from $300 to $500. Unless you're handy, you'll probably need a qualified plumbing or heating contractor to install the system. Installation will usually be less expensive in new home construction. Paybacks range from two-and-a-half to seven years, depending on how often the system is used.

17

Air Conditioning
Chilling Out

Have you ever sat at your desk feeling sweat streaks snaking down your back or lying in the smoldering heat struggling to sleep, praying for a cool breeze, your body percolating pools of perspiration?

Thank goodness for Willis Haviland Carrier (November 26, 1876–October 7, 1950), an American engineer who invented modern air conditioning and inadvertently changed the living conditions and politics of the population of the United States.

As with all modern appliances, the way you use your AC can vary greatly—depending on the size of your house, the climate in which you live, your energy costs, and how much you need to chill. On average, a room conditioner costs about twelve cents per hour to operate. A home AC unit, depending on the size of the home and the hours of use, will cost approximately twenty cents per hour.

FACTS AND FIGURES

In the early 1950s and 1960s, when air conditioning became readily available, it made living in the Sun Belt states of Florida, Texas, Arizona, New Mexico, Nevada, and California comfortable, producing a population shift and creating eighty-eight more Congressional seats that changed the political complexion of the United States.

The amount of energy the United States uses every year to power air conditioners is about the same amount consumed by the entire continent of Africa. On a hot day when the sun beats down on your home it can absorb as much as 90 percent of the sunlight's radiant heat.

About one-sixth of all the electricity generated in the United States is used to air condition buildings. Of 100 million homes in the United States about 84 percent have central air conditioning and another 23 percent have single AC room units. If just one household in ten bought EnergyStar-qualified heating and cooling equipment, it would prevent annual greenhouse gas emissions of 15 billion pounds, equivalent to the emissions from 1.3 million cars. According to the US DOE, heating and cooling systems emit over a half billion tons of carbon dioxide into the atmosphere each year, exacerbating the conditions of climate change. They also generate about 24 percent of the nation's sulfur dioxide, a chief ingredient in acid rain.

Home air conditioning can use up to 16 percent of total electricity consumed in summer, and in very hot climes can represent 60 percent of the utility bill during summer. The typical US homeowner spends 17 percent of their annual energy bill on cooling—about $170 to $375. Today's AC units use 30 to 50 percent less electricity than fifteen-year-old models. An air conditioner, when properly sized and installed, can save consumers 30 to 40 percent on cooling bills.

Room air conditioners last an average of nine years. Insist that a heating and cooling load analysis (Manual J or equivalent) be performed on your home to make sure that you are not buying a larger air conditioning system than you need. Always look for the EnergyStar label.

When looking for an AC unit, remember that each person contributes 400 Btus per room. However, if more than two people regularly occupy the room, add 600 Btus for each additional person.

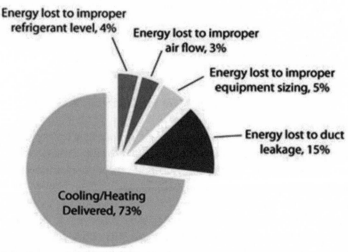

Figure 17.1.   HVAC energy loss.
Source: http://www.energystar.gov.

CENTRAL AIR CONDITIONING

Central air conditioning units' ratings are called SEER (Seasonal Energy Efficiency Ratio). The minimal rating for SEER is 13, with a higher number representing a higher efficiency rating. An efficient AC load calculation program, when you purchase a unit, takes into account many variables such as room-by-room calculations, proper ductwork, architectural features, including rooms with large, west-facing windows, shading, insulation and height of ceiling, walls, floors, air leakage, type of roof and the number of occupants, and square footage to be cooled. Using just the square footage of a home to size an air conditioner is an outdated method and will almost always yield an oversized system. Central AC can run from $0.34 to $1.60 an hour and can cost almost as much to operate as a furnace.

ROOM AIR CONDITIONING

Room-sized air conditioners come with an Energy Efficiency Ratio rating (EER). The higher the EER number, the better. Eleven or higher is excellent. An AC room unit used to cool an average-sized master bedroom (about 150 to 200 square feet) costs from five to fifteen cents per hour to run, depending on the size of your unit. If the room is very sunny, increase AC capacity by 10 percent.

Table 17.1. Room Air Conditioner Size

Room Size (square feet)	Room Air Conditioner Size (Btus per hour)
100–150	5,000
150–250	6,000
250–300	7,000
300–350	8,000
350–400	9,000
400–450	10,000
450–550	12,000
550–700	14,000
700–1000	18,000

Source: US Energy Information Administration

AIR CONDITIONER ASSISTANCE

Keep air conditioners free of obstructions inside so air can flow freely. Consider location of the unit. If mounting an air conditioner near the corner of a room, look for a unit that can send the airflow in the right direction. Turn off the furnace pilot light and other appliances during summer. This saves gas and heat. Utility companies will relight the pilot lights when asked at no cost.

Direct sunlight into the house will raise energy bills 20 percent. Close shades, drapes, doors, and windows when the AC is on. If the room is heavily shaded, reduce AC capacity by 10 percent. Installing solar screens and awnings on windows hit by direct sunlight will reflect back 60 to 70 percent of heat through sunlight before it can enter the house.

Turn off kitchen or bathroom exhaust fans when the air conditioning is operating. If the unit is used in a kitchen, increase capacity by 4,000 Btus. Open your windows in the evening or early morning to capture cool breezes and keep them closed during hot days. If your basement is livable, temporarily move downstairs on hot summer days. It is often 10° to 15°F cooler than the upstairs. While you are not at home, set the AC to about 82°F (28°C), or keep it off whenever possible, and use the timer on the AC so that it's not working needlessly while you are away.

When turning the AC back on, don't set the thermostat excessively low; it won't cool the house any faster. The recommended summer temperature setting while in the house is 78°F. Setting the thermostat each additional degree below 78°F will increase energy use by 3 to 4 percent.

Do not position heat-producing appliances, such as televisions or lamps, near the thermostat controls of the air conditioner. The heat they produce fools the thermostat and causes the air conditioner to run longer than necessary. Keep lights and appliances off when not in use; they also generate heat, making air conditioners run harder.

Completely closing room vents in a home with central AC reduces efficiency and makes the unit work harder. Partly close the registers in rooms where AC is not being used to decrease the air conditioner's workload. If your air conditioning equipment is older and less efficient, compensate by being extra careful about temperature settings, hours of operation, and filter condition.

Set the fan speed of central air conditioners on high except in very humid weather. Set the fan on central air conditioners to "on" rather than "auto." This will circulate air continuously, keeping the temperature more even throughout the house and aiding in dehumidification. Don't judge the efficiency of an air conditioner by the sound of the fan shutting on and off. The blower will continue to circulate cooled air up to fifteen minutes after the compressor has stopped. (The same holds true for a furnace.)

You've heard the saying, "It's not the heat; it's the humidity." Lowering humidity will help make your home feel more comfortable. Try setting your air conditioner above 78°F when using a dehumidifier combined with fans.

When it's humid, set the speed on low; you will get less cooling but more moisture will be removed from the air, which will make you feel cooler.

In architecture, passive cooling refers to a building that uses no energy-consuming technology or devices to help maintain a comfortable inside temperature. An example would be passively cooling a house outside via properly sheltering it from the sun, and utilizing reliable breezes to cool the air temperature.

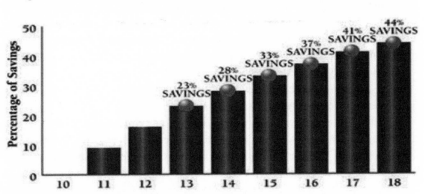

Figure 17.2. SEER cooling costs.
Source: trustmathis.com.

An AC unit will use 5 percent less energy when placed on the north side of the house, under shade, or behind trees and plants. Planting trees and shrubs for shade in the right place will lower the temperature of your house and increase the efficiency of your AC. One well-placed shade tree can reduce cooling costs by 25 percent.

Plant deciduous trees on the east and west sides of your home; in the summer, their broad leaves will shade your house, while in the winter bare branches won't stop the sun's warmth from reaching your walls.

Keep outside shrubs at least one foot away for adequate AC airflow, making certain that the air conditioner is not blocked by foliage or structures. A "free-flowing" air source makes the unit operate most efficiently.

MAINTENANCE

Air conditioners can lose 5 percent efficiency every two years. Commit to a preventive maintenance program of yearly inspections. An annual tune-up of an air conditioner by a service expert can improve the unit's efficiency by as much as 20 percent as well as lengthen performance life. Proper maintenance should be carried out by a HVAC professional. They should:

- Check for correct amount of refrigerant.
- Test for refrigerant leaks using a leak detector.
- Capture any refrigerant that must be evacuated from the system instead of illegally releasing it into the atmosphere. This is most often done by professionals.
- Check for and seal duct leakage in central systems.
- Measure airflow through the evaporator coil.
- Verify the correct electric control sequence and make sure that the heating system and cooling system cannot operate simultaneously.
- Inspect electric terminals, clean and tighten connections, and apply a nonconductive coating if necessary.
- Oil motors and check belts for tightness and wear.
- Check the accuracy of the thermostat.
- Clean the outdoor condenser coils and any filters every year with a strong stream of water to remove dirt, leaves, grass, etc. Occasionally pass a stiff wire through the unit's drain channels. Clogged drain channels prevent a unit from reducing humidity, and the resulting excess moisture may discolor walls or carpet.

At the start of each cooling season, inspect the seal between the air conditioner and the window frame to ensure it makes contact with the unit's metal case. Moisture can damage this seal, allowing cool air to escape from your house. Disposable AC filters that should be changed every three months are around $4 each, though you can recoup $20 to $40 of the cost of a permanent filter in as little as fifteen months. Check ducts—the average home loses 15 to 20 percent of cooling through leaking ducts. Keep your AC housing, coils, and fins clean and straight. During winter keep your portable room AC in a dry place and cover with a tarp.

While the tax benefits aren't as generous as they once were, you can still get tax credit worth 10 percent of the AC cost, up to $500. For complete qualification details, visit Web sites regarding state and federal tax credits for energy efficiency on the Internet.

PASSIVE AIR COOLING

Before plentiful energy and the machine age, designers came up with ingenious techniques for letting the forces of nature keep their buildings cool. Thomas Jefferson used passive cooling to keep Monticello comfy even in the blistering heat of August. Although designers are today relearning those techniques, despite advanced technology, passive cooling hasn't changed that much.

Passive cooling uses all natural processes and techniques of heat dissipation and modulation without the use of energy, or with as little energy as possible called "hybrid cooling systems." There are many passive techniques that are covered in different places in the chapter: green roofs, window films, etc.

No matter the climate or geographical region, passive houses stay at a comfortable temperature with minimal energy inputs. In fact, a passive house requires as little as 10 percent of the heating and cooling energy used by a typical building. Passively cooled houses costs about 8 percent more to build.

PRACTICAL SUGGESTIONS FOR HOUSE DESIGN AND POSITION

Check site for exposure to breezes and maximize cross ventilation. Ideally all summer easterly breezes should be directed through the home. Maximize the amount of daytime living space that faces north. Be sure to incorporate plenty of doors and windows into your home design, but be careful not to have them facing the west side. Large, well-designed eaves are generally all that is required to shade the northern elevations of single story houses. Group living areas along the north facing side and bedrooms along the south or east side.

Incorporate high-level windows and vents to draw the hot air out of a room. When placing ventilation openings, situate inlets and outlets to optimize the path air follows through the building. Windows or vents placed on opposite sides, but not necessarily across the building, give natural cross ventilation breezes. It is generally best not to place openings exactly across from each other and to minimize potential barriers. Make the outlet openings slightly larger than the inlet openings. Place the inlets at low to medium heights to provide airflow at occupant levels in the room. Also be certain that inlets for air movement are centered in the room. Because breezes come from many directions and can be deflected or diverted, designing windows and openings to collect and direct breezes is important.

MATERIALS AND INSULATION

Choose light-colored roofing and wall materials, including "cool paint." Cool paint coating systems represent a revolutionary concept in exterior wall coatings. Specially formulated to reflect the sun's heat, they can lower exterior wall surface temperatures by as much as 40 degrees when compared to traditional paints (lower exterior temperatures mean lower interior temperatures). Department of Energy's Oak Ridge National Laboratory demonstrated that "cool paints" can reduce a home's cooling costs by as much as 22 percent. Choose natural materials that are sustainably manufactured.

AIR CIRCULATION AND VENTILATION

Wind ventilation is the easiest, most common, and often least expensive form of passive cooling and ventilation. Wind ventilation is a kind of passive ventilation that uses the force of the wind to pull air through the building. Successful wind ventilation is determined by adequate fresh air for the ventilated spaces, while using little or no energy for active HVAC cooling and ventilation.

Ventilation carries heat out of the building as warmed air and replaces it with cooler external air. These breezes tend to occur in the late afternoon or early evening when cooling requirements usually peak. Cool breezes work best in open plan layouts. Even when there is no breeze, convection allows heat to leave a building via windows, roof ventilators, eaves, gables, and ceilings. Use casement windows to catch and deflect breezes from varying angles. Encourage airflow under floors and in basements. Wind can be steered by architectural features, such as casement windows, wing walls, fences, or even strategically planted vegetation. Place plants to funnel cooling breezes and filter strong winds.

SOLAR CHIMNEYS

The solar chimney is an invention that uses simple rule of heat transfer and provides ventilation. We all know that hot air rises. A vertical duct made at the roof of a building facing toward the sun is known as a solar chimney, and as it is exposed to sun the temperature inside the chimney rises. As the hot air begins to move upwards, it is exchanged by the cooler and fresher air through the vents and windows down in the building. The structure is usually constructed of concrete and glass, then insulated with a black metal absorber with a glazed outer surface in order to achieve high temperatures for efficiency of ventilation.

WINDCATCHERS

Windcatchers do just as the name suggests—architectural towers "catch" the wind to create natural airflow inside buildings. Used extensively throughout the Middle East, windcatchers function in one or more of three ways: Wind enters the chimney directly through a tall, capped tower with an opening to the prevailing wind, creating a downward flow of air. Dense hot air escapes out of the tunnel, while cool air from below fills the void, creating a natural indoor breeziness, or hot air is pulled in through a tunnel, which is then cooled in an underground space (sometimes with the use of water), which forces air in an upward motion through the tower.

PERFORATED DOUBLE-SKINNED EXTERIOR

Covering the exterior of a building with a "raised" perforated screen is another highly effective passive cooling technique. It allows natural daylight to diffuse through to provide illumination but shades the indoor spaces to avoid overheating. By putting four feet between the outer and inner walls of the building, natural air circulation is also created.

LANDSCAPE

Landscaping is an effective and attractive means of providing shading for your house. An effectively planned landscape will block out the hot summer sun, encourage warming sun to enter the house in winter, deflect the cold winter winds, and channel breezes for cooling in summer. A well-planned landscape can also reduce air conditioning costs by 15 to 50 percent, even more for small mobile homes.

In general, an ideal landscape plan would include trees to the east and west of the house to provide summer shading, with the area to the south of the house left relatively clear in order to allow solar heating in winter. Trees will be most effective if they shade east and west windows, where the most heat can enter, and also shade the roof. Large trees can also shade full walls, which can reduce the outside wall temperature from a very hot heat sink in full sunshine down to something more like the air temperature.

A fernery (a specialized garden for the cultivation and display of ferns) next to your home will work as a natural evaporative air cooler. Plant low shrubs and ground covers around the home to reduce reflected heat and glare. Plant deciduous vines around pergolas (a framework covered with trained climbing or trailing plants) to provide shading in summer. Large dense shrubs can be planted to channel cooling wind toward the home.

PERSONAL SUGGESTIONS FOR LIVING IN A HOT CLIMATE

Wear lightweight, light-colored clothing made of natural fibers. It will reflect heat and absorb perspiration, making you feel cooler. Use special blankets and sheets made of bamboo fiber, even wool, which aid in "wicking" or removing moisture from your body. Try using a Chillow, a cold-water-filled pillow that keeps your head cool while you sleep. Use a bed fan, a small, gentle fan that operates under the covers. Drink plenty of liquids. Plan cold meals with cold cuts, salads, etc. Take your shower during the middle of the day using cool water. Try to use as little hot water as possible. It adds heat and humidity. Use bath and kitchen vents to exhaust heat and moisture. Make sure your clothes dryer is vented outdoors. Keep both primary and storm windows shut when running the air conditioner. These lifestyle adjustments will help you adapt to the heat and aid in obtaining maximum efficiency from your air conditioning. These tips will also assist in avoiding brownouts and blackouts.

18

A House in Heat

The Cost of Keeping Cozy

Keeping the home heated and cooled used to be the largest expense of running a home. For decades "space conditioning" accounted for more than half of all residential energy consumption. Estimates from the most recent Residential Energy Consumption Survey (RECS) show that 48 percent of energy consumption in US homes in 2009 was for heating and cooling, down from 58 percent in 1993.

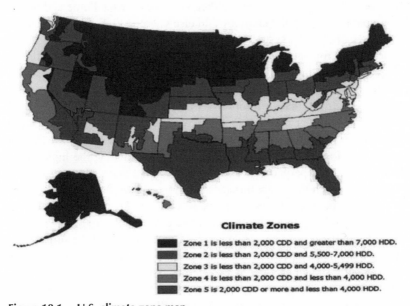

Climate Zones

Zone 1 is less than 2,000 CDD and greater than 7,000 HDD.
Zone 2 is less than 2,000 CDD and 5,500-7,000 HDD.
Zone 3 is less than 2,000 CDD and 4,000-5,499 HDD.
Zone 4 is less than 2,000 CDD and less than 4,000 HDD.
Zone 5 is 2,000 CDD or more and less than 4,000 HDD.

Figure 18.1.   U.S. climate zone map.
Source: US Energy Information Administration.

Still, what is warm to some is fevered to others. This ongoing war of house temperatures is not only contentious; it's counterproductive as it leads to thermostat wars. It's not difficult to keep the family comfy with some practical suggestions that will help avoiding getting hot under the collar about who controls the heat and the energy expense.

FACTS AND FIGURES

Most homes are heated from a central furnace (gas, coal, electric, etc.) via air ducts and registers that distribute the warmth. The annual fuel utilization efficiency (AFUE) rating that the US Department of Energy requires on a furnace indicates how efficiently the equipment is burning its fuel source and turning it into usable heat. The AFUE differs from the true "thermal efficiency" in that it is not a continual state or peak measure of heat efficiency but, instead, attempts to represent the actual, season-long, average efficiency a heater.

The American Council for an Energy-Efficient Economy (ACEEE) claims, "The single most important thing people can do to save energy in their homes is to make sure that their furnace is running efficiently." A cost-effective heating system starts with a good system design, efficient size, excellent insulation, economical appliances, and well-designed, tight construction practices, all of which affect operating costs. An AFUE of 90 percent means that 90 percent of the energy in the fuel becomes heat for the home and the other 10 percent escapes up the chimney and elsewhere. AFUE doesn't include the heat losses of the duct system or piping, which can be as much as 35 percent of the energy for output of the furnace when ducts are located in the attic, garage, or other (uninsulated) spaces. For gas or propane, in mixed and cold climates a rating of 95 AFUE or better is recommended.

An all-electric furnace or boiler has no flue loss through a chimney. The AFUE rating for an all-electric furnace or boiler is between 95 and 100 percent. The lower values are for units installed outdoors because they have greater heat loss. However, despite their high efficiency, the higher cost of electricity in most parts of the country makes all-electric furnaces or boilers an uneconomic choice. New furnaces are more efficient than older equipment (of ten years or more) by as much as 30 percent. According to California's Pacific Gas and Electric, a forced-air furnace can cost up to $1.85 per hour to run, depending on the size and location of your home and the furnace's age, making it the most expensive appliance in the house. Lowering the thermostat 2° F can cut as much as 5 percent off the heating bill.

Most heating and air conditioning (HVAC) units can last approximately twenty years and furnaces have been known to last up to thirty years when they have been well maintained. Conventional heating systems in the United States are responsible for a billion tons of carbon dioxide, and about 12 percent of the sulfur dioxide and nitrogen oxides emitted by the nation yearly. If just one in ten households used current technology to upgrade their inefficient heating systems, we could keep 17 billion pounds of pollution out of the air annually.

Heating equipment is the leading cause of home fires during the months of December, January, and February, and is a close second to kitchen fires the rest of the year. Each year an estimated 54,900 home heating equipment fires were reported to US fire departments, resulting in 220 deaths, 1,120 injuries, and $502 million in property damage.

The new federal minimum energy conservation standard in the northern region is 90 AFUE (started May 1, 2013), and 80 AFUE in the southern region. The southern region includes Alabama, Arizona, Arkansas, California, Delaware, District of Columbia, Florida, Georgia, Hawaii, Kentucky, Louisiana,

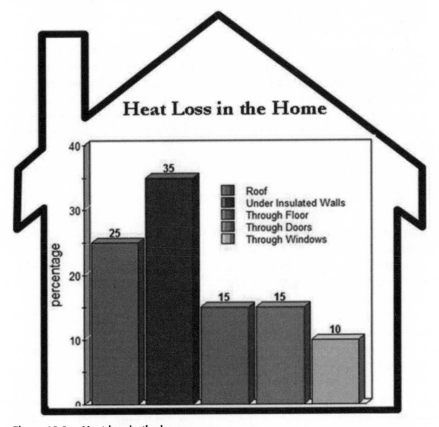

Figure 18.2.   Heat loss in the home.
Source: Provided by the author.

Maryland, Mississippi, Nevada, New Mexico, North Carolina, Oklahoma, South Carolina, Tennessee, Texas, and Virginia. The northern region consists of Alaska, Colorado, Connecticut, Idaho, Illinois, Indiana, Iowa, Kansas, Maine, Massachusetts, Michigan, Minnesota, Missouri, Montana, Nebraska, New Hampshire, New Jersey, New York, North Dakota, Ohio, Oregon, Pennsylvania, Rhode Island, South Dakota, Utah, Vermont, Washington, West Virginia, Wisconsin, and Wyoming.

SIMPLE SUGGESTIONS TO COMBAT THE COLD

Adjust for the reasonable comfort level of your family. Don't be an energy hog, but you don't have to live like a cave-dwelling monk either. Those who are comfortable dialing back the thermostat are able to reduce their heating fuel consumption substantially, as the heating system does not have to maintain a large temperature differential or heat the whole house.

Save energy by getting under comforters and using thermal blankets that envelop you in a pocket of air warmed by your body. Pull on sweaters and sweat suits before cranking up the heat. Try a heated throw, mini electric blanket, or an electric heating pad, especially for two. Or, instead of an electric blanket, go to bed with a hot water bottle. Share body heat—cuddle with loved ones, including pets, to keep warm. Indulge in hot beverages such as cocoa, tea, broth, coffee, or a hot toddy. Pump yourself up with a little vigorous exercise.

THE HEAT-EFFICIENT HOUSE

Keeping the temp at 68°F is comfortable for most people. Turn the thermostat down to 55°F before going to bed and when away from home. Try to "sleep cold," turning down the thermostat to the low-60°s or mid-50°s, or even turning the furnace off at night. Turning the thermostat down from 70° to 55°F for eight hours can cut heating costs as much as 30 percent. It doesn't take more energy to bring a house back to the desired temperature than to maintain it at that temperature. Remember to turn off any heater when not in use. Keep doors, especially the garage door, closed during the winter. Cold air from underheated rooms can escape into the rest of the house, reducing the effectiveness of all your insulating and weatherizing.

If you have a forced-air furnace, do not completely close heat registers in unused rooms. Furnaces are designed to heat a specific square footage of space and can't sense if a register is closed. It simply will continue working at the same or harder pace. Place humidifiers and dehumidifiers away from walls and bulky furniture. These appliances work best when air circulates freely around them.

Be sure to keep furniture and draperies away from radiators, vents, and electric baseboards, leaving at least a three- to five-inch clearance from a heating unit to ensure circulation. Keep curtains and blinds closed at night to keep cold air out, but open them during the day to let warm sunlight in. If you have hardwood or tile floors, add area rugs to help keep feet warm.

Inexpensive plastic deflectors can direct air under tables and chairs or downward. If you have a hot water or steam heat system, buy or make a reflector to place behind the radiator to reflect heat back into the room. A piece of cardboard wrapped in aluminum foil works fine. Use heat-generating appliances (dishwasher, washing machine, clothes dryer) in the cooler evening hours. This will help heat the home in the winter and ease the air conditioner's job in the summer.

Most furnaces installed prior to 1992 are only 65 percent efficient, compared with newer furnaces, which report at least 80 percent efficiency. Fully weatherize and insulate your home before replacing your furnace. If you have room air conditioners, either take them out in the winter or cover them well. They tend to be poor insulators.

TYPES OF HEATING SYSTEMS

Forced-Air Systems

A forced-air system, fueled by natural gas, propane, oil, or electricity, is by far the most common type of central heating method used in North American homes that can be filtered, humidified, and dehumidified. The heating (and cooling) system relies on plenums (heat collectors), ductwork, vents, or registers.

HVAC contractors use various calculations to determine furnace sizes for homes, but they can be hard to understand—so how about a "rule-of-thumb" estimation to pick the right size for your home? For cooler climates (check out climate zones below), a very broad estimate of furnace sizing is to select one that generates 40 to 45 Btus per square foot. At 40 to 45 Btus per square foot, you'd need an efficient 100,000- to 112,500-Btu furnace to heat your 2,500-square-foot home. Many homes have only one thermostat monitoring the system, resulting in some rooms being warmer or cooler than others, and you typically have to heat and cool the entire home or open and close registers (remember the tip about registers) rather than just the room you're using.

Gas Heaters

Although gas furnaces are more efficient than oil and electric furnaces, that efficiency comes at an initial price—gas units can be priced between 20 to 30 percent higher than the same size oil, coal, or electric furnace, depending on the needs of your home.

Gas Heater Pros: Gas generally costs less than electricity and typically has the highest energy efficiency. Natural gas has the fewest emissions of any home heating fuel, hence lessening the impact on the environment. Natural gas furnaces are cheap to maintain. A gas furnace heats up to higher temperatures than an electric one.

Gas Heater Cons: Gas furnaces cost more than oil, coal, and electric alternatives. The gas furnace has a shorter lifespan than one powered by electricity. Natural gas is flammable and powered by fossil fuels. Gas furnaces also require ductwork in walls. Furnace fans are often noisy, and moving air can distribute allergens. Installation involves technical skills and specialized tools. Gas furnaces require filtration and regular maintenance.

Your home must be vented. Defective heating sources that burn fossil fuel can release colorless, odorless, tasteless, and deadly carbon monoxide. As a result, an estimated 200 to 500 deaths and 15,000 visits to the emergency room occur each year in the United States due to carbon monoxide poisoning from defective heating sources. By the way, this is a very good reason to install an inexpensive carbon monoxide detector in your home.

Maintenance: Heating contractors say simple dust and dirt are the cause of almost half of all their service calls. Check the gas pilot safety system and clean if needed. Check the motor, fan, and blower operation. Check the condition, tension, and alignment of any fan belts, and adjust as required. Clean burners and settings for proper combustion and ignition. Check gas piping to the furnace. Check vents at least twice a year.

Change filters—they're cheap—every other month during winter; pushing air through dirty filters makes your systems work harder, using more energy. Dirty filters can also contribute to indoor air pollution, which at times can be 25 to 90 percent worse than outside air. Have your natural gas heating system inspected once a year. A $50 to $100 annual tune-up can help reduce your heating costs by up to 5 percent.

Electric Furnace

An electric furnace is a simple electric heating element that warms the air. It can be a space heater for a single room or a heat source for the whole house.

Electric Furnace Pros: An electric furnace will last for twenty to thirty years. You will initially pay less for an electric furnace than for a gas, oil, or coal furnace, but they are costly to operate. An electric furnace requires very little maintenance. They do not create concern about carbon monoxide poisoning or the possibility of a fuel leak that could cause an explosion. They are quiet while operating. Electric furnaces are easy to install, basically "plug and play."

Many cities or states offer incentive programs to homeowners who install electric furnaces in an attempt to reduce in-house emissions. Some utility companies will offer a cheaper electricity rate to those who run their home with electric heat. However, check your power company's source of fuel—if they burn coal or fuel oil you're not cutting down on greenhouse gas emissions.

Small electrical space heaters are far more economical than gas furnaces for heating small areas. They are safer and more durable than the gas furnace. Electric furnaces require less attention and have more issues with efficiency rather than safety, and troubleshooting maintenance issues are easier.

Electric Furnace Cons: Electric furnaces are more expensive to operate than natural gas furnaces. It can cost three times as much to heat water with electricity as it does with gas, and they take longer to heat a room. Electric rates vary greatly across the United States, so it is important to do research on local kWh prices with different utilities. The fuel efficiency of electric heating (converting a resource to produce electricity) is around 30 percent, according to the DOE.

Maintenance: Keep your furnace properly inspected to save 5 to 10 percent in energy costs annually. Don't hesitate to call a pro if you believe the heater is not acting correctly.

Fuel Oil

This petroleum product is mainly used for heating fuel in the north and eastern part of the United States. Diesel is a type of fuel oil.

Fuel Oil Pros: Oil provides more heat per Btu than other heating sources. Oil furnaces are regularly and easily serviced by the delivery company (a service contract is required), but maintenance is more extensive due to dirt and soot build-up—chimneys must be cleaned and the oil filters changed frequently.

Oil furnaces cost less than gas furnaces, but efficiency is lower and fuel prices are higher than with gas systems. Oil furnaces offer efficiency ratings of 80 percent and higher for energy use. A number of companies are now offering heating oil blended with biodiesel, allowing their customers to reduce their dependence on foreign oil. The biodiesel blends also produce less pollution than pure heating oil.

Fuel Oil Cons: The highest levels of fine particles, sulfur dioxide, and other pollutants are produced in neighborhoods where many residential and commercial buildings burn No. 4 or No. 6 oil. Prices can fluctuate. As of 2014, an oil furnace serves as one of the most expensive ways to heat a home due to the high cost of heating oil, over $1,000 or more than natural gas annually. An on-site storage tank is required and oil must be delivered. Fuel oil is extremely volatile as well.

Maintenance: Oil-fired forced-air furnaces have greater maintenance requirements than gas furnaces and should be serviced every year. Home oil tanks should be replaced every twenty years.

Regular maintenance should include:

- Inspecting oil tank, piping, and tubing for leaks.
- Maintaining HVAC air filters that reduce the amount of dust that is blown around the house and also protect the heating equipment.
- If you see black soot on the heating registers, call a service technician.
- If you smell combustion products in the home, call a service technician.
- If your furnace fails to run, press the reset button. This may be located on the flue pipe near the furnace or on the burner. You should only press this one time. If the furnace still fails to ignite, call a service technician.
- Pressing the reset button repeatedly will cause raw oil to squirt into the burner chamber. If you do not have an automatic reset button, this procedure is dangerous.

Table 18.1.   A Comparison of Current Energy Costs

	US Home Heating Residential Fuel Prices 2014–2015		
Fuel Type	*Recent Price (USD)*	*Units*	*Source & Comments*
Natural gas	$10.21 [1]	K cu ft [2]	US EIA 49% of homes use natural gas
No. 2 home heating oil	$2.80	US gallon	US EIA 6% of homes use No. 2 oil
LPG/propane	$1.83	US gallon	US EIA 6% of homes use propane
Electricity	$0.1246 (12.46 cents)	kWh [3]	US EIA 4% of homes heat with electricity
Firewood	$230	Full cord	Web survey of vendors Feb. 5 2015; 2% of US homes heat primarily by wood
Other			1% of homes use other heating methods
Pellet fuel	$5.22	40-lb. bag	Walmart Price quoted 5 Feb. 2015; US Tractor Supply quotes $5.29
Coal	$53.00 to >$11.55	Ton	US EIA Coal prices range by area and coal type, including coal SO_2 levels; Btus per ton also varied from 12.5K Btu/pound to 8.8K Btu/pound where prices roughly also track Btu differences Note: these prices will vary by individual geographic area or market

Source: Courtesy of Carson Dunlop Associates

Radiant Heating Systems

Objects that are in the direct pathway of these systems absorb heat immediately. Once they heat up, they radiate it to other objects in the room. Radiant heating systems involve supplying heat directly to the floor or to panels in the wall or ceiling of a house using electrically heated water, electric elements, fossil fuels, biomass, and solar.

There are three types of radiant floor heat: radiant air floors (air is the heat-carrying medium), electric radiant floors (embedded coils), and hot water (hydronic) radiant floors.

Radiant Air Heating Pros: Radiant heat uses wires or pipes (no ductwork) to get the hot water or electricity to each area of a home and these wires and pipes take up very little space. A radiant system is nearly silent, clean, comfortable, there are no ducts to clean, it's efficient, and requires minimal maintenance. Radiant heat can be delivered by floor heating panels, floor heating coils, baseboard heaters, and kickspace heaters. This type of system works by turning cold surfaces hot and keeping the heat distribution comfortable.

Radiant Air Heating Cons: Because air cannot hold large amounts of heat, radiant air floors are not cost-effective in residential applications and are seldom installed. Electric radiant floors typically consist of electric cables built into the floor. Systems that feature mats of electrically conductive plastic are also available, and are mounted onto the subfloor below a covering such as tile, which makes installation maintenance problematic as the heating elements are in the floor or walls. This system is expensive to install and not too energy-efficient because of the relatively high cost of electricity, electric radiant floors are usually only cost-effective if they include a significant thermal mass, such as a thick concrete floor, and if your electric utility company offers time-of-use rates. Radiant systems may also require their own separate network of ducts.

Radiant Heat Hot-Water System

This system uses hot water in small pipes, which is circulated and vented to produce heat in floor radiators, floors, and baseboards.

Radiant Heat Hot-Water Pros: The system is energy-efficient and can pay for itself if fuel cost is low. Radiant systems for ceilings or walls are far more efficient than floor systems. The new system can be controlled room-by-room, great for people who disagree on the perfect room temperature. The system can respond quickly to changes in heating needs. It operates quietly and invisibly. Radiant heating systems offer a gentle and comfortable temperature. You never have to worry about your children or pets getting burned by this system.

Radiant heating is environmentally friendly and energy-efficient. Home-owners can save up to 30 percent, and commercial property owners up to 60 percent on their heating bills. Many people find radiant hot-water heating find more comfortable than forced hot air. Hot-water systems take up less room because the water circulates in small diameter pipes. It is more efficient because it doesn't have to travel though ducts.

Radiant Heat Hot-Water Cons: Radiant systems are usually more expensive to install than forced-air, and they are not easily adapted for air conditioning or cooling. Water leaks are rare, but can result in serious damage. Maintenance, which can be problematic since the heating elements are in the floors or walls, should be performed by a professional. Baseboards should remain unobstructed, which may be difficult for people with pets and children. Radiant floor heat is greatly affected by floor coverings, which makes the system run hotter, which in turn creates pumping power for cooling requirements to skyrocket.

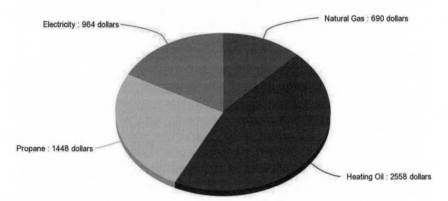

Figure 18.3.   The best annual bang for your energy buck.
Source: Provided by the author.

Hydronic Coil

A hydronic coil is a heat exchanger that warms a small metal coil using hot water produced by the burning of fuel (gas/propane/oil) in a boiler, from either a tank or tankless system. Air is then forced over the coil and warmed before being pumped back into the home via forced air.

Hydronic Coil Pros: A hydronic system can be used with any kind of heat delivery package you want in a device—hot water baseboard, panel radiators, radiant floor/wall/ceiling heat, and hydro-air using a hot air delivery system with ductwork. The system provides quiet and gentle heating. Also, the heated water can be put to other uses such as providing hot potable water sent to pools or spas, and to melt ice and snow from sidewalks and driveways, saving money. The price for a hydronic system is comparatively low.

Hydronic Coil Cons: The system is not widely used as it generally doesn't have a duct system and cannot control indoor air quality. The system is also prone to infiltration as stray heat can sneak into or out of the system. Many ducting systems are incompatible with a hydronic system or upgrades. A hydronic system cannot be used in conjunction with air conditioning.

Maintenance: It depends upon the type of system. With a forced-air system, it is important to change the furnace filters on an annual basis. If the fan coil becomes dirty, it should be cleaned according to the manufacturer's recommended procedures. Baseboard systems need routine cleaning and vacuuming to ensure that the convective fins are free from dirt and lint. Radiant floor and ceiling systems have no need for maintenance except for the routine upkeep of the boiler or water heater, which requires routine maintenance as recommended by the manufacturer. Also, it is important to regularly inspect the water pressures in the circulation loops. Most systems are equipped with a pressure gauge that reads the pressure of the water loop.

Heat Pump

By drawing heat from the air or from the ground, heat pumps employs the same basic refrigeration-type cycle used by an air conditioner or a refrigerator. That simply means that when a refrigerant is used, the temperature of the refrigerant drops a lot so the cold outdoor air is actually warmer when it comes in contact with the outdoor coil of your heat pump. And, as we know, heat likes to move from warmer objects to cooler objects. Once the heat from the air gets into the refrigerant, it's just a matter of bringing it into the house and then transferring it into your home's air.

Heat Pump Pros: Heat pumps are considered very efficient, delivering nearly double the energy in heat than the energy they consume, according to the US DOE. While conventional heaters have efficiencies of around 80 percent, heat pumps can have efficiencies of 100 percent continually. A heat pump will also turn on and off less often than a gas furnace. The system can also be used in cooling, just as any central air conditioning system, working in reverse in summer by expelling the warm air outside.

Heat Pump Cons: Heat pump systems tend to be somewhat ineffective in any climate where the outdoor air temperature falls near or below freezing on a regular basis. Many homeowners report that the heat generated by a heat pump created in their home during the winter months feels cold. Consequently, they are not suitable for very cold climates unless used with a backup source of heat. The heat produced by heat pumps isn't as intense as the heat produced by a gas or oil-burning furnace.

Maintenance: If you use your heat pump on a regular basis or even peri-odically, you should change the filter every one to three months. Keep fans and coils clean and free from debris, and have your heat pump inspected by a professional once every year or two. If the unit isn't working, try resetting its motor. Check the pump ignition system for problems, and make sure you don't have a tripped circuit breaker or blown fuse.

Solar Power

The best example of inexhaustible, free, nonpolluting radiant heat is the energy that comes from our solar system's star. Active power is produced via photocells that change light from the sun into electricity, used in solar panels, pocket calculators, etc. The savings over time completely outweigh the expense and this type of power—either active or passive—is one of our best choices for alternative energy.

Solar Power Pros: After costs of installation, it's free. That means saying goodbye to that expensive electric bill every month and for the rest of the life of your home. Over time, this will save you tens of thousands of dol-lars. Technological improvements are bringing down the cost and variety of solar power continually, and many companies will lease you the equipment, reducing the initial cost. They are low maintenance as residential panels only require cleaning a couple times a year. Some solar manufacturers offer war-ranties for twenty to twenty-five years with their panels.

Solar energy is virtually soundless. Other renewable sources, such as wind turbines, can be very noisy—something to consider if young children are in the house or if you simply enjoy peace and quiet. Generating your own solar power means you are not as dependent on utilities and the electric power grid to provide your electricity.

Besides generous state and federal rebates and tax breaks, there are some states with a program called "net metering" that essentially turns your meter backwards giving you a credit on your utilities or selling the extra energy that you have generated to the other companies, easing pressure on the grid and utility companies.

Solar Power Cons: The manufacturing, transporting, and installation of a solar system involves producing pollutants. The sun doesn't shine brightly 24 hours a day. Some locations have trees or taller buildings that could shade your roof. Excessively high outdoor temperatures, pollution, storms, and weather can reduce efficiency of the system. Since solar energy runs off the sun, you may need to invest in other sources of electricity or large household batteries (which cost about $3,000 at present) for nighttime or during bad weather.

Although solar panels are installed on the roof, space can be an issue. If your roof isn't compatible, try shared solar panels that allow you to generate green electricity via a "solar garden" that is central to the community and not on your own roof. Unfortunately, solar energy is not cheap. For the average home in the United States, active solar might cost from $10,000 to $30,000 to install. If you typically spend $2,000 per year on electricity, it will take a good fifteen years to get back your investment monetarily—but you'd be making an altruistic effort on the part of the Earth.

Maintenance: Photovoltaic (PV) panels only need to be cleaned periodically so that dirt and debris do not reduce efficiency.

Geothermal Energy

This system doesn't make heat—it moves it by absorbing heat stored in the ground through the water that circulates in an underground loop. Below the frost line it always stays around 50°F, so when heating or cooling, you are more than halfway to your goal. The geothermal unit, which acts as furnace and air conditioner, uses refrigerant and the temperate water from the underground pipes to heat or cool air. This air is carried to the ground source heat pumps where it's concentrated and then sent as warm, comfortable air throughout the home. Heat can be obtained in low intensity at a shallow depth, which makes it perfect for the heating of the home.

Geothermal Pros: Geothermal (Earth heat) power is extremely reliable and, unlike wind and solar, the geothermal power source never varies. The source will always be available and has a lower rate than nonrenewable resources such as fossil fuels. A geothermal energy system can cut cooling and heating costs by 20 to 80 percent. The actual amount that you will save is dependent on several factors, which include the amount of energy used and the efficiency rating of the heat pump installed. A ground source heat pump may pay for itself in a period of two to ten years.

As the technology continues to improve and become more widely available, the costs will go down and, over time, the initial installation costs will be covered by the energy savings that you receive. Geothermal energy also has the smallest carbon footprint of any of the major power sources.

Geothermal Cons: Geothermal energy is still a relatively new concept for private homes and relatively expensive to install compared to the cost of traditional furnaces or air conditioning units, up to $30,000, but there are tax breaks and rebates available from your Uncle Sam. However, if you do not have the extra funds specifically for this purpose, you may find the cost to be a financial burden. Electricity is still needed to power the heat pump that makes the entire system work, so the system is not pollution free if your power source is created by fossil fuels. Quite a bit of land is required to have it properly installed, on which a grid is established. Where the system can be installed is extremely location-specific. Finally, there is a minimum temperature requirement of at least 350°F required for the system to perform at optimum levels. Figure on about ten to twelve years for investment payback.

Maintenance: A geothermal heat pump is a high performance piece of equipment. The most important hint is to keep your air filter clean, and every couple of years have it inspected by a professional.

Space Heaters

Most space heaters are convection heaters, meaning they rely on the circulation of air to heat a room. Ceramic heaters feature a ceramic disc heating element and fan to distribute warm air evenly and efficiently. Micathermic heaters combine the processes of convection and radiant heat. Radiant (glowing) heat is felt almost immediately by the occupants of a room, while convection or rising heat warms the surrounding air. Radiant heaters are the best choice in rooms where people can remain within the line of sight of the heater. Quartz heaters are called direct object heaters. They don't warm air, but transfer heat to people and walls, furniture, etc. They are ineffective outside of ten to fifteen feet. Space heaters can also run on fossil fuel.

You can determine how large an area a portable heater is equipped for by its wattage output. As a rule of thumb, you'll need roughly ten watts of heating power for every square foot of floor area in the room. This means that a 1,500-watt heater can be the primary heat source for an area measuring up to 150 square feet.

One of the cheapest ways to lower your energy bill is to use thermostat-controlled electric space heaters. You wouldn't, for example, start the furnace up just to heat one room. Such a space heater reduces the amount of electricity consumed and switches power off and on when needed. However, if there is no thermostat for your heater, then an oil-filled heater is advisable as it retains a lot of residual heat and will continue to give off warmth. The cheapest overall to run is a kerosene or propane heater, but they are used primarily outdoors. They also present added hazards as the fuels are flammable and can produce toxic gases.

Space Heater Pros: Using space heaters and turning off the furnace when you're not home can save up to $1,000 per year. Space heaters cost around ten to twenty cents an hour to run, as opposed to approximately $1.85 for your furnace, but can be costly in the long run.

Convection heaters are known for their ability to heat entire rooms efficiently and for long periods of time via a heating element (like electric coil, oil, or electric wire). Most models incorporate fans to circulate warm air across entire rooms. Fanless space heaters reduce the number of dry spots in your room and don't recirculate dust and other allergens throughout a room—a great benefit for allergy and asthma sufferers. Radiant space heaters are best for spot heating because they deliver focused warmth to areas directly in front of the heater. Because of this, they're popular in offices, bedrooms, and other small rooms. Ceramic heaters are popular for small spaces such as children's bedrooms and spaces with pets because they are safe to touch. An advantage of space heaters is that they are portable and can be left in rooms that are unventilated.

Space Heater Cons: Prices can be high. A space heater can range from around $30 for a basic personal heater to more than $2,000 for an elegant electric fireplace.

Fossil fuel heaters use materials such as alcohol or kerosene that create a flame within a glass bulb to create heat. These are mostly used for camping. Electric or fuel-powered space heaters can be a real hazard if they are defective or used improperly. Chemical, alcohol, or fossil fuels are very flammable and toxic so when employing them, make sure you have a good supply of fresh air by cracking a window open.

Ventless gas fireplaces should be used with caution, as they produce pollutants that are released into the air, so use a carbon monoxide detector. Make sure the space heater is not placed in a heavy traffic area, where it might be bumped or knocked over. However, most modern electric space heaters have a "trip" switch that will turn off heaters that have fallen over.

Leave at least three feet (one meter) of space on all sides and above the heater from anything that could burn. Do not use the heater to dry damp articles like clothing or towels. This is a fire hazard. The Consumer Product Safety Commission reports two of every three home heating fires in the United States are attributed to space heaters, which cause 57,300 fires and 270 deaths every year.

Maintenance: This depends on the type of space heater you use. Keep them clean, dusted, and change the filters. Fuel heaters should have their wicks and burners cleaned.

CALCULATING THE RIGHT SIZE FURNACE

Figure the total square footage of your home by measuring and multiplying the length and width of every room. Determine the zone of your home by referring to a United States government climate zone map (see below). Each of these zones is defined by a specific color and a heating degree day or cooling degree day number (see below), or HDD and CDD.

Degree days are based on the assumption that when the outside temperature is 65°F, we don't need heating or cooling to be comfortable. Degree days are the difference between the daily temperature mean, high temperature plus low temperature divided by two. If the temperature mean is above 65°F, we subtract 65 from the mean and the result is a cooling degree day. If the temperature mean is below 65°F, we subtract the mean from 65 and the result is a heating degree day.

For every one HDD or CDD, the outside temperature makes an indoor environment one degree too hot or too cold to be comfortable, meaning a building will have to use heat or air conditioning to compensate. These numbers refer to the energy demand of the climate and can help determine how much you'll utilize your HVAC. Many furnaces will also be labeled to show what zone they're suitable for.

WHEN IT'S TIME TO REPLACE YOUR FURNACE

Energy-efficient upgrades and a new high-efficiency heating system can often cut your fuel bills and your furnace's pollution output in half. Upgrading your furnace or boiler from 56 to 90 percent efficiency in an average cold-climate house will save 1.5 tons of carbon dioxide emissions each year if you heat with gas, 2.5 tons if you heat with oil.

Certain telltale signs indicate it's time to consider replacing heating and cooling equipment, or improving the performance of your overall system.

It may be time to call a professional contractor to help you make a change if:

- Your heat pump or air conditioner is more than ten years old.
- Your furnace or boiler is more than fifteen years old. An EnergyStar furnace is 15 percent more efficient than a conventional older furnace. If you have a boiler, consider replacing it with an EnergyStar-qualified boiler that is 10 to 15 percent more efficient than an older model.
- Your equipment needs frequent repairs and your energy bills are going up.
- Some rooms in your home are too hot or too cold.
- Your home has humidity problems.
- Your home has excessive dust. Crawl spaces and basements distribute them throughout your house. Sealing your ducts may be a solution.
- Your heating or cooling system is noisy.

REBATES AND INCENTIVES

For state and federal tax incentives and rebates, always check with your appliance retailer, the Internet, or local officials.

19

The Bathroom

A Whopping Water Waster

In the "day," families often had multiple kids and adults living in one house with only one bathroom. To get a shower, they had to make a reservation and on school mornings, getting to the bathroom was always chaos and almost physical combat. For the boys of the house it was simply easier to relieve themselves outside, much to the detriment of the shrubbery, but to the benefit of the gals.

For most of us the bathroom is the last bastion of privacy, a great place to catch up on reading or thinking (makes one wonder where the location of Rodin's "The Thinker" was), and the room is the butt of many jokes.

It's also a place that uses a large amount of energy and is the main consumer of water indoors, making it a target-rich area for conservation that translates into money saved.

Curiously, even though a majority of people claim they try to conserve water in the bathroom, only one in four is buying low-water-consumption products, and very few people simply turn off the faucet when brushing their teeth.

And the idea of saving 4,000 gallons of water a year by buying a water-conserving toilet gets an overwhelmingly positive response—but only if the commode is at the right price.

FACTS AND FIGURES

It is estimated by the EPA that of the trillion gallons of water used in US households yearly, most of it is wasted in the bathroom. We spend billions of

147

dollars making water drinkable and then use only 10 percent of it for drinking and cooking and we flush most of the rest down the toilet or drain.

More than 40 percent water used in the average American home occurs in the bathroom, with nearly 35 percent of that being flushed, 40 percent used in showers and baths, 15 percent coming from faucets, and 10 percent for leaks. Americans use 1.2 trillion gallons of water taking showers each year. If just 1 percent of American homes replaced an older toilet with a new low-flow, efficient toilet, the country would save more than 38 million kilowatt-hours of electricity—enough electricity to supply approximately 43,000 households for one month.

A leak caused by a faulty flush valve in a toilet tank can waste as much as 10 gallons of water an hour, typically costing more than $200 per year. Water heating is the third-largest energy expense in the home, accounting for between 13 and 25 percent of energy costs. A steady leak of hot water and its heating bill can run up to $25 for gas or $75 for electricity per year.

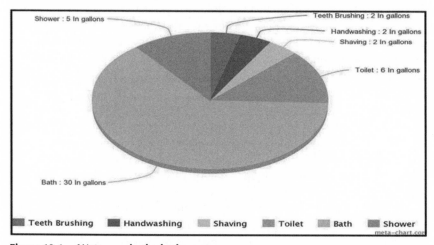

Figure 19.1.   Water use in the bathroom.
Source: Information courtesy of the U.S. Environmental Protection Agency.

PRACTICAL SUGGESTIONS: SHOWERS AND SHOWERHEADS

Pre-1992 showerheads have flow rates of 5.5 gallons per minute (gpm). Therefore, if you have old fixtures you might want to replace them. A water-efficient showerhead can reduce water consumption by up to 40 percent. Federal regulations mandate that new showerhead flow rates can't exceed more than 2.5 gpm of water pressure or 80 psi for maximum water efficiency.

If your shower fills a one-gallon bucket in less than 20 seconds, replace the showerhead. Standard showerheads use 2.5 gallons per minute and also require energy to heat the water. A showerhead leaking at ten drips per minute wastes more than 500 gallons per year. That's enough water to wash sixty loads of dishes in your dishwasher.

Shower better by replacing showerheads with WaterSense-labeled models; replacing just one showerhead can save the average family 2,900 gallons of water annually, the amount of electricity needed to power the home for thirteen days, and more than $70 in utility bills. If everyone in the United States could manage to use just one less gallon of water per shower every day (about 30 seconds), we could save some 85 billion gallons per year.

WaterSense-labeled models are certified by the EPA to be high-performing, available in many styles and price points, and some utilities even offer rebates. Water-conserving showerheads are inexpensive, easy to install, and can save a family of four, showering fifteen minutes every other day, 17,000 gallons of water a year and cut up to 12 percent of your water bill. Changing out an old showerhead and replacing it with a new low-flow showerhead that reduces the flow rate to 1.5 gallons per minute can lower the cost per shower to $0.91 from $2.10, or save approximately $1.19 per shower. Showering twenty times a month is, on average, a monthly savings of $23.80 per family member.

There are two basic types of low-flow showerheads: aerating and laminar flow. Aerating showerheads mix air with water, creating a misty spray. Laminar-flow showerheads form individual streams of water. Laminar-flow showerheads are best for humid climates because they won't create as much steam and moisture as aerating ones.

If you have hard water (water with high mineral content), which makes soap hard to lather and leaves a filmy residue, clean aerators and showerheads by soaking them for a few minutes in vinegar, or a product such as CLR, regularly to reduce deposits and build-up. Always turn water pressure down when adjusting temperature in the shower.

As a sidelight, the Haier PowerPad, a new product from China, is a device that captures the energy contained within the water that runs off our bodies every morning in the shower, and returns 15 to 20 percent of that energy back to the hot water tank. It's expensive (about $600) and hasn't been reliably tested in the United States at this time.

A HEALTH AND SAFETY NOTE

The heavy, cloying, chemical smell of a new shower curtain is actually VOCs (volatile organic compounds that off-gas) that many claim are associated with a range of health conditions. A healthier alternative is a shower curtain made from mold-resistant products such as hemp, glass or plastic doors, or washable fabric curtains.

One of the most common accidents in the home is falling into open toilets and slipping on wet floors, so use slip-proof rugs, decals, and always keep the seat down.

PRACTICAL SUGGESTIONS: BRUSHING AND WASHING

Use a waterless, non-antibacterial soap when washing hands and use cold water when brushing teeth as the temperature makes no difference in hygiene but will cut the energy bill. To save water and time, consider brushing your teeth while in the shower.

A family of four that "water watches" when brushing and washing can save a minimum of 15,600 gallons a year, let alone the power to heat it. Saving energy in a household can simply involve changing habits. Say you're a person who always washes your face before brushing your teeth. To save a bit of energy and water, try brushing your teeth first before you wash your face, using cold water until it heats.

PRACTICAL SUGGESTIONS: BATHS

Baths should be a luxury item. A ten-minute shower will use about 15 to 20 gallons of hot water, while filling a bathtub will use 40 to 60 gallons. When running a bath, plug the tub before turning the water on, and then adjust the temperature as the tub fills up. And fill it half as full as you usually do to save 10 to 15 gallons. A hot bath can use 15 gallons less than a long (30-minute) shower. Heaters that reheat bath water cost about $150. However, many find these not too effective, especially for the cost.

PRACTICAL SUGGESTIONS: FAUCETS (FOR THE KITCHEN, TOO)

Faucets account for more than 15 percent of indoor household water use, and a large part of that can be from leaks. Ten percent of homes have leaks that waste 90 gallons or more per day. Common types of leaks found in the home include worn toilet flappers, bad gaskets, dripping faucets, and other leaking valves. All are easily correctable. And according to IBM, a faucet that drips one drop per second would waste 27,000 gallons of water annually. A home with modern WaterSense-faucets could use that water to flush for six months. An efficient low-flow fixture can save 1,000 gallons a year, saving up to 2 percent on the water bill.

Leaky faucets can be reduced by checking faucet washers and gaskets for wear, and replacing them if necessary. When replacing a faucet, look for the EPA WaterSense-approved label.

The average bathroom faucet flows at a rate of two gallons per minute. Turning off the tap while brushing your teeth in the morning and at bedtime can save up to 8 gallons of water per day, which equals 240 gallons a month. If you think that it's really not all that much, multiple that times the number of people in your house, your neighborhood, your city, county, state, then the country. Letting just your faucet run for five minutes uses about as much energy as letting a 60-watt light bulb run for fourteen hours.

A faucet aerator is often found at the tip of modern indoor water faucets. Aerators can simply be screwed onto the faucet head to create a nonsplashing stream and often deliver a mixture of water and air, shape the water stream, save water and reduce energy costs, reduce faucet noise, and ultimately determine the maximum flow rate of a faucet.

Aerators are inexpensive to replace and they can be one of the most cost-effective water conservation measures. Aerators cost about $2 and take about two minutes to install. When replacing an aerator, take the replacement to the store with you to ensure a proper fit. New kitchen faucets come equipped with aerators that restrict flow rates from 0.5 to 2.5 gallons gpm. For maximum water efficiency, purchase aerators that have flow rates of no more than 1.0 gpm.

Some aerators even come with shut-off valves that can stop the flow of water without affecting the temperature. Properly aerated faucets can reduce a sink's waterflow by 30 percent or more without sacrificing performance. Billions of gallons each year could be saved by simply retrofitting the country's 222 million bathroom sink faucets with aerators.

COMMODE FACTS AND FIGURES

The toilet was not invented by Sir Thomas Crapper, but the first flushing toilet was patented in 1819 by an employee of his. The single greatest achievement in defeating disease is the modern toilet and plumbing.

Americans use 422 million miles or 26 billion rolls of toilet paper a year, enough to travel to the sun and back more than four-and-a-half times and just the paper rolls alone could fill the Empire State Building twice. Every

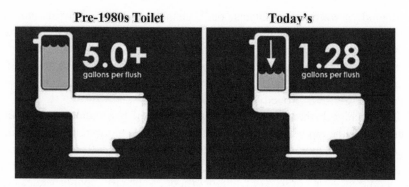

Figure 19.2. On the left, a pre-1980s toilet; on the right, today's high-efficiency commode.

Source: www.wikipedia.org (fair use).

day Americans flush more than 4.6 billion gallons of water down the toilet, representing 30 percent of home water use.

Toilets dating from 1992 and earlier use between 3.5 to 7 gallons per flush. Newer, high-efficiency toilets use less than 1.3 gallons per flush—at least 60 percent less water per flush.

Toilet leaks can waste as much as four to five gallons of water per minute and it's estimated that 20 percent of all toilets leak. A leaking toilet can waste about 200 gallons every day. Leaking toilets comprise nine out of ten complaints most utility companies receive concerning high water bills. If everyone in the United States flushed the toilet just one fewer time per day every day we could save a lake full of water about a mile long, a mile wide, and four feet deep. If 1 percent of American homes replaced their older, inefficient toilets with WaterSense-labeled models, the country would save more than 38 million kWh of electricity—enough to supply electricity to more than 43,000 households for one month and more than one billion gallons of water a year.

PRACTICAL SUGGESTIONS

Most of the western half of the country is suffering a severe drought. So think about California's drought mantra, "If it's yellow, let it mellow; if it's brown, flush it down." Upgrade toilets older than 1992 with water-efficient models that cost less than $100. Installing a low-flow toilet can save up to 37 percent more water (5.4 billion gallons per day), and save up to 18 percent on the water bill. If every home in the country installed a low-flow toilet, the daily dollar-volume savings could reach $11.3 million, or more than $4 billion per year in the United States. For older toilet upgrades, consider installing an early-closing flapper valve, which prevents a part of the tank from emptying.

A cheap trick to reduce the amount of water used for each flush is to insert a displacement device, such as a brick or a plastic container, in the tank, and fill the container with sand, gravel, or water.

Dropping your tissue after blowing your nose, etc., in the trash instead of flushing it will save water. Conserve energy and help the environment in the bathroom by using recycled toilet paper, petrochemical-free personal care products, organic and environmentally friendly cleaning products, and compact fluorescent light (CFL) vanity light bulbs.

COMPOSTING COMMODES

A composting toilet is a dry toilet that may be used as an alternative to flush toilets in situations where there is no suitable water supply or waste treatment facility available. The composting toilet contains different chambers into which it separates the liquid and solid waste. It allows all the liquid to evaporate. The solid waste is held in either one or several containers, where it is allowed to compost for up to a year. Europe long ago adopted the "urine separation" toilet, a combination of a regular commode and a composting toilet that diverts urine to a storage tank while composting the solids.

DETERMINING IF YOUR TOILET IS TAKING A LEAK

If there is water on the floor around a toilet, your toilet is leaking (or someone has a very bad aim) and will require a wax seal also—more about that later. If you have to jiggle the handle to make a toilet stop running, it's leaking. Any sounds coming from a toilet that is not being used are sure signs of leaks. If you have to hold the handle down to allow the tank to empty, or the chain or strap has to be tailored so the flapper valve can close, you have a leak. If you see water running over the top of the overflow tube in the tank, you have a leaking refill valve.

If you are unsure whether or not water is running over the top of the overflow tube, sprinkle talcum powder on top of the water in the tank and you can clearly see whether or not it is. If you can see water trickling down the inside of the toilet bowl long after it's been flushed, it is leaking. If water drips out of the refill tube into the overflow pipe, it's leaking!

Put dye (instant coffee, food dye, dehydrated fruit drink mix) in your tank. If there is any colored water in the bowl, you've got a leak. If a toilet turns the water on for fifteen seconds or so without you touching the handle, it is leaking. Draw a pencil line in the tank at the waterline. After thirty minutes, check the waterline. If the water level has fallen, you have a leak. Turn the water off to the toilet before going to bed. In the morning, check the water level. If there's about an inch in the bottom of the tank the leak is due to either a bad stopper, flapper, or a damaged flapper seat (located under the flapper).

If the tank is almost entirely empty, the problem is a damaged gasket under the flush valve (the hole in the bottom of your tank). This means the tank will have to be separated from the bowl in order to get to the connections. New washers and Teflon pipe tape are inexpensive ways to stop leaks and save more than a drop in the bucket. Manually turning off the valve supplying water to the toilet and drying every area around the unit, then turning the shut-off valve back on should enable you to visually see where any condensation and leaks are coming from. Some water companies furnish free "leak kits" for customers.

When considering things you can do to improve home water conservation, keep in mind this quote from Jerry Yudelson, environmental author and water activist, "If you're planning on dramatically cutting the water use of your home, it's always wise to do a detailed water audit first, to find out what is driving your water use, then with the results start to tackling no-cost/low-cost measures first. Plan on taking some time to get everything under control. As with energy use, start with behavioral changes (such as not running water while brushing your teeth, taking shorter showers, etc.), then moving to basic conservation measures such as choosing WaterSense appliances and fixtures, and only then moving to 'active' strategies such as installing drip irrigation, reducing lawn area, collecting rainwater, recycling graywater, etc." Let's try to not have our well run dry.

20

The Kitchen
The Efficient and Economical Family Center

If the bedroom and bathroom carry an innate need for privacy, the kitchen is a multitasking traditional space for family gatherings, and a spot where people naturally gravitate during get-togethers. There are few things more comforting that a warm, steamy, aroma-stuffed kitchen, oven cooking, pots bubbling, people eating together, or sitting around the family table chatting—however, the kitchen also uses the second largest amount of energy in the house, a site where many appliances are on duty 24/7. Consequently, it's a good place to snoop for savings in energy and resources.

FACTS AND FIGURES

The kitchen consumes from 17 to 20 percent of a home's energy. So the more ways you can reduce energy use, the more you'll conserve, and the money you'll save can be used to stock the pantry in the homiest room in your house. It's often said that the kitchen is the heart of the house—but be careful not to get heartburn, as three in ten home fires start in the kitchen, more than any other room in the house.

By the way, if everyone boiled only the water they needed to make a cup of tea instead of filling the kettle every time, we could save enough electricity in a year to run nearly half of the street lighting in the country.

OLD FRIDGES

The power to run a refrigerator costs many times its purchase price over its lifetime. Even modern, "efficient" refrigerators can use up to 600 kilowatt-hours per year, the amount of energy it takes to light up 10,000 incandescent light bulbs. Refrigerators consume about a sixth of all electricity in a typical American home, using more electricity than any other single household appliance, and cost about $110 a year to operate. A separate freezer can cost up to $8 a month.

Today's refrigerators use 60 percent less electricity on average than twenty-year-old models that cost consumers an added $4.7 billion a year in energy costs. At present federal law requires a maximum refrigerator energy use of

Table 20.1.   Your Average Monthly Appliance Cost

Appliance	Typical Wattage	Estimated Hours	Estimated Kilowatts	Estimated Cost
Air Conditioner (12,000 Btu)	1500	200	300	$23.40
Air Conditioner (36,000 Btu)	4500	200	900	$70.20
Blender	385	2	.8	$0.06
Bug Zapper	40	300	12	$0.94
CD, Tape, Radio, Receiver Station	250	60	15	$1.17
Clock	3	730	2.2	$0.17
Clothes Dryer	5000	17	85	$6.63
Coffee Maker (auto-drip)	1165	4	4.7	$0.37
Compactor	400	10	4	$0.31
Computer (w/monitor and printer)	365	75	27.4	$2.14
Convection Oven	1500	8	12	$0.94
Curling Iron	1500	5	7.2	$0.56
Dehumidifier (20 pints, summer)	450	360	162	$12.64
Dishwasher (dry cycle)	1200	25	30	$2.34
Dishwasher (wash cycle)	200	25	5	$0.39
Disposal	420	60	25.2	$1.97
Electric Blanket	175	180	31.5	$2.46
Fan (attic)	400	71	28.4	$2.22
Fan (ceiling)	80	150	12	$0.94
Freezer (automatic defrost, 15 cu ft)	440	334	147	$11.47
Freezer (manual defrost, 15 cu ft)	350	292	102.2	$7.97
Fry Pan	1200	10	12	$0.94
Garage Door Opener	350	3	1.1	$0.09
Hair Dryer (handheld)	1000	10	10	$0.78
Heat Lamp	250	5	1.3	$0.10
Heat Tape (30 ft, winter)	180	720	129.6	$10.11
Heater (auto engine, winter)	1000	180	180	$14.04
Heater (portable)	1500	40	6	$4.68
Heating System (warm air fan)	312	288	89.9	$7.01
Humidifier (winter)	177	230	40.7	$3.17
Iron	1000	5	5	$0.39
Jacuzzi (maintain temp, two people)	1500	93	139.5	$10.88

Source: US Energy Information Administration

940 kWh per year. The leading-edge eco-refrigerator uses only 240 kWh per year for a full-size unit. When it's time to retire the old fridge, check with local utility companies or refuse companies. Many have free recycling programs.

NEW FRIDGES

Purchase refrigerators with the freezer on either the bottom or top, which are 16 to 25 percent more efficient than side-by-side models. Bottom freezer models use approximately 16 percent less energy and top freezer models use about 13 percent less than side-by-side. Buy the right size for your needs. Too large a refrigerator may waste space and energy. One that's too small can mean extra trips to the grocery store. Your best bet is to decide which size fits your needs then compare the EnergyGuide label on each so you can purchase the most energy-efficient make and model.

A new, more efficient model will pay for itself from the energy savings alone compared to an old-style, inefficient refrigerator, which may cost as much as $280 a year in electricity in areas with high electrical rates. A ten-year-old refrigerator uses up to 75 percent more energy than a new EnergyStar model and uses 1,300 kilowatt-hours per year, producing roughly 2,000 pounds of carbon dioxide—the same amount from burning 105 gallons of gasoline. Replacing a ten-year-old refrigerator with a newer, EnergyStar model will save $135 to $440 a year and the energy saved by recycling an old refrigerator is enough energy to run an efficient refrigerator for eight months. EnergyStar.gov has a calculator to help you determine how long it'll take for your new refrigerator to pay for itself. Assuming that your old fridge is from 1980–1989, and measures about 20 cu. ft., you'll save $150 a year operating a new EnergyStar fridge. Assuming you can pay $900 or less for the replacement, payback time is six years away.

Look for a refrigerator with automatic moisture control. This prevents moisture accumulation on the cabinet exterior without the addition of a heater. This is not the same as an "anti-sweat" heater that prevents condensation on the refrigerator cabinet and will consume 5 to 10 percent more energy than models without this feature. The anti-sweat should only be on during the summer.

It's nice to belly up to your refrigerator to get ice and water—but you'll pay extra for that convenience. Although icemakers and water dispensers are convenient and reduce the need to open the door, these convenient items will increase your refrigerator's energy use by 14 to 20 percent, or about $20 per year.

A 10 percent refrigerant leak can decrease the efficiency of a refrigerator or freezer by 20 percent. Ten minutes spent once a year to clean a refrigerator's coils will save more energy than sitting in the dark for one hour every day for a year.

Chest freezers are typically more efficient than upright freezers, because they're better insulated and cold air doesn't spill out when the door is opened. Home bar refrigerators aren't very efficient, can use as much energy as a full-sized refrigerator, and can generate up to 300 pounds of carbon dioxide (CO_2) each year, depending on their efficiency.

Running one efficient refrigerator is cheaper than running two older ones. Don't use old refrigerators as "spare" or "garage coolers." An extra appliance can add more than $100 to energy bills every year. Plus, old models can be a safety hazard for small children who can become trapped in them.

MAINTAINING YOUR COOL

Check the temperature. Refrigerators should be kept between 38° and 40°F and freezers at 0° to 5°F. One that is 10°F colder than necessary can use 25 percent more energy per month. To check refrigerator temperature, place an appliance thermometer in a glass of water in the center of the refrigerator and leave for twenty-four hours.

Try to keep your refrigerator full. Cold food acts as an insulator to prevent lost heat. When the refrigerator is empty the compressor works harder. Fill empty space and reduce energy by filling plastic containers with water, which will reduce the cost of ice making and dispensing.

Glass conducts and holds cold better than other materials. Storing food in glass containers keeps it colder longer. The more cold the refrigerator or freezer can maintain, the less it needs to produce. Cover liquids and wrap foods stored in the refrigerator. Uncovered foods release moisture, making the compressor work harder, and might leave unpleasant odors and encourage fungus and mold growth. Placing covered warm leftovers in the refrigerator won't significantly affect energy use, but first cool hot items on a counter so the compressor won't have to work as hard cooling hot food. Move items from the freezer to the refrigerator a day before use. This decreases energy use and helps the compressor work less.

Label items in the refrigerator or freezer for quick identification and keep more frequently grabbed foods and beverages up front so that you don't have to keep the door open too long. Don't ponder the contents as keeping the door open can lose up to 30 percent of the cooled air in a short time. Place refrigerators and freezers away from heat sources and direct sunlight. If you have to put a heat source close, place a sheet of foam insulation between the source and the refrigerator. For every degree above 70°F surrounding your fridge, it will use 2.5 percent more energy. Also, allow at least one inch of space on each side of your refrigerator or freezer to allow good air circulation.

Always unplug the refrigerator before defrosting. A manual defrost refrigerator uses half the energy of an automatic defrost model but must be defrosted regularly to stay energy-efficient. Defrost manually when there is more than one-quarter inch thickness of ice, or at least twice a year. Use a hair blow dryer or pots of hot water to loosen ice. But do not use anything sharp as you can puncture coolant lines.

Make sure your refrigerator door seals are airtight. Place a piece of paper half in and half out of the refrigerator door. If the paper pulls out easily, the door latch may need adjustment, the seal may need replacing, or you might consider buying a new unit. Make sure the door automatically swings shut. If not, prop up the front of the refrigerator with a spacer or shim (a thin and often tapered piece of material).

During an emergency if the power is off, keep your refrigerator door closed and open it only when absolutely necessary and the contents will remain cool for up to five hours without added ice.

FACTS AND FIGURES

Cookware

Ever notice the efficiency of one pan over another? That's because pans and skillets made from different metals conduct heat differently. Glass and ceramic baking dishes retain heat well and can lower cooking temperatures up to 25°F and there are always the fave raves of cast iron, stainless steel, and copper.

When Teflon gets above 300°F, the coating can break apart and emit toxic particles and gases. This has been linked to thousands of pet bird deaths and an unknown number of human illnesses each year. Because Teflon coated pans are tough to take care and present health concerns, many people are changing to cast iron, enameled, or ceramic cookware.

Thermolon nonstick coating is a patented ceramic technology that has been hailed as the next breakthrough in nonstick cookware, as are Scanpan Greentek pans, which are said to use a "clean and green" nonstick compound in their coating. Then there are the Gotham Steel and Red Copper pans touted on TV. A little research shows that they are not what they are hyped to be.

Stainless steel is a great cooking surface but tends to be a bad heat conductor so it is combined with aluminum or a copper core to help distribute heat nicely. Stainless steel pans are much more expensive than other types, but they require less maintenance and, when used properly, they're effectively nonstick. Waterless cookware is a uniquely designed, surgical stainless steel made of several layers of metals that provide thorough conduction of the heat.

Waterless cooking tends to preserve most of the nutrients in the food, and the natural flavor is not lost or diluted.

Cast iron pans are made to last and are inexpensive. For $15 to $40 a variety of sizes are available that will last forever. Cast iron requires more time to warm up and needs seasoning or curing before it performs well and it is easily cared for. Enameled cast iron is another option that is more expensive than cast iron, but it doesn't need any seasoning. It is made from heavy cast iron, but its surface is smooth and holds heat well.

The thermal conductivity of copper is about five times better than the thermal conductivity of iron and more than twenty times better than that of stainless steel and conducts, distributes, and stores heat very well. Food inside a copper pot remains warm much longer than in a pot made of stainless steel. Copper is a soft metal and expands when heated; the bottom of a thin-walled copper pot can deform when heated, consequently it is used mostly layered with other metals. Bacteria will not survive on copper. Copper cookware can be quite pricey, but when properly cared for will last a lifetime.

HOME ON THE RANGE AND OVEN

Twenty years is the average lifespan for stoves and ovens. The US DOE estimates that cooking accounts for 4.5 percent of the energy used at home. All appliances have two costs—the purchase price and the operating cost.

Newer ovens have high insulation, tighter-fitting oven door gaskets, and hinges to save energy. These include self-cleaning models that use less energy for normal cooking because of additional insulation levels. However, new ovens and stovetops—also called kitchen stoves and ranges—have no federal energy regulations, so they don't carry EnergyGuide labels or EnergyStar recommendations. Remember that an electric oven might need a 220- to 240-volt outlet.

Use a microwave for reheating and defrosting, especially in small portions as they are 70 percent more efficient than conventional ovens. Slow cookers and pressure cookers are far more efficient than regular stovetops or ovens for long cooking periods.

PRACTICAL SUGGESTIONS

Place a pan on the burner before turning the burner on. Use only the minimum amount of heat and water needed to cook the meal. Cover pans and keep oven doors closed while cooking to prevent heat loss. Every time the oven door opens it loses 25°F of heat. Covering a pot of water will bring it to a boil in half the time it takes uncovered. Use a good thermometer to get an accurate reading on oven temperature. Remember that convection ovens distribute heated air more evenly than ordinary ovens, so cooking time and cooking temperatures can be reduced, cutting energy use on average 30 to 35 percent.

Check for seals on oven doors. Moisture or "sweat" on an oven door may mean you may have a faulty door gasket and a tear or a crack can be an energy vampire. Keeping the oven clean increases efficiency and lessens kitchen pollution as a heavy grease build-up on the oven interior will cause the oven to smoke, and may even cause a fire. Keep the grease plates under range burners clean to reflect heat more efficiently. Use the oven's self-cleaning feature immediately after cooking if the oven gets greasy while the oven is still hot. This will reduce a lengthy warm-up time.

Preheat the oven only when necessary, and then keep the preheating time to a minimum. Unless baking breads or pastries, it may not be necessary to preheat the oven at all. Schedule oven use. For example, bake several items at the same time on the same day.

Don't cover oven racks with foil; it blocks the flow of hot air. Food cooks more quickly and efficiently when heated air can circulate freely. Stagger pans on upper and lower racks to improve airflow. This seems obvious, but don't cook with the oven door open. And never use your oven as a source of heat as it is dangerous for many reasons, including being a source of children's burns; ranges or cook tops, with or without ovens, account for 61 percent of home cooking fire incidents.

FUEL CHOICES

Natural Gas (NG)

When purchasing a natural gas range, buy one with a piezoelectric ignition (one that causes a small spark to autoignite a burner). Pilot lights that are on continually in a gas range can consume up to 50 percent of the annual energy use of a range. Cooking with a gas range is about half the cost of cooking with electricity as ovens and ranges offer immediate heat. A newer gas range with an automatic start only costs about $2.35 a month operate. Around 58 percent of American households cook with electricity, but gas cooking is becoming more popular. When cooking on a gas burner, use a moderate flame setting to conserve gas. Remember that a blue flame means the gas stove is operating efficiently. A yellowish flame indicates an adjustment is needed.

When using fossil fuels, carbon monoxide and combustion are always a danger. Be careful of leaks. It's best to call your utility company if you smell gas or a leak is suspected. A harmless chemical called mercaptan is added to give gas a distinctive odor. Most people describe the smell as similar to rotten eggs. This also might sound obvious, but you'd be surprised about the fires and injuries caused by people looking for gas leaks with a lighted match.

Propane

It's primarily used in rural areas, as fuel for specially converted vehicles, in RVs, and in backyard barbeques. Propane will only work with special gas burners and jets and comes in tanks, which are filled, measured, and sold by the gallon. One gallon should run a 12,000 Btu cooktop burner, comparable to a gas burner, for about seven hours. A typical home equipped with propane heating and cooking appliances can use over 1,000 gallons of propane per heating season. Costs will vary depending on location and supply, but overall, natural gas is less expensive than propane.

Electric Ranges and Ovens

Electric ranges and ovens on average will cost about $6 a month to operate (depending on location, use, and cost of electricity). Most electric units take time to heat standard electric coils and fall well below high performance energy efficiency. There are a number of new types of burners for electric cook tops on the market: glass top units, solid disk elements, radiant elements under glass, halogen elements, and induction elements.

Solid disk elements and radiant elements are mounted under glass, making them easy to clean, but they take longer to heat up and use more electricity, compared to electric coils.

Halogen cook tops use powerful bulbs filled with a halogen gas to create radiant heat under a ceramic glass. The food cooks because of radiation from the bulb itself and conduction between the ceramic cook top and the pot. This uses less electricity than a standard coil element, but only if you have very flat pans that maintain good contact with the burner. Otherwise, you'll lose heat. Since the cooking surface is smooth glass, it is easy to clean.

Induction elements are the most energy-efficient technology using 90 percent of their energy for cooking. By comparison, a gas burner typically uses 55 percent, while a standard electric range uses 65 percent. Induction elements use electromagnetic waves to turn the bottom of the pot into an active heating surface. They provide accurate temperature control while keeping the smooth cook top surface cool. An induction element can boil water up to 50 percent faster than a regular stove.

Turn off your electric burners several minutes before the allotted cooking time is up. The heating element will stay hot long enough, called residual cooking, to finish the cooking without using more electricity.

Make sure stovetop electric coils work properly. A worn-out element is a real power drain. If you need new ones, buy quality. The best on the market can save as much as one-third of the energy used when cooking on top of the stove.

On electric stovetops, use only flat-bottomed pans that make full contact with the element. A warped or rounded pan will waste most of the heat. Match the size of the pan to the heating element; more heat will get to the pan and less will be lost to the surrounding air. A 6-inch pan on an 8-inch burner will waste over 40 percent of the energy.

INDUCTION OVENS

Induction units, at this time, are mostly used in Europe and haven't caught on here yet. Induction relies on an electromagnetic field via a "burner" to heat iron or steel cookware and can heat water to boiling almost immediately. Because the burner does not heat, but transfers energy, the burner is always cool. The induction cooktop technology gives a far more efficient transfer of energy than a gas flame or heated electrical element. It is electrically powered and allegedly uses 84 percent of the power it consumes for cooking, but they are expensive.

The biggest drawback to induction cooking is that it only works with cooking vessels made of magnetic materials. Cookware must be compatible with induction heating; glass and ceramics are unusable, as are solid copper or solid aluminum cookware. Enameled steel cookware works well with induction cooking. In situations in which a hotplate would typically be dangerous or illegal, an induction plate is ideal, as it creates no heat itself. Induction cookers are safer to use than conventional cookers because there are no open flames or heated coils.

CERAMIC RANGES

Ceramic cook tops are easily cleaned, but also easily scratched. Ceramic glass cook tops have halogen elements as a heat source located under the ceramic glass units (either gas or electric). They deliver instant heat, respond quickly, and are easy to clean, but when the characteristic redness of the top disappears the cooktop is still hot and dangerous. Aluminum- or copper-bottom pots and pans should not be used because they leave marks that can be hard or even impossible to remove. Painted or enameled pots and pans are another no-no because they can stick to and damage the ceramic surface. Special care and cleanser is needed.

SOLAR OVEN

The first known western solar oven was built by Swiss naturalist, Horace-Bénédict de Saussure, in 1767. Solar box cookers became popular in the 1970s when people began to be more energy conscious and looked for ways to harness the sun's energy.

A solar oven or solar cooker is a device that uses nonpolluting sunlight as its energy source. Because solar cooking depends on sunlight, cooking times will vary based on location, weather conditions, the seasons, and time of day.

The most obvious attractions to solar cooking are the cost of the fuel and materials and ease of construction. A reliable solar oven can be made from everyday materials such as cardboard, wood, metal, or plastic and costs very little.

A typical solar oven is a medium-sized rectangular box with a clear cover than allows the sun to enter and heat the cooking chamber. The most important element in using a solar cooker in the winter is the brightness (or intensity) of the day, not the outside air temperature. The use of removable reflectors available on some models can help magnify the sun's rays on partly cloudy days or during the winter months when the intensity and angle of the sun is lower.

Solar ovens maintain a steady temperature between 210° and 260°F in most areas. Because of the heat generated, they compare to an electric slow cooker for their ability to roast foods slowly over low heat for long periods of time. Because there is no open flame, they are safe to use in areas where a campfire is not permitted. They are portable and lightweight, which makes them ideal for camping, boating, picnicking, and hiking. Solar ovens can also be used during power outages. Very simple do-it-yourself directions can be found on the Internet or at a library.

BUILD YOUR OWN SOLAR COOKER

Remember that food is cooked in a solar oven not just by sunlight, but also by the ultraviolet rays of the sun.

- Get a cardboard box at least 16 inches × 16 inches. Use black construction paper (or black paint) placed at the bottom of the box along with a rack.
- Place a smaller box inside and then fill the void with crumbled newspaper filling for insulation. Make sure there are gaps between the newspapers. Those gaps will store the warm heat in the air pockets.
- Use tinfoil to cover the four sides in the inner box using the insulation as a wall from the outside box. Use clear tape if necessary to secure the foil.
- The next step is to make the reflectors. Cover the top of the box (which will fold over the top to close the box) with tinfoil. It is best to keep at a 45 degree angle.
- Next, use either a heavy plastic, or glass cut to the size of the opening of the box. The more exact it is the less hot air will escape increasing the efficiency of the cooker.
- The oven will work best during peak sunlight hours during summer.

THE MIGHTY MICROWAVE

Microwaves are a type of electromagnetic waves. They're absorbed by water, fats, and sugars, where they're converted directly into heat, so they cook from the inside out, not by external heat. Microwave energy can heat or cook food in a fraction of the time needed to cook with conventional ovens. In the United States they cost between five and ten cents per kWh to operate.

For warming small amounts of food, a microwave oven can save a third of the power of a conventional electric stove, but it uses twice the energy to thaw frozen foods. An electric burner uses about 25 percent less electricity than a microwave to boil a cup of water, although the microwave is more efficient at reheating foods. Running empty microwaves wastes energy and is not good for the machine.

Microwaves with display clocks use more energy to power the clock 24/7 than they do to heat up food. Switch the clock off when not in use.

Metals reflect and arc microwaves. Don't use metal containers in a microwave as they will produce sparks which can cause fires and burnouts. Anything wrapped in foil won't cook properly as the foil reflects the microwaves. Very thin metallic foil such as fast food containers and aluminum foil can be used inside a microwave, but it has to be placed in the center well away from the sides of the oven so as to reduce discharge and sparking. If sparking occurs, turn the oven off and stop using foil as it will eventually damage the oven.

ELECTRIC TOASTER OVENS

A toaster or convection oven uses one-third to one-half as much energy as a full-sized oven. The upper and lower heating elements in a toaster oven are only about 750 watts each. For broiling, only the top is used. In convection baking, both are on.

If you're going to buy a toaster oven, select one with a convection heating feature. It doesn't require much additional electricity to run the small fan, but moving hot air bakes foods faster. Models with electronic controls are more precise, but manual controls are quicker to set. A basic toaster oven (at 1,500 watts) is going to cost about 12.75 cents/hour on highest heat.

COOKERS UNDER PRESSURE

This isn't your grandma's pressure cooker anymore with the weighted "jiggle-top" hissing-and-spitting pressure regulator that everyone was afraid might blow a meal into the ceiling. The newer style is a closed system, uses spring valves, and won't explode.

Using a pressure cooker that cooks food at a higher temperature and under pressure reduces cooking time dramatically and energy use is cut by 50 to 75 percent compared to conventional methods. The savings can add up quickly when comparing a pressure cooker to hours in a slow cooker or in the oven. A pressure cooker can save seven to ten cents per meal, about $2.17 a month. A good quality stainless steel pressure cooker is a long-term investment that will last for twenty to thirty years or longer and pays for itself in energy savings. Modern pressure cookers are silent, 100 percent safe, and very user friendly.

MAINTENANCE

A pressure cooker should be thoroughly inspected before use and the cooker should be clean, inside and out. There should be no sign of warping, dents or dings, or any other damage to the rim of the cooker or lid of the pressure cooker. The gasket should fit snugly in its place in the lid. Remove and examine the gasket. The gasket should be in good condition with no signs of cracking, tears, or other deterioration such as gumminess or brittleness. Replace the rubber/silicon parts at the first sign of deterioration.

When using a jiggle-top pressure cooker, always check the vent pipe to make sure it is clear and open. On a valve-type cooker, lift or turn the valve to make sure it moves freely and the inside connecting screw is tight. Periodically check the handles and tighten the screws as necessary.

DISHING THE DIRT ABOUT DISHES

Dirty dishes pile up faster than promises to clean them. We can't help enforce dishwashing duties, but we can promise to help you use less energy and save some change when you do.

Buy the appliance size that fits your needs. Larger dishwashers are more expensive to buy and operate. The family dishwasher lasts about ten years and washes over 25,000 dishes per year for a total of 250,000 dishes in its lifespan.

Eighty percent of the energy running a dishwasher is used to heat water to about 140°F, although 120°F will do the job. Most dishwashers have a heating element that is used to heat the water in the sump. Some dishwashers have an "Energy Saver" switch that disables the internal heating element during the wash cycle. Use dishwasher short cycles, mid-cycle turn-off, and other such features designed for energy conservation in dishwashers for everything but the dirtiest dishes. This can save up to 25 percent on hot water and electricity bills.

Dishwashers use almost 40 percent less water and energy than washing by hand, which costs about sixty-three cents a load compared to around twenty cents for a dishwasher. A modern dishwasher generates up to one pound of CO_2 per wash.

Dishwashers are classified as compact capacity and standard capacity. Compact models use less energy, but they also hold fewer dishes. Having to run a compact dishwasher several times to clean your family's dishes will result in greater energy use. If you have a ten-year-old dishwasher, you're paying an extra $40 a year on your utility bills compared to owning a new EnergyStar-qualified model. A dishwasher built before 1994 wastes more than ten gallons of water per cycle. A new, EnergyStar-qualified dishwasher will save, on average, 1,300 gallons of water over its lifetime.

TYPES OF DISHWASHERS

Standard Size Dishwasher, Installed

Dishwasher types are influenced more by capacity than style and the most common is the standard size 24 inches.

Pros: Best for convenience, features, and style, and offers best value.

Cons: Requires plumbing and electrical hook-up, uses cabinet space, which could be used for storage.

Standard Size Dishwasher, Portable

While a portable dishwasher may not appeal to all, it's the next best thing to an installed unit. If you rent, constantly move, or installing is not possible, a portable dishwasher, standard or compact, is the way to go. The top of a portable dishwasher can also add a handy workspace in the kitchen.

Pros: Good variety of features, best nonpermanent option, and can wheel out of sight.

Cons: Must be wheeled to faucet for hook-up, faucet inaccessible while dishwasher is running. Can be costly.

Countertop Dishwashers

More suitable for a two-to-three-person household, the countertop dishwasher is an economical choice that offers dishwashing convenience with a temporary hook-up. But most are heavy and bulky to place and they should be on a stable cart, counter, or table close to the sink.

Pros: Ideal for a couple or very small family, cheap models, easy to use, temporary hook-up.

Cons: Bulky, heavy, and needs counter space and faucet hook-up.

PRACTICAL SUGGESTIONS: DISHWASHING

Scrape, pre-rinse, or soak only the most stubborn food residue. Modern dishwashers are very efficient and will remove those tenacious food remains. Clean dishwasher drains and filters to ensure efficient operation. Use a cold wash, unless it's absolutely necessary to use hot water for your dishes. Cold water uses much less energy and will get your dishes just as clean and hygienic.

When not in use, switch off the appliance rather than leaving it on standby. Lower the water-heater thermostat in dishwashers that have booster heaters. It will help save on energy. If you have to wash by hand, don't let the water run while rinsing. Fill one sink with wash water and the other with rinse water.

Avoid using the "rinse hold" on your machine for just a few soiled dishes. It uses three to seven gallons of hot water each use. Let your dishes air dry;

if you don't have an automatic air-dry switch, turn off the control knob after the final rinse and prop the door open slightly so the dishes will dry faster.

Avoiding one load of dishes saves enough power to run a 100-watt light bulb for half a day. And replace one of these old dishwashers with EnergyStar-rated model and save enough money to pay for dishwasher detergent all year.

KITCHEN FANS

Range hoods should ventilate to the outside of the house and not simply re-circulate and filter the cooking fumes. This is especially important with gas ranges. Keep ducts as free of grease as possible. Be careful about the sizes of fans as well—too large a fan can waste energy and cause combustion gases to backdraft into the house. This can be a major problem with large downdraft ventilation fans used with some cooktops and ranges. Range hood exhaust vents normally have a gravity damper. When the exhaust fan is on, it has enough pressure to force the damper open to expel the fumes. Once the fan is turned off, gravity closes the damper.

GARBAGE DISPOSALS

Never put hands or finger in a garbage disposal unit. Even if the motor doesn't accidentally start up, the cutting jaws are sharp enough to cut fingers. Once a year, put about dozen ice cubes with a cup of rock salt down the disposal, grind them up, and flush with cold water. This will help sharpen the blades and remove build-up from the inside of the disposer. Run a lime, orange, or lemon peel through the system for safe, easy, and natural deodorizing.

MORE PRACTICAL SUGGESTIONS: KITCHEN

Save gallons of water and compost vegetable food waste instead of using the garbage disposal. Using hot water wastes energy and can melt fats, which makes it easier for them to clog the disposal mechanism and your pipes when congealed, one of the biggest problems with pipes and municipal sewers. Run the disposal with cold water, which also helps to keep the mechanism cool while running.

To prevent stoppages, remember to run water during use and for at least fifteen seconds after. Pour a cup of vinegar into the sink drain and let it sit for about one hour, then flush down with very hot water. This will help to remove scale build-up.

Check city ordinances if you have a septic system; some towns and cities do not allow garbage disposals to be installed where there are septic systems.

Wash fruits and vegetables in a pan of water instead of running water from the tap. Don't use running water to thaw food. Defrost food in the refrigerator for water efficiency and food safety, or leave in a pot of cool water.

Soak pots and pans instead of letting the water run while you scrape them clean. Think about installing an instant water heater near the kitchen sink to avoid running the water while it heats up. And save any water while a faucet is on.

Remember what a famous chef said about the kitchen, "It should always be open."

21

The Laundry Room

Clean Your Clothes, Not Your Wallet

A great byproduct of doing laundry is the aromatherapy and caress of clean and dry washed things. Who hasn't luxuriated in the simple pleasure of a warm towel when coming out of the shower, the feel of a heated sweatshirt on a brisk day, and crawling in between clean sheets at bedtime?

Although everyone loves clean clothes, remember that the washer and the dryer are high-end uses of water and energy. But you can take some of the pinch out of pinching pennies, saving energy, and making laundry day feel even cleaner in and out of the pocketbook.

FACTS AND FIGURES

There are newer, tougher federal standards requiring all new washers made to use less water and energy. That means the newest EnergyStar-qualified washing machines will use 25 percent less energy and 40 percent less water than washers not carrying the EnergyStar.

Americans do about 35 million loads of laundry each year, using about 140 million gallons of water. The American family of four washes about 400 pounds of laundry per year, using around 10,000 to 12,000 gallons of water, doing about four to eight loads per week at between 6 and 15 pounds per load—depending on the size of your machine. An estimated 84.1 million households have top-loading washers with agitators, 24 million of which are more than ten years old and inefficient. A ten-year-old washer is four times less efficient than a new one and can cost $135 extra a year in consumer expense and more than $9 billion in extra energy and water. A front-loading washer's lifetime is about ten years, a top-loading washer lasts about fourteen years, and a dryer's lifespan is about thirteen years.

It costs approximately forty cents to wash and twenty cents to dry a load of laundry at home. Washers use as much water as two showers per load (25 to 50 gallons), and 90 percent of the energy is used to heat water. Efficient standard washing machines use less than 25 gallons of water per load. Many EnergyStar-qualified washing machines and dryers will use over 50 percent less water and energy for each load of laundry. Some models will use as much as 64 percent less water and 75 percent less energy. These can mean more than $500 in energy savings over the course of the appliance's lifetime. Capacities of front-loaders and high-efficiency (HE) top-loaders keep increasing, with some washers handling up to 28 pounds of laundry.

Clothes washers have a significant impact on water and sewer costs. The national average for water and sewer costs is estimated to be $2.84 per 1,000 gallons. This brings the estimated total cost for water and sewer over the life of the clothes washer to around $660 (based on eight loads of clothes a week for fourteen years).

Replacing in-unit apartment washing machines with a common-area laundry room can save more than 8,000 gallons of water per apartment per year. A burst washing machine hose can spill 650 gallons of water per hour and is one of the top homeowner's insurance claims, resulting in an average $4,000 to $6,000 in damages.

An exercise bike has been invented with a lithium-ion battery that collects energy as you pedal and is hardwired to a front-loading machine. Twenty minutes' effort is said to give you one cold cycle wash without drawing power from the grid, along with a good workout.

WHAT KIND OF WASHER?

Top-Load Washers

Newer top-loaders with center-post agitators typically cost less and wash the fastest, but performance can be mediocre. The washer's tub in a top-loader sits vertically in the machine and has an agitator in the middle that churns the water and clothes together, forcing water through the items.

Pros: Top-loaders cost less and allow for additions and adjustments anytime throughout the wash cycle, though you should always wait for the drum to stop spinning before reaching inside. High performance top-loaders can save up to 28 gallons of water per load with 68 percent less energy usage and can save an average home up to $900 over a ten-year lifespan in utility costs.

High-efficiency top-loaders hold more laundry and use less water while extracting more of it. That cuts drying time, saving energy and money. With top-loaders it is easy to judge how much laundry to drop in. Top loaders are basically uncomplicated so they are less likely to break. For added life, consider getting one with a stainless steel wash drum.

Agitator-free top-loaders can tie clothes in knots and aren't good at cleaning medium to heavily soiled clothes. Overall top-loaders are much more reliable, but generally use more water and detergent. A plus is that they don't require bending down to load and unload.

Cons: Because the spin mechanism in older top-loaders is slower than front-loaders, their cycle is longer and uses more energy. Older top-loaders can use from 45 to 55 gallons of water per load, which has to be heated, using more energy. In top-load machines, the tub must fill before the load will start.

Front-Load Washer

Pros: The front-loading machine's greatest advantage is its energy efficiency. It uses gravity as the drum turns to wash the clothes in a small pool of water, sprays the clothes clean, and spins at about 1,000 rpm, saving up to 12,584 gallons of water a year over an old top-loader spinning at 650 rpm, significantly reducing the amount of water and energy needed for the cleaning process. The higher spin speeds on a front-load washer can lead to a shorter time in the dryer because it leaves less water in the clothing.

An EnergyStar front-loader will use 50 percent less energy and 35 percent less water than top-loading washers. But with front-loaders and high efficiency (HE) top-loaders you may have to make a few changes in the way you do laundry. Most front-loading washers can be stacked with a companion dryer to save space. There's no agitator in a front-loading machine, making it easier on laundry, and there's more room for dirty clothes—and larger loads (like blankets) means fewer loads.

Cons: The design, however, isn't very convenient and requires lots of bending with wet clothes, which strains the back. Front-loaders can be difficult to keep clean. They may gather mold, trapped in the seals around the door, which can lead to problems with mold and may smell musty unless kept clean and dry.

Front-loading units tend to vibrate, which can lead to unwanted noise, especially if the machine sits in the main living area of the home. These machines are also more complex than top-loaders, which means higher maintenance costs. Front-loading washers may cost several hundred dollars more than their top-loading counterparts.

Table 21.1.   Cost Comparison: Top-Loader vs. Front-Loader

	Top-Loader	Front-Loader
Cost per Load/Washer	$.85	$.32
Cost per Load/Dryer	$.50	$.46
Total Cost per Load	$1.34	$.78
Total Cost per Load Month (approximately 32 loads)	$44.00	$25.00
Total Cost per Year (approximately 400 loads)	$525.00	$305.00

Source: USEIA.

COMBO WASHER-DRYER/PROS AND CONS

A washer-dryer combo unit can wash and then dry laundry in one machine. Most washer-dryer combos have very small capacities from an 8 to 15 pound wash load and a drying load of about 7 to 9 pounds. Because of their compact nature, nonpermanent hook-up, and ease of installation, they are a great choice for closets, bathrooms, RVs, cottages, boats, condos, apartments, or wherever there is little space. Most combos are ventless, which means no exterior dryer venting is required, and they plug into a standard electrical wall outlet. However, they do need access to water intake and a drain. Many models have wheels and connection kits available for a portable to-the-kitchen-sink operation. These washer-dryer models cost about the same as buying a separate washer and dryer.

PRACTICAL SUGGESTIONS

Replacing a pre-1994 clothes washer will save $200 to $300 a year. A low-flow washer uses 6,000 gallons a year, half as much as an old washer, saving up to 12 percent on the water bill. Look for a clothes washer with a low water factor. The water factor is the number of gallons per cycle per cubic foot that a clothes washer uses.

Use hot water only for very dirty clothes; otherwise always use cold water in the rinse cycle. Many clothes can be washed in cold water, saving 6 percent or more on the bills, a savings of fifteen cents per load, or from $30 to $100 a year. Washing laundry in cold water saves energy, and will also cut from 500 to 2,500 pounds of CO_2 emission a year.

If the washing machine shakes, it's unbalanced. All legs should be on the ground and evenly balanced. If they are not, the machine's mercury switch won't work properly and can shut off water flow and leave clothes in a pool of dirty water. Experiment with using the delicate cycle. It uses far less energy. Use the pre-soak or soak cycle when washing heavily soiled garments instead of washing them twice.

Choose washers with adjustable temperature and water controls. Adjust the water level to the size of your load. Wash full loads to maximize your money, but do not overload the machine or you'll lessen efficiency. For smaller loads, use the proper setting. The same amount of electricity is used whether washing a partial or full load.

To keep the drum spinning smoothly, use only high-efficiency (HE) detergent. The suds that are created by non-high-efficiency detergents will wreak havoc on the drum and drive system. *Consumer Reports* recommends the high-efficiency (HE) detergents, or one of the new "dual-use" detergents, suitable for all machines. Too many bubbles make the machine work harder and use more energy. Buy items such as laundry detergent (try biodegradable) and fabric softener in bulk or in concentrated form with minimal packaging. Almost all conventional detergents contain phosphates, which cause lasting damage to natural water systems.

Whenever possible, buy powdered detergent over liquid detergent. Liquid detergent is mostly water and costs a great deal more in terms of energy and waste packaging and transportation. As an inexpensive substitute for fabric softener, use one-half cup of white vinegar with two drops of your choice of an essential oil. Not a trace of detergent residue will be left in your clothes, and the essential oil will cancel out the vinegar smell and give your laundry a nice aroma.

Table 21.2. Cost Comparison: Wash Cycles

Water Wash	Rinse Setting	Electrical Use	Cost per Load
Hot/Warm	4.5 kWh	$.88	$265.00
Warm/Warm	3.5 kWh	$.53	$206.00
Hot/Cold	2.8 kWh	$.42	$165.00
Warm/Cold	1.9 kWh	$.29	$112.00
Cold/Cold	.03 kWh	$.04	$16.00

Source: USEIA.

This table doesn't factor in the cost of water. The average price of water in the United States is about $1.50 for 1,000 gallons.

MAINTENANCE

Cold-water washing is fantastic for conserving energy, but it can add to the build-up of residue in various parts of the machine. Front-load washer users report that an occasional hot water wash can blast away some of the leftover soap and grime from cold-water washing.

Inspect the basket after each cycle because smaller items such as socks can easily become stuck to a front-load washer's basket. Front-loading washers need to be completely empty after each cycle. Neglecting this step could result in yet another source for potential mold. It may also leave the foul smell of a wayward sock.

In front-loading machines, leave the dispenser drawer out, leave the door open when not in use, and regularly run the machine cleaning cycle to prevent mold. Manufacturers suggest replacing hoses every three to five years, regardless of wear, as a broken hose is a disaster. Drain hoses if temperatures below freezing are expected.

For a family of four with relatively high use, the washing machine should be cleaned once a month. Use a quart of bleach and a quart of white vinegar:

- Fill the washer with hot water and add the bleach.
- Run the machine in wash cycle for one minute and let it sit for one hour.
- Then run the machine for a full cycle. Empty the washer.
- Fill the washer with hot water and this time add the vinegar and mix for a minute.
- Let the vinegar sit for an hour then let the cycle complete and drain.
- This should take about two hours and costs less than $3.

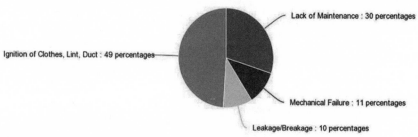

Figure 21.1.   Causes of dryer failure.
Source: Provided by the author.

DRY YOUR CLOTHES, NOT YOUR RESOURCES

There are two basic kinds of dryers and two basic ways to power them: spin and tumble, powered by gas or electricity. All dryers work the same way—they tumble clothes through heated air to remove moisture.

FACTS AND FIGURES

The energy efficiency of a clothes dryer is measured by a term called the energy factor. It's a rating somewhat similar to miles per gallon for a car— the lower the better. In dryers, it's the measure in pounds of clothing per kilowatt-hour of electricity. The minimum energy factor for a standard capacity electric dryer is 3.01. For gas dryers, the minimum energy factor is 2.67.

Over its expected lifetime of ten to eighteen years, the average clothes dryer will cost approximately $1,530 to operate. A dryer is typically the second- or third-biggest electrical appliance after the refrigerator and the furnace, costing about $3.25 to $14.50 a month, accounting for up to 12 percent of the electricity used in a typical household. Electric dryers use roughly 1,800 to 5,000 watts of electricity per load. On average, drying a load a day costs roughly $70 per year.

The EPA estimates that all residential clothes dryers in the United States annually consume about 43 billion kilowatt-hours of electricity and 445 million therms (a unit of heat equivalent to 100,000 Btus of natural gas), leaving carbon dioxide emissions of 32 million metric tons.

Choose a dryer with a large capacity drum, even if you don't think you need all that space. Clothes will dry faster in a large-capacity dryer. It's more economical to dry full loads, but don't overpack the dryer because clothes need breathing room to tumble properly. Look for a dryer with a cycle that includes a cool-down period, sometimes known as a "perma-press" cycle. In the last few minutes of the cycle, cool air, rather than heated air, is blown through the tumbling clothes to complete the drying process, which reduces energy use as well as wrinkles. Overdrying clothes can make them stiff, crumpled looking, difficult to iron, and wastes energy. Choose dryer features that have a moisture sensor that automatically shuts off the machine as soon as your clothes are dry

SPIN AND TUMBLE DRYERS

A spin dryer rotates the clothes at a high speed and centrifugal force removes any water from the clothes. Consider the rotational speed spin dryer, which ranges from 2,500 to 3,300 rotations per minute. The greater the speed of the spin dryer, the more efficient it is. Spin dyers are much better than tumble dryers and only use about 400 watts of power.

Tumble dryers contain a rotating tumbler and an electric powered heater that heats the air that is drawn through the clothes to dry them. Tumble dryers can dry clothes within minutes because they heat much faster, but they use about 2,400 watts of power. Tumble dryers are most often used in commercial applications.

Engineers are working to develop dryers that use microwaves to dry clothes, but at this time they are not practical. One reason is that they cannot handle metal like rivets, zippers, etc.

VENTED OR CONDENSER DRYERS

Vented dryers expel hot damp air via a venting pipe through an open window or with an outside wall with a vent from it. A tumble condenser clothes dryer will send the damp air into a condensing chamber where it is turned into water and collected in a tank. The tank must be manually emptied (it is a good idea to do this as part of the dryer maintenance plan when you clean the lint filter).

GAS, ELECTRIC, OR SUN?

Think about putting up a clothesline and use free solar heat as a dryer. See below for suggestions about creating various alternatives.

Electric dryers use heating coils to supply heat and are the most expensive way to dry clothes. Electric dryers operate on a 120- to 240-volt current. Smaller units use 120 volts, the ordinary household current.

Gas dryers use a gas burner to create heat, but otherwise they operate the same as an electric dryer. They require a gas hookup, with proper connections and safe venting of the gas's exhaust. In most areas, gas dryers will cost less to run over their lifetimes.

Gas dryers tend to be more energy-efficient than electric ones, averaging about twenty cents per load as opposed to about forty cents per load. EnergyStar gas dryers could reduce CO_2 emissions by at least 30 percent when compared with standard electric models.

DUELING DOLLARS: GAS VERSUS ELECTRIC

The initial cost of the average gas dryer is between $50 to $100 more than an electric dryer, plus the labor costs required to install it. However, operating a gas dryer will cost around $20 a year less.

An electric dryer just has to be plugged in—but to a 220-volt outlet. So if there is none handy, an electrician will need to install one.

- Propane gas dryers use about 15 to 25 gallons of per year, or about $105 a year depending on the current cost of propane.
- Electric Dryer Cost per load (1 hour) = 6.72 kWh × $0.0998 = $0.67
- Gas Dryer Cost per load (1 hour) = .25 therms × $0.6179 = $0.16

The above depends on the cost of the energy to run the appliance and how much it's used.

MAINTENANCE AND PRACTICAL SUGGESTIONS

Clean the lint filter because the dryer takes longer to dry when it's trying to push air through lint—this can mean 30 percent more energy use. Once a month, use a vacuum cleaner's fine nozzle to suction the lint slot or screen. According to the US Consumer Product Safety Commission, more than 15,000 fires are sparked every year by clothes dryers. Lint and other debris can build up in your dryer vent, reducing air flow to the dryer, backing up dryer exhaust gases, creating a fire hazard.

A cold basement is the worst place for a dryer as using cold incoming air takes more energy for the dryer to heat it up. The warmer the place you can put the dryer, the better. Leaving clothes in a dryer too long causes them to wrinkle. Throw a wet towel in and dry again.

Make sure the dryer is plugged into a receptacle suitable for its electrical needs as overloaded receptacles can cause blown fuses or tripped circuit breakers. Turn off the dryer when leaving the home. Turn off the dryer before going to bed at night.

Wash and dry very early in the morning or at night to avoid peak load charges, especially if your utility imposes a demand charge (based on the amount of electricity you demand at one time).

Dry one load of clothes immediately after another. This will minimize heat loss, reducing warm-up and drying times, but don't add wet items to a load already drying. Try to keep like fabrics in the same load, so they will all dry at the same time.

Install an air diverter on an electric dryer to vent the warm exhaust into the home in the winter if humidity is not a problem. This diverter should not vent near the dryer or the furnace. Never vent a gas dryer into the house, as its exhaust may contain toxic byproducts. In the United States, law mandates all gas dryers be vented to the outdoors.

Check the outside dryer exhaust vent periodically. If it doesn't close tightly, replace it with one that does to keep the outside air from leaking in. This will reduce heating and cooling bills. Dryer vents should be made of rigid metal. Flexible plastic vents can be damaged by high heat, age, and contact with other objects. Accordion type vents (metal or plastic) can crimp and are also more likely to trap lint. The vent should be run as short a distance as possible, never more than twenty-five feet in a straight line. All vents should discharge directly to the home's exterior, never a crawl space, attic, garage, chimney, or other room.

Recent research from the University of Washington has revealed that fragrance components in some liquid clothing detergents, fabric softeners, and dryer sheets were found to infuse the vented air with hazardous pollutants, including two known carcinogens.

Gas dryers should be installed, serviced, and inspected by authorized service/repair persons.

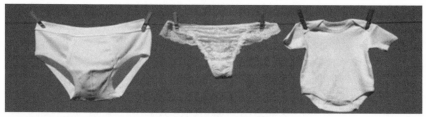

Figure 21.2.   Practical suggestions: Letting it all hang out.

LET IT ALL HANG OUT

When hanging clothes, start closest to the clothesline tightening device. This maximizes the length for hanging clothes. Be sure all attachments and connection points are tight and secure, and check them frequently to ensure they remain that way. Be careful not to overload a pulley clothesline.

Hang towels vertically, folding the tops over the line about three inches. If the towel has a band, that's a good place to fold over. Use clothespins at each side and one in the center of the towel to keep the towel's shape. When you bring the dried towels in, toss them in the dryer and turn the setting to "Air Dry" for five minutes. You will have soft fluffy towels that will smell outdoor fresh but still feel like they were dryer-dried from the start. Use fabric softener for line drying, particularly towels, but if you're using liquid, try using half the amount.

Jeans and slacks should be hung by their bottom hems. This prevents shrinkage and helps pull out wrinkles. Children's play clothes or work pants should also hang flat-legged on the line, two clothespins on each ankle edge. For dressier items pinch and hang with the two legs seams together, finger creasing down the center to smooth. Hang upside down and pin right at the very bottom hem at each side. Shaping and smoothing wrinkles at hanging time will result in a just-ironed look when they dry.

Shirts should be hung upside down at the side seams; fold about 3 inches of material over the clothesline and pin. Close zippers and/or bottom buttons so the shirt hangs flat. Smooth wrinkles or creases to give them a finished look. Socks hung by the toe-tips rather than by the ankle will keep their shape. Hanging sheets folded in half side-to-side makes a nice center crease. Pillowcases hung from their closed end, hems down, keep their shape better and will allow air to circulate inside them. Hang delicates on hangers wherever convenient. You might want to hang them out of direct sunlight when possible to avoid fading. To prevent wrinkles, fold items as they're taken off the lines.

COMING UP WITH A GOOD (CLOTHES) LINE

Sometimes low tech or no tech is the best tech. A good example is the low-tech "solar" clothes dryer: a clothesline. The cheapest clothes dryer is the sun and you can save 100 percent of your clothes drying energy cost by simply hanging your clothes up to dry. And it will reacquaint you with the aroma of sundried laundry and the use of an earlier alternative technology that still works just fine.

FACTS AND FIGURES

Always check homeowner associations for rules and local regulations that restrict the use of clotheslines. Using a clothesline instead of a dryer can save from $200 to $1,500 a year, depending on the size of your family and how much you use a dryer.

If possible, keep your clothesline away from trees and overhanging wires so you can avoid tree sap, bird droppings, and unforeseen electrical problems—all counterproductive to clean clothes. Plan for the clothesline to run as close to north and south as possible. This will give your clothes the best amount of sunlight.

Figure out what kind of clothesline you want. An umbrella clothesline has some advantages; it doesn't take up a lot of room and can be removable, which makes it a good choice for a small yard. The old fashioned T-bar clothesline (see below) with a pulley requires more space, but has the advantage of allowing more air movement through your clothes, letting them dry faster.

To install a clothesline, you'll need a shovel or a posthole digger, a hammer, a saw, a knife, and a hand wrench or ratchet wrench to drive in screws or lag bolts.

THE T-BAR

All the parts, the hardware, and the cement are inexpensive and available at any home improvement center:

- Two 4 × 4s, length of ten feet. Obtain insect and weather resistant, pressure-treated wood or cedar and redwood.
- Two 2 × 4s, length of four feet. They will come in eight-foot sections.
- Two bags of posthole cement or concrete.
- Two 2 × 4 sheet metal hanging brackets.
- Two metal or plastic pulleys (with hooks and eyebolts kit).
- Length of line (however long you want the clothesline).
- Several 12 penny (4-inch) nails.
- Four 2-inch screws or lag bolts.
- Clothesline adjusters or "jaws."
- Clothespins.

HOW TO INSTALL A T-BAR

Almost all set-ups mean digging a couple of holes, unless you can string a (static) line between two existing structures. Before you start your posthole digging, make sure you know where your underground utility lines are located. Poking a hole in a gas line or digging up a cable can ruin your whole day. Better to ask companies before you run into a problem.

A T-bar clothesline requires two postholes (unless you're going to attach one end to the house or a tree, etc.). If you live in an area where the ground freezes in winter, dig down below the frost line. Three feet should be enough (you'll need a slightly longer 4 × 4), even in the coldest climates. It's also a good idea to try to make the bottom of the hole slightly wider than the top—this helps prevent any movement of the base if frost moves the ground.

Try to position your finished clothesline so it's about two or three inches above the head of the person who uses it most. The height should be comfortable enough so that a user doesn't have to be constantly reaching above the head to hang clothes.

Dig the hole position for your posts and then fill the hole around your posts with dry concrete and then just add water. Be sure to poke around into the cement to make certain that moisture gets into all parts of the hole. It's better to be a little too wet than too dry. Use a level to ensure your post is straight and "on plumb" in all directions. Let the cement dry for at least 24 hours.

For the T-bars that sit atop your posts, the easiest way to install them is to place each two-by-four (the four-inch side up) across the top of the posts, anchoring them with nails. Then screw the two-by-four sheet metal brackets (hangers) with two-inch screws or lag bolts securing them to the posts. Screw in the hooks or eyebolts into the crossbars two feet away from the middle on each side. Attach the two metal clothesline pulleys via the hooks or eyebolts on the two-by-fours.

You'll need enough clothesline length to make a complete circle between each post plus a couple of extra feet for insurance. You'll have to choose between cotton, vinyl, or polyester line. Do not use line that will rust. Each type has its strong points. Ask hardware store personnel.

Cotton is inexpensive, but tends to stretch and sag over time. Vinyl-coated wire is probably the strongest, but not as easy to work with. Nylon or polyester are strong, but more susceptible to sun damage.

Install the clothesline by threading it through both pulleys; connect the ends of the lines. After connecting the lines, install a clothesline adjuster by pulling the rope through the clothesline device's jaws. The clothesline will remain tight as long as the jaws continue to grip the rope and prevent it from sway backing, which allows a line to sag in the middle.

Now for the test. It shouldn't be too tight or difficult to pull the line easily. It shouldn't be so loose that it will sag or twist around in the breeze. You'll need some clothespins to hang your damp laundry.

HOW TO INSTALL AN UMBRELLA CLOTHESLINE

If you are installing a removable umbrella line, you need to install a piece of plastic pipe slightly wider than the laundry pole into your hole. Dig the hole at least two to three feet deep.

Cover the bottom end of the tube, put it into the hole, cover the hole with cement, and add water, making sure the plastic tube sticks well up out of the ground so you can straighten it. Once the cement has set up you can cut the tube off at ground level, thus removing a hazard that someone might trip over, but still have a sturdy support for the pole.

This type of clothes dryer unfolds like an upside-down umbrella. It can also be folded up and removed from the ground, leaving only the plastic pipe in the hole.

RETRACTABLES

They can be attached indoors between two walls, or outside connected to fences, two posts, or two trees. You can find single lines of different sizes and weights and even a multiline model. Before you select a retractable line, think of how you plan to use it. Single lines will not support heavy towels or linens well. If you plan to use it often, select a heavier gauge line or a multiple strand clothesline for better support of wet items.

Of course, do not hang clothes if there is danger of a lightning storm—you will be a perfect conductor and target for a bolt from above.

22

Recycling the Circular Fan

Being Breezy

Overhead fans were not only sexy in tropical settings in films like *Casablanca* and *Key Largo*, they were also the best air conditioning available at the time. They're still an enchanting and economical part of decor, and all fans, even the lowly desktop office fan, can help stretch your energy bill dollars where air conditioning is concerned.

Overhead fans not only dress up a room, they can circulate warm air trapped against ceilings in winter, and because of the wind chill factor, can make you feel 3° to 8°F cooler in summer. Because air moved by fans carries heat away from the body, fans can be used in tandem with air conditioners. This allows you to lower the workload for your AC while saving energy and lowering toxic emissions from power plants.

A fan creates a breeze that helps by replacing hot, humid air with cooler, drier air that flows around the body and allows for evaporation which makes you feel cooler.

FACTS AND FIGURES

Americans buy close to 20 million fans a year. The DOE states that 60 percent of all US households have ceiling fans. Ceiling fans are cheaper than you might expect—as low as $30 at home improvement stores. A typical 36-inch, 48-inch, or 52-inch ceiling fan uses about 55, 75, or 90 watts of electricity, respectively, at top speed. A super-efficient ceiling fan costs approximately $12.61 per year to run based on a usage of six hours per day. By contrast, it costs $1.21 per day to run a 6,000-Btu room air conditioner.

The air at the ceiling of a room is 15°F warmer than that on the floor, so fans are used to balance heat distribution in a room. Using ceiling fans instead of the air conditioner can save up to $438 a year. Ceiling fans can cut a home's energy use up to 40 percent in the summer, and 10 percent in the winter. Small box fans are very inexpensive to buy and cost only pennies an hour to run.

EnergyStar ceiling fans move air 20 percent more efficiently than standard models due to efficient motors and improved blade design. EnergyStar ceiling fans with light kits are about 50 percent more efficient than conventional fans. Light units and the light kits produce about 75 percent less heat, and save more than $15 per year in utility costs. Remember that fans cool people, not rooms—be sure to turn them off when leaving.

PRACTICAL SUGGESTIONS

Fans should spin counterclockwise in the summer to suck hot air up, and spin clockwise in the winter to push warm air down—the direction can be changed via a switch on the fan. Ceiling fans run on the same energy as a 75-watt compact fluorescent lamp (CFL) light bulb. Ask for fans that have more than one speed and work in reverse, with blades that are angled at least 10 percent. Buy a 36- to 42-inch ceiling fan for rooms that are twelve-by-twelve feet. For rooms around twelve to eighteen feet, use a 48- to 52-inch fan. For larger rooms, use multiple fans. For fans that may come in direct contact with water, such as on the front porch or patio, purchase a fan with a UL "wet" rating. These fans will have features such as sealed/moisture-resistant motors, rust-resistant housing, stainless steel hardware, and all-weather blades.

Rooms with high ceilings are the best candidates for fans. For optimal cooling, the fan should be installed eight to nine feet above the floor. With cathedral type ceilings, the fan may look better if it hangs ten to fourteen feet high.

Ceiling fans should be centered in the room with a minimum of 18 inches clearance between the wall and the blade. For ceilings nine feet tall or taller, use a "down rod" to bring the ceiling fan down to the proper height above the floor. Subtract nine feet from ceiling height for rod length. Install a ceiling fan in the largest room of your house. This will allow you to lower the setting on your air conditioner 3° to 6°F, which will save up to 25 percent on energy to cool the home. When looking for a fan, as with any appliance, look for EnergyStar-rated merchandise.

IN THE SUMMER

If you don't have an exhaust fan in the kitchen, cool the room by setting up a portable fan. The fan not only cools the air, but can also help move odors out of the kitchen and out a window or into an exhaust fan. Smaller fans work well in smaller rooms.

When installing a fan in a bathroom or any humid location, purchase a fan that has been UL listed with a "damp" rating. The trick is to have one fan blowing in at one window and the other blowing out at another window. This two-fan trick works in hard-to-cool rooms on a third floor or in a hot, stuffy attic.

IN THE WINTER

In winter, run your fan in reverse to recirculate the warm air throughout your house. By setting your thermostat lower, you'll save on heating costs as the fan provides even, comfortable temperatures throughout the room. High ceilings trap heat, so use a fan to move heat from high places to lower heights where it can be used.

IN GENERAL

A fan complements the AC, so if the air conditioning suffers a breakdown, there is backup in the form of a ceiling fan. Fans keep insects and flies at bay. Paddle fans are safe since they are usually installed over the ceiling and are therefore away from the reach of kids and pets. Fans offer a great variety in terms of looks, designs, themes, and sizes.

CHOOSING THE RIGHT SIZE

Ceiling fan blades can range from 29 to 72 inches. To determine the appropriate size ceiling fan and quantity of fans you will need, measure the room and use the table below.

Table 22.1. Ceiling Fan Chart

Room Size	Rooms	Blade Size
Up to 75 sq. ft.	Bathrooms, hallways, breakfast nooks	29 to 36 inches
76 to 144 sq. ft.	Small bedrooms, kitchens	36 to 42 inches
145 to 225 sq. ft.	Bedrooms, kitchens, dining rooms	44 to 48 inches
226 to 400 sq. ft.	Standard bedrooms, family rooms, dining rooms	48 to 54 inches
Over 400 sq. ft.	Great rooms or large areas	52 to 72 inches

23

Efficient Appliances
Domicile Devices

People will use anything, especially appliances, to the final gasp and then try to repair them to last just a little longer. Duct tape is one of man's best friends. As frugal as some people are, they don't understand that it is costing more time and money in the long run than if new energy-efficient devices were bought and the old stuff recycled.

The question of whether we need all the extras and accessories is a fait accompli—which means that we love and are going to buy more gadgets. What Tom Brokaw calls the "Greatest Generation," the parents of the Baby Boomers, learned hard lessons about using things until they broke and about recycling during wars and the Great Depression. Ironically they also became instigators of the throwaway society, and the next generations have followed in the wake of their flotsam and jetsam.

FACTS AND FIGURES

There are an estimated 600 million appliances at work in American households. We spend more than $15 billion a year on new appliances, which account for about 17 to 20 percent of household energy consumption (excluding the furnace) with refrigerators, clothes washers, and clothes dryers at the top of the consumption list, followed by all the dozens of devices and gadgets that we surround ourselves with.

The United States uses 56 percent less energy today than we would if we didn't have energy-efficient technologies and policies. That's fifty-two quads of energy (a quad is a unit of energy equal to 10^{15} or a short-scale quadrillion Btus) saved per year—the same amount of energy needed to power twelve mid-sized states for a year. If all households followed efficiency recommendations for appliances, the total US energy consumption could be reduced by 11 percent and national carbon emissions by more than 7 percent over ten years, or about 62,000 metric tons each year.

Buying EnergyStar appliances saves up to 30 percent on electricity bills for our devices. Americans spend the equivalent of 17 percent of their monthly mortgage or rent on technology and devices. Overall, energy efficiency is saving the American government, its citizens, and businesses more than $500 billion a year in avoided energy costs.

Some 80 percent of homeowners fail to do any appliance maintenance, according to studies by Sears. Appliances that perform the same tasks may look alike, but they can vary greatly in terms of purchase price, energy efficiency, and operating costs. Look for EnergyGuide labels, the bright yellow and black tags you'll find on appliances. Each manufacturer follows federal standards when testing their appliances. The Federal Trade Commission then uses this information to calculate the energy efficiency of different appliances and their operating costs. The EnergyGuide label shows the results of these tests and how the appliance compares to other similar models. By the way, everyone can qualify for the EnergyStar federal tax credits on appliances regardless of income.

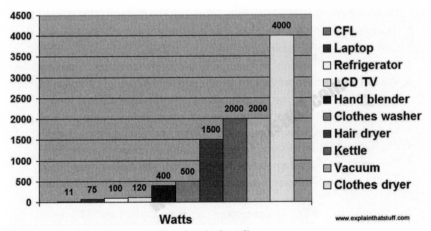

Figure 23.1. Energy consumption of typical appliances.
Source: www.explainthatstuff.com (fair use).

PRACTICAL APPLICATIONS

Remember that there are two appliance costs: the purchase price and the cost of operation. In many cases, you may actually save money in the long run by buying the more expensive but more energy-efficient model. Think about the fact that you'll be paying that second price tag every month with your utility bill for the next ten to twenty years. Replace inefficient appliances, even if they're still working. An aging appliance, large or small, could be costing more than you think, not only in the utility bill but also by using excess energy that creates greenhouse gases.

Each label contains the following information to help you compare options:

- Name, model, and size.
- Additional features.
- Estimated yearly operating cost.
- Range chart showing the least and most efficient models' yearly operational cost and where the model you're looking at compares.
- Estimated yearly energy usage in kilowatt-hours.
- Optional: EnergyStar logo certifying it as eco-friendly.

Check out publications and consumer review Web sites and publications for appliance ratings and reviews. The Federal Trade Commission (FTC) requires an EnergyGuide label to be attached to these new appliances:

- Refrigerators and freezers.
- Dishwashers.
- Clothes washers.
- Central air conditioners.
- Room air conditioners.
- Water heaters (some types).
- Heat pumps.
- Furnaces and boilers.
- Lighting products.
- Fluorescent lamp ballasts.
- Plumbing products (some types).
- Televisions (manufactured after May 10, 2011).

According to a FTC spokesperson, certain appliances, like ovens and certain heating equipment, have been found to have insignificant differences between like-sized products and are not rated. By the way, the FTC is a five-person, bipartisan panel appointed by the president that works in conjunction with the DOE to investigate new products, update information on older ones, add new products, and remove others. It has a unique dual mission to protect consumers and promote competition as well as to develop policy and research tools through hearings, workshops, and conferences. For specific room-to-room appliances go to https://www.energystar.gov/products.

Check for the highest energy factor number when comparing different models. The EnergyStar label is designated by the Environmental Protection Agency and means that the appliance meets federal energy use requirements. Check for the Underwriters Laboratory (UL) mark, the single, most-accepted safety certification in the United States.

Choose the capacity that's right for your family. It doesn't pay to purchase a unit that's too large or too small. Measure the space the appliance will occupy to ensure fit in terms of size and style. Be sure that there's enough room to open the doors or lids fully, and enough clearance for ventilation.

Many heating and cooling manufacturers offer significant rebates during sales promotions and off-season sales when dealers may charge less for installation. Check for floor models or for minor imperfections such as a minor dent, scratch, or last year's model, or go to outlet stores—it may mean a discount. Look for special offers such as cash rebates, low-interest loans, or other incentive programs used to encourage buyers to purchase energy-efficient appliances.

To find rebates in your area, use the EnergyStar Rebate Locator Web site: http://www.energystar.gov/index.cfm?fuseaction=rebate.rebate_locator.

Go to the DOE EnergyStar page for information about products for home and office: http://www.energystar.gov/index.cfm?c=products.pr_find_es_products.

Don't forget to ask about warranties, service contracts, delivery fees, and installation costs. Be sure to choose a reputable and knowledgeable dealer. A good dealer should be able to help calculate energy savings and an appliance's payback period, and to offer you choices in brands and prices.

Investigate new technologies carefully. Some innovations, such as convection ovens or argon-filled windows, may save energy and make life more convenient while others might merely be expensive cosmetic enhancements.

LIFE OF A DEVICE

If your appliances are nearing the end of their expected lifespan, you may want to plan ahead. Always pay particular attention to energy efficiency and the choices that will save you money.

Table 23.1.   Life of a Device

Appliance	Lifespan
Air conditioner (room sized)	10 to 15 years
Compactor, trash	5 years
Dehumidifier	10 years
Dryer	10 to 15 years
Dishwasher	10 to 15 years
Electric range	15 to 20 years
Exhaust fans	10 years
Freezers	10 to 20 years
Garbage disposal	10 to 15 years
Gas range	15 to 20 years
Hand dryer	10 to 15 years
Humidifier, portable	10 years
Microwave	10 years
Refrigerator	10 to 15 years
Swamp cooler	10 years
Washing machine, gas	15 years
Vacuum cleaner	10 to 20 years
Whole house vacuum system	20 years

Source: US Energy Information Administration

OLD-SCHOOL ENERGY-SAVING APPLIANCES

Cut down on electricity use by replacing these electrical kitchen appliances and give yourself a hand with a:

- Hand can opener
- Coffee grinder
- Juicer
- Mixers and hand beaters

24

Standby Power

The Energy Vampire

Have you ever seen the workers in reflective vests standing by the roadside getting paid for supporting their shovels? That's how standby energy works. It's the energy used by some appliances when they are turned off but still plugged in. While this standby power sometimes provides useful functions in remote controls, clock displays, and timers, in other cases it is simply wasted power as a result of leaving electronic devices plugged in and on. The devices causing this waste are referred to as energy vampires because many gadgets are slowly sucking money from your economic artery while providing little or no useful function.

FACTS AND FIGURES

But what the heck, what can a few minor appliances cost? Wake up and staunch the bleeding. The number of products with standby power consumption is growing rapidly in both quantity and diversity and should be monitored because they cost money and resources, waste power, and contribute to pollution.

The average American household has approximately twenty-five consumer electronic devices in the home and the amount of energy used by these products in standby mode costs the average US household more than $100 per year. On a national basis, standby power accounts for a billion kilowatt-hours of annual US electricity consumption, or more than $21.5 billion annually. Standby power consumption equals the output of seventeen one-megawatt power plants (120 billion kWh), enough to power approximately 115.5 million US households for a year.

If a machine has an external power supply (power cords with blocky power adaptors), LED lights, a remote control, or any sort of continuous display, your appliance is using standby power. For most appliances, only 15 percent of the power is used in operation and 85 percent of the power used is consumed while on "standby." Although the power needed for functions such as displays, indicators, and remote control functions is relatively small, the large number of devices that are continuously plugged in results in energy usage of around 5 to 12 percent of total residential consumption. Research suggests that new, more efficient devices will lower that usage to 1 percent. Over the eighteen-year life of most household appliances, standby energy costs around $2,000.

Some devices that constantly consume power are:

- Transformers for voltage conversion.
- Many devices with "instant-on" functions (like TVs) that respond immediately to user action without warm-up delay.
- Devices that can be "awakened" by remote control.
- Devices that can carry out some functions even when switched off, such as computers, or devices with electrically powered timers.
- Uninterruptible power supplies (UPS), essentially batteries that have to be kept charged and can provide power to equipment in the event of power problems or outages.
- Cordless telephones and answering machines.
- Security systems and fire alarms, transformer-powered doorbells, programmable thermostats, motion sensors, light sensors, built-in timers, and automatic sprinklers.

Standby Pros: This may enable a device to switch on very quickly (instant-on) without delays that might otherwise occur. Standby power may be used to power a display, operate a clock, etc., without switching on to full power. Battery-powered equipment connected to main electricity can be kept fully charged. Standby power can keep batteries on computing devices charged allowing them to function without plugging in.

Standby Cons: Up to 90 percent of standby power is wasted. Electricity is often generated in power plants by burning hydrocarbons (oil, coal, gas) or other substances that release substantial amounts of carbon dioxide and other pollutants such as sulfur dioxide, which produces acid rain. Standby power use is roughly responsible for 1 percent of global carbon dioxide emissions or about 50 million tons per year. Standby power can be as high as 10 to 15 watts per device, occasionally more. In the average US home, consumers waste about 50 watts of standby power an hour. Each device, especially older

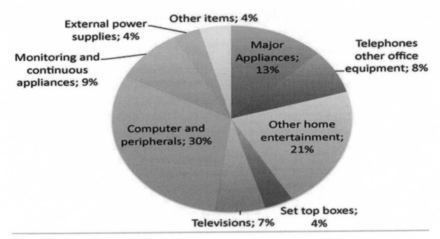

Figure 24.1. Total standby power use in various appliances.
Source: standby.lbl.gov.

ones, could cost $10 annually. Unfortunately, some devices will lose memory when standby electricity is shut off.

PRACTICAL SUGGESTIONS: CUTTING OFF THE JUICE

Reduce your electricity bills by as much as 10 percent by unplugging appliances or making sure they are switched completely off. Using a power strip and switching it off is a convenient way to save electricity coming from multiple appliances. Do be careful. Certain devices use standby power to retain configuration settings and information and unplugging them will cause these settings to be lost.

When buying new appliances, ask or look for low-energy standby products (look for the EnergyStar label). Consider buying energy-saving devices or devices that offer a genuine off switch. Many machines with an off switch still use standby power. Ask questions and do some research before purchasing. Replacing battery-powered devices (such as cordless phones or rechargeable razors) with corded alternatives not only cuts down on the standby power required to charge the battery, but also reduces energy lost in inefficient battery charging and discharging.

Switching devices on or off on a regular schedule can even be automated. Timers, or activity sensors, can be used to turn off standby power to devices that are not being used. You can always get "techie" and buy a low-cost wattmeter to measure the standby (and other) devices in your home. Not only might you be surprised by the information, you may even recoup the cost of the meter in energy savings.

California became the first place in the world to introduce mandatory standby requirements for various electronic devices. The new standards require a low-cost wattmeter to measure a 90 percent reduction—from 5 watts to 0.5 watts—in standby power drawn by external power-supply cords for things like laptops and cell phone chargers. Researchers suggest that an informed and aggressive approach can reduce standby use by about 30 percent in the near future.

The Power List

The Nonrenewables

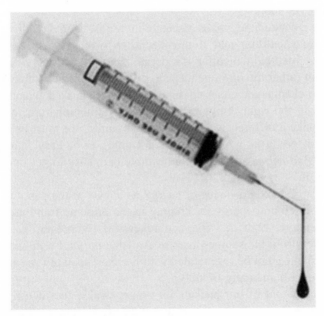

Figure 25.1. Fossil fuel fix.
Source: Provided by the author.

From the Bronze Age to the age of fossil fuels to the age of alternative energy, our need and hunger for more power is insatiable. Since the industrial age, we have glutted ourselves and are now paying the piper—in pollution. Energy is the building block of society and we are going to need ever-increasing sources to run civilization. By 2050, we will need almost 50 percent more. Our compact with the power plants is that we turn on the switch and the power comes on. We take it for granted until the power goes off.

Today we face the challenge to find clean and safe sources of energy. We can't have civilization with energy, but with it comes side effects. How we define and meet our needs may be how we define our world.

Petroleum products—like many other substances such as food, medicine, even sunlight—may be necessary, dangerous, and potentially fatal when overindulged in or misused. Humans are hooked on petro-products. Breaking any bad habit takes time, effort, perseverance, and some sacrifice. Kicking petro dependency won't be accomplished in a day; we're still on a fossil fuel high and hangover.

Take a look around your home; anything you touch produces a carbon fingerprint—whether in supplying power to your plugs, in manufacturing, or in transportation. And it's bound to stay that way for a long while. That's one of the reasons it's so important to conserve. Another great reason is that it will save you money.

Kicking a dependency takes a change in mindset and a readiness to alter behavior for a healthier goal. Remember when tobacco was an accepted part of everyday life? Now nicotine is a pariah. Darwin didn't say the strongest survive, but rather the intelligent species that are most adaptable to change. It's time to change and clean up our act, our fuel, and our planet. Ordinary people doing the right things in extraordinary situations create the action that will make a difference. To paraphrase Gandhi, we must be the change we wish to see in the world. But it's not going to be easy. Someone else said that "Bad habits are like a comfortable bed; easy to get into, but hard to get out of."

In exchange for the sources of energy we chose in the past, we have received pollution and energy uncertainty in the present. There are two basic types of energy, nonrenewable and renewable. Nonrenewable energy is energy taken from the sources that are available on the Earth, but in limited quantities that cannot be regenerated within a short span of time and are generally not environmentally friendly.

What comes out of our pockets for nonrenewable fuel doesn't take into account secondary costs like the damage to the environment, the pollution of water, climate change, or the overall health of people and our planet. Fossil-fuel power plants dump their waste gases into the atmosphere at no cost to themselves but at a great cost to the environment. In some places the water table is in jeopardy due to waste dumping, fracking, and toxic water from refineries, agricultural, and manufacturing runoff.

Nonrenewables such as coal are cheap. Loads of nonrenewables are readily available and their industries receive massive subsidies from Congress to the tune of $54 billion from 2002 to 2008. In contrast, nonpolluting renewables received $18 billion. We should be "detoxing" and moving away from fossil fuels in favor of clean, sustainable sources. In 2013, carbon dioxide accounted for about 82 percent of all US greenhouse gas emissions. However, many high-tech and clean power sources are not yet up to speed for widespread use by the masses.

The next two chapters are meant to inform you about the choices for power. Our goals should be to conserve energy first, then to support, create, and consume sustainable sources of energy produced by low- or even zero-pollution facilities. Petroleum products are going to be around for some time—almost everything you use, wear, or eat comes from petroleum in one way or another. We are fossil-fuel junkies and it's time to start kicking the habit.

FACTS AND FIGURES

Of all the energy harnessed since the industrial revolution (around 1760), more than half has been consumed in the last two decades, and we have probably consumed more energy since 1900 than in all of human history prior to that. The total US residential energy demand is for about 10 quadrillion Btus each year, though conservation has saved approximately $150 billion off the nation's annual energy bill.

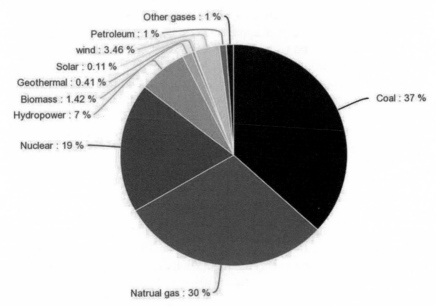

Figure 25.2. Primary sources of energy.

In 2012, the United States generated approximately 4,054 billion kilowatt-hours of electricity. About 65 percent of the electricity generated was from fossil fuel (34 percent attributed to coal and the rest to natural gas and petroleum). By the year 2050 it's estimated that we will require twice the energy we consume today. The US Census Bureau projects that in the next thirty years the US population will grow by 100 million. A spurt of this magnitude could threaten to wipe out the progress made from power efficiency programs and technological advances.

ELECTRICITY

US households average about 11,000 kWhs annually, which tallies in at $2,000 to $3,000 on average per household for electricity each year, depending on cost, size of house, and location. For example, costs in northwest communities near hydropower dams are as low as two cents per kilowatt-hour. New York's Consolidated Edison at 26 cents per kilowatt-hour is powered by natural gas, and the most expensive major utility is in Hawaii and costs approximately 37 cents per kWh.

Startlingly, only about 35 percent of electricity produced by power plants reaches consumers. The rest is lost through transmission lines across the power grid. A brownout occurs when a power utility's voltage is reduced by trying to produce over the capacity of a plant, and a blackout is produced when it exceeds 15 percent over capacity, or through an accident.

The United States receives approximately 84 percent of its energy from fossil fuels and those power plants are responsible for 67 percent of the nation's sulfur dioxide emissions, 23 percent of nitrogen oxide emissions, and 40 percent of man-made carbon dioxide emissions. Other energy sources are in trouble for different reasons. Hoover Dam, the largest reservoir in the United States, produces the bulk of Nevada's electricity and is in danger, within a decade, of not having enough water to produce power because of a mega-drought.

THE OIL APOCALYPSE—NO FREE LUNCH

Petroleum is the most profitable product in history. Fossil fuels represent the lion's share of our energy base and we still have substantial resources. The overall price of petroleum is becoming much higher than we bargained for—not just at the pump, but also on the planet.

CRUDE OIL

Oil was formed from the remains of marine plants that lived millions of years ago, even before the dinosaurs. Originally these organisms took carbon dioxide out of the atmosphere. Over time these remains became covered by layers of sand and silt where pressure and heat changed them into the hydrocarbons and other organic compounds that form crude oil and natural gas. When heated and combined with oxygen, they release energy and also that stored CO_2, a greenhouse gas.

Coal still powers almost 40 percent of the country, about 900 million tons per year, although its use is declining. That represents about 30 percent of total US carbon dioxide emissions.

The United States consumes an average of about 19.4 million barrels of oil per day. About 25 percent is imported. The resources for easily found and processed crude oil peaked in 1970. Assuming that our rate of usage remains constant, we will run out of easily excavated and processed conventional oil deposits in 2045. But, as far as other sources of oil, the United States has enough raw materials (petroleum and natural gas) for another one hundred to two hundred years, although it is expensive to mine and process and is a particularly "dirty" source of oil.

Crude oil is produced in thirty-one states and 3,500 offshore rigs in US coastal waters, overseen by only sixty-two federal inspectors. While spills from ships are the most well-known sources of oil in ocean water, more water gets contaminated from natural seepage coming from the ocean floor.

A "barrel" (42 US gallons) of crude oil produces slightly more than 44 gallons of petroleum products with gasoline production making up 45 percent of crude oil usage.

OIL SHALE

Oil shale, an organically rich, fine-grained sedimentary rock, contains significant amounts of kerogen (a solid mixture of organic chemical compounds) from which oil is extracted. The energy potential for shale gas is incredible, but the process of refining and using it causes pollution. It is among the fastest-growing energy sources in the country. In 2000, shale gas represented 1 percent of natural gas supplies in the country. Today that number is 30 percent and rising. However, by 2040, oil shale and oil tar sand will be responsible for 75 percent of all greenhouse gases.

Canada and the United States have the world's largest deposits of oil shale. The US government controls 72 percent of all US oil shale acreage. Oil shale can be hard to mine and expensive to refine. A new technology, called "in-situ" or heat extraction mining, has emerged that may begin to tap oil shale's potential. When the oil shale technology is perfected, it could yield a billion barrels per square mile over an area covering more than a thousand square miles, or a trillion barrels, almost four times Saudi Arabia's oil reserves. The price to retrieve the oil is estimated at $90 per barrel at present, but the industry claims it could lower costs by a third. If so, it would become the largest and most inexpensive source of oil on the planet.

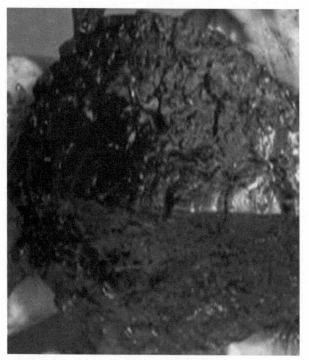

Figure 25.3.   Photo of oil tar sand.
Source: https://www.desmog.ca.

OIL TAR SAND

Oil tar sands are a combination of clay, sand, water, and bitumen, which can be mined and processed to extract refined oil. The bitumen in tar sands is usually obtained using strip mining or open pit techniques. Tar sand is expensive to refine and presents environmental issues as it is detrimental to human health and the environment. The EPA and the Sierra Club claim that tar sand oil creates the dirtiest emissions, up to 82 percent more than average crude oil.

Oil tar supporters want to build the Keystone XL pipeline beginning in Canada and traversing the United States to the Texas gulf in order to transport tar sand oil for refinement. The US Energy and Commerce Committee calculated that the pipeline could import three million barrels a day, which would add the carbon equivalent of "18 million passenger vehicles to the roads" and bring in "the dirtiest source of transportation fuel currently available" that would erase the benefits of new motor vehicle standards to reduce pollution. A barrel of refined oil tar produces more than 82 pounds of greenhouse gases, while conventional US crude makes only 45 pounds.

Canada's oil tar project now befouls the atmosphere with about 37 million added tons of toxic emissions a year, more than the emissions generated by the state of Montana. Canada has enough oil sand reserves to power the United States for one hundred years, although in a free market economy there is no guarantee that any fuel produced or imported to the United States from Canada will be sold to US consumers, easing our need for fuel.

FUEL OIL

Fuel oil is obtained from petroleum distillation and includes any liquid petroleum product that is burned in a furnace or boiler for the generation of heat, or that is used in an engine for the generation of power.

Sixteen of the largest ocean freighters in the world that use fuel oil produce more sulfur byproducts than all the cars in the world. Fuel oil power is also more expensive than coal to produce.

Most new oil furnaces have annual fuel utilization efficiency (AFUE) ratings between 80 percent and 90 percent, while their natural gas counterparts boast ratings between 89 percent and 98 percent. Although gas furnaces are more efficient than oil furnaces, that efficiency comes at a price—gas units are more expensive than the same size oil furnace. Oil furnaces are primarily used in the eastern part of the United States. For the most part, they are efficient, but can be expensive depending on the fluctuating cost of fuel and the policies of the supplier. Some oil companies offer price ceilings or guaranteed seasonal prices, which can make oil furnaces competitive with natural gas.

Older oil-fired furnaces produce at a seasonal efficiency of about 60 percent. This means for each dollar you spend on oil, you're getting sixty cents worth of heat into the home.

COAL

Coal is a combustible, black or brownish-black sedimentary rock composed mostly of carbon and hydrocarbons. It is the most abundant fossil fuel produced in the United States. The United States holds 28 percent of all coal reserves, or nearly 262 billion tons, which is estimated to be enough to last 250 years. In 2008, the United States consumed 1.12 billion tons of coal, making it the second-largest consumer of coal in the world after China. Coal is found in thirty-eight US states, under about 13 percent of the nation's land area. It is mined in twenty-six states, including Texas (the largest producer). The amount of explosives used in Earth removal in West Virginia mines is equal to one Hiroshima-force atomic bomb a week.

Coal accounts for about 39 percent of US total energy production and 25 percent of total energy consumption. It also accounts for approximately 94 percent of the nation's fossil energy reserve. There are approximately 600 coal-generating facilities and 1,100 manufacturing facilities using coal in the United States, according to the US Energy Information Administration (EIA). There are plans to build more than 150 new coal-fired power plants over the next several years.

One half-tons of coal could provide enough energy for one household for one month, and the United States burns about 5.5 tons of coal annually.

Coal Pros: Coal is cheap; it's the most affordable source of fuel per million Btus, averaging less than one-quarter the price of petroleum and natural gas. Coal is called a necessary evil as it is the only source of energy that is sufficiently abundant in production to keep up with our enormous and ever-growing appetite for energy. It is also possible to "clean" coal by carbon sequestration and underground coal gasification (where it is left in the ground, converted to gas, and then brought to the surface). But the process is expensive and has not yet come into productive use.

Coal Cons: The waste and landfill from coal found in valleys and rivers in West Virginia is about the size of Delaware. A typical coal plant generates about three tons of ash per second and produces a total of 1.7 billion tons of carbon dioxide annually, which is the primary man-made cause of global warming, according to a host of scientists. The carbon sequestration system proposed by the Carter administration, forty years ago, is prohibitively costly. The cost of carbon sequestration and decarbonizing our power plants is estimated at $1 trillion, according to a Massachusetts Institute of Technology study.

Although coal ash has not been classified as a toxic substance, it produces more radioactive waste than nuclear power plants and contains mercury, lead, arsenic, asbestos, and heavy metals and other toxic substances. Burning coal is a leading cause of smog, acid rain, and toxic air pollution, exacerbating lung ailments and making people more susceptible to chronic respiratory diseases. The Obama administration has classified greenhouse gases and carbon dioxide emissions, but not coal ash, as health hazards. The coal industry insists that coal ash is not toxic, although they use stringent safety precautions when moving, processing, or handling it. And coal ash waste never decays or decomposes.

COAL-TO-LIQUID (CTL) TECHNOLOGY

CTL is a process that can be used to turn coal into a synthetic gasoline or diesel fuel used in the transportation sector as well as raw materials for industrial products. One hundred pounds of coal will get as far as one tank of gasoline. CTL is an expensive process that also releases large quantities of heat-trapping carbon pollution into the air.

CTL Pros: It is a mature and economically viable technology and it reduces dependence on foreign oil. However, coal-based liquid fuel only becomes viable when the per-barrel price of oil exceeds the $45 to $50 range. CTL processes can also easily be converted to hydrogen fuel cell production plants once fuel cell technology becomes more viable.

CTL Cons: The fuel derived from CTL produces more than twice the amount of carbon dioxide emitted by conventional hydrocarbons. Even with carbon sequestration, any emissions benefits over conventional fuel appear negligible at best, and reliance on coal as a transportation fuel would increase the other environment stresses associated with coal mining.

NATURAL GAS

It used to be thought of as a useless byproduct of oil drilling but is now considered a viable option to other fossil fuels. It has been used in the United States since 1949 and, for the first time, natural gas is now the number one power source in America.

Natural gas can be used for many things, like powering cars, heating homes, cooking, and generating electricity. Thirty states currently mine for natural gas. Louisiana has 10,000 natural gas wells. Major producing reserves are also found in the Rocky Mountains and Texas. In addition, significant natural gas comes from offshore production in the Gulf of Mexico. Pennsylvania contains nearly 500 trillion cubic feet of gas in one deposit—enough to power all American homes for fifty years.

The US DOE predicts that 900 of the next 1,000 power plants built in the United States will use natural gas. New York Con Edison's "Big Alice" power plant burns 9 million cubic feet of natural gas every hour. The natural

gas industry claims that new restrictions on drilling and fracking could result
in the closure of one-third of the gas wells in the United States, dropping
domestic natural gas production, causing a rise in prices, and losing the US
government revenue amounting to four billion dollars per year.

Natural Gas Pros: It is huge resource in the United States. The natural gas
is still relatively cheap, and will remain that way for a long time due to its
abundance. The DOE estimates the supply in the United States at 1.8 trillion
barrels, enough for close to one hundred years. The United States produces a
quarter of the Earth's natural gas and North America supplies 99 percent of
the natural gas consumed in the United States.

The natural gas deposits in Alaska are enormous—enough to support all of
the United States' natural gas needs (at current consumption rates) for more

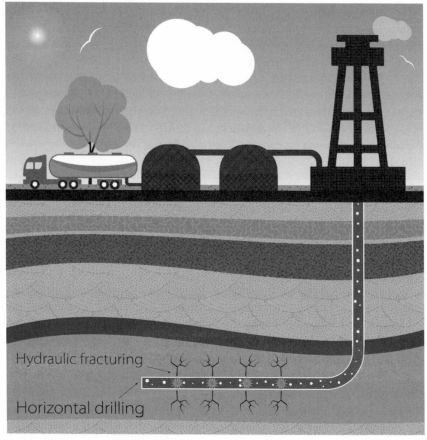

Figure 25.4.   Natural gas well head.
Source: www.huffingtonpost.con/infot.

than a decade, but at present there are no cost-effective means to move the natural gas to the lower 48 states.

Of all the kinds of furnaces available, the most efficient are powered by gas, at more than 95 percent efficiency. Natural gas furnaces will produce 35 to 50 percent fewer GHG emissions than employing energy from power plants fired by other types of fossil fuels.

Natural gas emits 45 percent less carbon dioxide than coal and 30 percent less CO_2 than fuel oil. It does not produce ash or residue. The use of natural gas can slow the progression of climate change while allowing the United States to meet alternative energy goals. Natural gas plants are also relatively cheap to build, and they can be scaled easily to meet energy demands. Because of this, natural gas is expected to be the baseline energy source of choice for the foreseeable future. The natural gas industry employs about 1.2 million people.

Natural Gas Cons: There's some risk attached to using natural gas, however, as accidental fires, explosions, or carbon monoxide poisoning can occur if appliances are not properly operated and maintained. US fire departments respond to an estimated annual average of more than 2,000 home fires involving natural gas, causing $48 million in damages. Natural gas still emits carbon dioxide when burned and contains 80 to 95 percent methane, a greenhouse gas (GHG) three times more potent than carbon dioxide. Finally, concentrated sources of natural gas require long distance transmission and transportation.

WHAT THE FRACK?

Hydraulic fracturing, or fracking, is a mining technique that creates fractures deep within the Earth, which are then highly pressurized with water and chemicals used to pump natural gas to the surface. Many scientists state that fracking and natural gas should be a bridge, not a solution, to reducing our dependency on fossil fuels.

Pros: Fracking stabilizes energy prices while producing an inexpensive and abundant fuel source. The oil industry assures that fracking will supply large reserves for future use, which increases the potential of energy independence and security. It has lowered the cost of generating electricity by gas to about the same as coal.

Fracking creates economic growth through access to convenient and cost-efficient fuel, and by stimulating jobs and the economy. Natural gas is also an important chemical feedstock used in the production of all manner of plastics and other chemicals, with applications from consumer packaging to medicine.

Cons: It is a controversial technique that is undergoing intense investigation concerning damage to water tables, the leaking of flammable gas into homes, damage to plants and illness in animals, and the possible creation and amplification of earthquakes, especially in Oklahoma, a large user of the technique, and now the earthquake capital of the United States, according to *Time* magazine. Companies that frack do not have to divulge the toxic chemical cocktails they use due to the "Halliburton Loophole" legislation that came about as a result of the efforts of Vice President Dick Cheney's Energy Task Force while he was CEO of Halliburton, an important exponent of the extracting technique.

There is evidence that fracking pollutes the water table with carcinogens making waste water disposal is a big challenge. There is concern that "reclaimed" water that still contains toxic chemicals is being sold to water-starved farmers in California.

A 2011 EPA report estimated that 70 to 140 billion gallons of water are used to fracture 35,000 wells at about 50,000 to 350,000 gallons of water per well. This represents the annual water consumption of approximately sixty cities each with a population of 50,000 people and is a drain on drought-stricken states.

Because natural gas is so relatively cheap and plentiful it hampers the development of zero-carbon alternatives, such as solar and wind power. The "dash for gas" may also slow the decarbonization of the electricity system.

If wells are not properly capped, too much methane is vented—a gas more destructive to the atmosphere than carbon dioxide—negating the environmental benefit of natural gas.

The impact on local economy and tourism might be jeopardized by damage to the environment and pollution of land and water. Residents of areas where fracking takes place also have concerns about the effect that the consistent use and the number of heavy vehicles and equipment has on their daily lives.

PROPANE

If you live in a rural area, own an RV, drive a propane-powered vehicle, or have a gas barbecue, you're familiar with propane. Propane is an abundant fuel, obtained through the refining of crude oil or the processing of natural gas.

Pros: The United States is one of the largest propane manufacturers in the world producing more than 90 percent of our own propane. It comes in a liquid state (in tanks) and when used changes from a liquid to a gas. It is a nontoxic, colorless, and odorless gas. Similar to natural gas, an identifying odor is added so it can be readily detected. Propane gas is not harmful to soil and water.

Propane exhaust creates 60 to 70 percent less smog-producing hydrocarbons than gasoline, 12 percent less carbon dioxide, about 20 percent less nitrous oxide, and 60 percent less carbon monoxide. It also cuts emissions of toxins and carcinogens such as benzene and toluene by up to 96 percent.

Cons: Like all fossil fuels, it is flammable and should be used with caution. Propane suppliers can be difficult to find. The cost of propane is more than natural gas due to the added cost of refining, and it doesn't burn as clean as natural gas. Some people even claim that it can taint the taste of barbecue. Lastly, in freezing weather it shrinks in volume.

METHANE

Methane is the major component of natural gas. According to the US Geological Survey (USGS), 100 to 300 million Tcf (trillion cubic feet) of methane exists globally in hydrate form—most of it in the ocean floor bound with water, ice, and rock—representing more energy than all other fossil energy resources combined, according to the DOE.

Livestock produces manure and when decomposing, it also gives off methane gas similar to garbage. The abundant methane gas from rotting trash at landfills can actually be mined for methane and then burned like natural gas to power turbines to produce electricity. Energy produced by methane costs about half as much as the energy from natural gas, but building a landfill methane project is twice as expensive.

North Carolina utilities only pay about three cents per kilowatt-hour for electricity produced by landfills (with subsidies from an environmental group) and have enough methane being mined to provide 700,000 homes with electricity, with enough untapped gas to power 700,000 more. Some scientists are suggesting using human and animal waste and/or the leftovers from farm production, putting them into a big tank, and then letting it ferment anaerobically to produce methane biogas.

Methane makes up about 31 percent of the energy produced in the United States. Natural gas locked up in methane hydrates could be the world's next great energy source—if engineers can figure out how to extract it safely.

Like the federal government, states have also turned their regulatory attention to methane emissions—especially California following the Aliso Canyon disaster which released an estimated 97,100 metric tons of methane into the atmosphere. By that measure, the Aliso Canyon leak produced the same amount of greenhouse gases as 1,735,404 cars during a year.

Pros: It's estimated that methane could fuel 3 million homes in the United States. The EPA believes that one medium-sized methane gas landfill could provide power for 3,000 households. There are at least 600 landfills nation-wide. Using landfill gas as another source of energy reduces the release of landfill methane into the atmosphere and slows the accumulation of greenhouse gases.

Also according to the EPA, a three-megawatt landfill gas project producing electricity generates the environmental equivalent of removing 25,000 cars from the road, planting 35,000 acres of trees, or preventing the use of 304,000 barrels of oil.

The Energy Research and Development Administration (ERDA) study on municipal solid waste found that methane recovery from wastewater treatment could supply ten to fifteen times the amount of energy average cities use for providing municipal services.

Cons: Methane, if not handled properly, is very volatile. The US EPA has documented explosions or fires caused by migrating landfill methane gas. Mining can cause environmental damage and methane is especially difficult to mine and extract underwater as it can explode, kick-starting tsunamis by causing seafloor slumping.

It exists in hydrate (solid compound in which a large amount of methane is trapped) deposits 3,000 times more concentrated than in the atmosphere. Releasing even a fraction of this amount would amplify climate change enormously. If methane is inhaled, it can displace oxygen in human lungs and can essentially poison and cause death.

Over a twenty-year period, methane is estimated to have a warming effect on Earth's atmosphere 84 times that of carbon dioxide and causes more damage to the environment than CO_2 as it is 21 times more effective at trapping heat.

Methane is a far more potent GHG than carbon dioxide on a per-unit basis. Total annual global emissions of carbon dioxide dwarf those of methane so lawmakers and regulators have historically focused their regulatory efforts on limiting CO_2 emissions. This year the EPA is finalizing a set of standards that will reduce methane, volatile organic compounds (VOCs), and toxic air emissions in the oil and natural gas industry.

EFFECTS OF BURNING FOSSIL FUELS

Once emitted, GHGs can remain in the atmosphere for a long time from approximately ten years to thousands of years, depending on the type and amount of gas. Approximately 85 percent of US greenhouse gas emissions result from energy created by fossil fuels. Many scientists credit climate change to the abundance of GHGs in the atmosphere, which deflect heat back onto the planet.

The United States has 5 percent of the global population, uses 25 percent of the world's resources, and contributes 20 percent of global greenhouse gases from burning fossil fuels. It releases toxic GHGs that include:

• Carbon dioxide (CO_2).
• Carbon monoxide (CO).
• Sulfur dioxide (SO_2).
• Nitrogen oxides (NOx).
• Volatile Organic Compounds (VOCs).
• Particulate matter (PM).

Lead and various air toxins such as benzene, formaldehyde, acetaldehyde, and butadiene may be emitted when some types of petroleum are burned. All of these byproducts have negative impacts on the environment and human health.

Since the industrial revolution, about 250 years ago, more than 551 billion tons of carbon have been burned, making the world's atmospheric concentration of carbon dioxide 100 parts per million higher than it has ever been. Scientists claim that a new device, which is small enough to fit inside a shipping container, will be able to capture a ton of CO_2 per day from the air. Unfortunately, it would take hundreds of millions of these devices to suck up all the planet's excess carbon emissions, and the initial cost of the device is roughly $200,000 per unit.

ATOMIC ENERGY

The first US nuclear plant was in Shippingport, Pennsylvania, online from 1957 until 1982. Construction began on the first new nuclear plant to be built in the United States since 1977 in 2013 in South Carolina. The United States is the largest producer of nuclear power, but it provides for less than 10 percent of our energy needs. Vermont is the leader in nuclear power usage, followed by Connecticut, South Carolina, and New Jersey. There are sixty-five nuclear power plants in the United States, with 104 operating nuclear reactors that generate a total of 798.74 billion kWh, or about 19.8 percent of electricity used. Close to 15 percent of the world's power is nuclear—with minimal problems.

NUCLEAR POWER

There are two basic types of nuclear energy being used and experimented with for sources of power: nuclear fission and nuclear fusion. Fission occurs

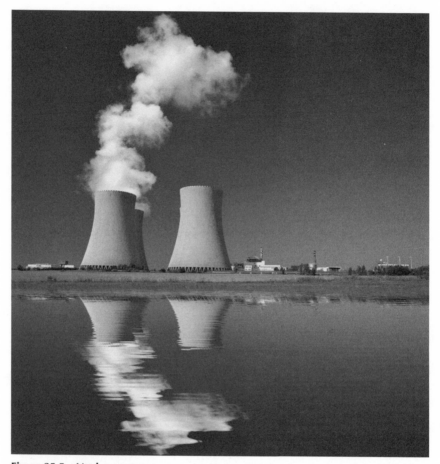

Figure 25.5   Nuclear power.
Source: U.S. Environmental Protection Agency.

when uranium atoms are split apart in a chain reaction and part of the original mass is converted into huge amounts of heat. This is used for heating a boiler that produces steam, which runs turbines and ultimately produces electricity.

The main drawbacks are the possibility of meltdowns in older plants and the radioactive byproducts that have to be transported to safe facilities for storage—which brings out the NIMBY (Not In My Back Yard) and BANANA (Build Absolutely Nothing Anywhere Near Anything) in many of us.

Fusion, on the other hand, is the holy grail of atomic power. To create fusion, hydrogen atoms must be heated to very high temperatures (100 million degrees), ionized (forming a plasma), have sufficient energy to fuse, and then be held together long enough for fusion to occur.

The sun and stars do this through gravity. More practical approaches on Earth are energy sources that hold the ionized atoms together so that fusion occurs before the atoms can fly apart. It's a relatively stable reaction, generating little or no radioactive waste. In addition, there's no chance of a reactor disaster since there is no chain reaction. Better yet, because fusion produces no radioactive waste material, it's useless as a weapon, causes little or no atmospheric pollution, and the byproduct is harmless helium.

Unfortunately, at present fusion takes more energy to create than it generates, making it economically unfeasible. A practical and productive technology is probably decades away.

One pound of enriched uranium is equal in energy to 3,000,000 pounds of coal, and produces no GHGs in the process. A single two-gram uranium fuel pellet has the same energy value as three barrels of oil. Based on a cost of $3,000 for 453 grams, the two grams are worth about 675 barrels of oil. Therefore, uranium fuel is cheaper than oil by at least a factor of 20. However, the cost of traditional nuclear reactors runs about $8 billion, making big-time taxpayer dollars necessary.

ATOMIC POWER PARANOIA

Unfortunately, nuclear power has a bad-boy reputation caused by its use in weapons of mass destruction, by its depiction in the film industry, and by the problematic fallout of some power plant troubles. A reactor meltdown would have to occur every two weeks to make nuclear power as deadly as the routine emissions from coal-fired power. The main danger of a nuclear chemical spill or accident is during shipping of fuel or waste. No such spills have ever happened in the United States. To date, no workers or members of the public have died as a result of exposure to radiation due to a commercial nuclear reactor accident at a US power plant. Nuclear wastes are neither particularly hazardous nor hard to manage relative to other toxic industrial wastes. The amount of nuclear waste each person generates in a lifetime would only be about two liters.

Still, no one wants nuclear waste stored in their state. As a result, there are more than 50,000 tons of uranium soaking in pools next to US reactors, waiting for a permanent home.

Spent fuel still contains 96 percent of the original uranium, 1 percent of plutonium, and also about 3 percent of fission waste products. The reusable uranium and plutonium can be processed into new fuel such as mixed-oxide (MOX) fuel that has incredible energy potential. Just one MOX fuel pellet (about one-quarter inch long and thick) is equal to one ton of coal.

At the present rate of use, there are about fifty to seventy years left of known uranium-235 reserves, which power nuclear power plants that are economically recoverable. New technology and an increased need for reserves could fuel more production.

Another type of nuclear energy is fusion, the exact opposite of fission. The best example of fusion is our solar furnace, the sun which fuses hydrogen into helium, producing energy in the process. Fusion doesn't create runaway chain reactions, will not cause "meltdowns," and doesn't produce weapons-grade byproducts or radioactive waste. Among other things, the bad news is that it is incredibly expensive to create in that it requires temperatures of at least 100 million degrees (Celsius), hotter than the core of the sun, so the amount of energy you'd need to put in to produce that kind of heat or pressure is much, much higher than what you get out in usable energy.

Fusion Pros: The hydrogen fuels used are almost limitless; a single gallon of seawater could produce as much energy as 300 gallons of gasoline, and require only about one-millionth of the mass of fuel needed to produce the same amount of energy as coal. Fusion is clean energy, and does not produce GHGs. The products of a fusion reaction are not radioactive, thus there are no nuclear waste problems.

Fusion is not a chain reaction, therefore it can be stopped at any time and there is no threat of a meltdown making safety risks associated with its storage and handling minimal. It may also be the most cost-efficient of all nonpolluting power plants.

Fusion Cons: The temperatures and pressures needed to sustain fusion make it a very difficult process to control. Although both the United States and the European Union, along with other countries, support fusion research, it has stalled for the past twenty years.

Fission Pros: Fission produces lots of energy derived from small amounts of fuel. Radioactivity of spent fuel is low. Waste can be reduced by using new reactors along with recycling and reprocessing, although the radioactive half-life (the amount of time required for a quantity to fall to half its value) of spent fuel is still 24,000 years. Nuclear technology is also known, safe, and reliable. It produces significantly fewer greenhouse gases. Many people with environmental concerns, including Stewart Brand (of *Whole Earth Catalog*), are taking a friendlier and closer look at nuclear power as a feasible option. And according to the History Channel, beer has thirteen times more radioactivity than the water that cools a nuclear reactor.

Fission Cons: Nuclear fuel sources are finite. Power plants are also expensive to build; subsidies and large loan guarantees will be needed. Byproducts can be long-lasting and unhealthy. We must also keep in mind that the development of enriching processes in fission leads to nuclear weapons capabilities. Plants also need to be protected, as they could be targets for terrorism.

26

The Renewables

Energy that Keeps on Keeping On

The energy gifts that keep on giving because they will never give out are called renewables. They are derived from natural resources such as the sun, Earth, wind, and water; they do not harm the environment by their use nor do they bring with them the extra hidden costs of damage to the health of the people.

THE SUN

The sun is the primary source of all life and most of the resources on Earth. It is our solar system furnace with a core temperature of 27 million degrees Fahrenheit. It produces 120,000 terawatts of energy daily, more than ten times all the energy used on planet Earth every day. There is enough solar energy available to fulfill all our energy requirements now and forever. Solar power is the second fastest-growing energy technology in the world, but the key is developing technologies that efficiently convert solar power into energy in a cost-effective and storable manner.

FACTS AND FIGURES

The source of our light, warmth, and life come from a yellow dwarf star 93 million miles away. Our sun is called a yellow dwarf because it is yellow in color and, as far as stars go, it is small. However, the sun still spans a million miles across and a million Earths could fit inside. Its power is created by nuclear fusion.

It takes about eight minutes for the light or "photons" emitted by the sun to get to the Earth. In one second the sun generates all the power that mankind has ever used—it radiates 380 billion-billion megawatts of energy per second. The sun is our most sustainable, cheap, and nonpolluting resource and is the purest form of renewable energy. It can be active, as in photovoltaic cells that produce electricity, or passive as with sunlight used to heat water.

Studies have shown that annual energy costs can be reduced by as much as 80 percent by using different solar energy methods. The United States is the most technologically advanced country in solar power technology, but only ranks fifth in solar power utilization. However, according to the US Energy Information Administration (USEIA) solar use grew by 418 percent from 2010 to 2014. The Department of Energy estimates that by the year 2030, at least 10 percent of all homes will be powered by the sun. Total financial investment in solar technology grew by 172 percent from 2004 to 2008.

A medium-sized home solar energy system that generates approximately 800 to 1,000 kilowatt-hours a month would cost about $10,000 before the 30 percent federal tax credit and other rebates offered by individual states or utility companies. Several factors have to be considered, but many systems pay for themselves within seven to fourteen years. Although there are approximately one million homes using solar energy, solar power accounts for less than 1 percent of the energy produced in the United States.

The Ivanpah BrightSource's solar thermal system in California's Mojave Desert is currently the largest solar plant in the world. Its 170,000 solar

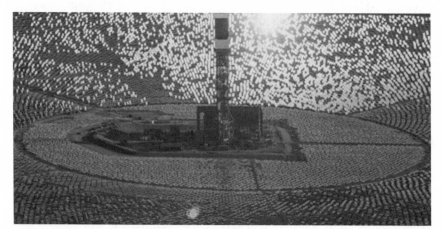

Figure 26.1. The Ivanpah BrightSource's solar thermal system in California's Mojave Desert.
Source: www.brightsourceenergy.com.

panels, each measuring 70 square feet, gather sunlight and focus it on three towers filled with water, raising the water temperature to more than 1,000°F. This produces steam that spins turbines, which generate electricity and supply power to 140,000 homes in southern California.

With 300 days a year of harvestable sunlight, Arizona and Colorado are poised to become the Persian Gulf of solar power. The largest solar roof is on a Toys "R" Us warehouse in New Jersey; the 5.38-megawatt system creates enough energy to power 700 homes, produces more than enough energy to power its 1.3 million-square-foot building, and sells the surplus.

Solar Pros: As a fuel source, solar power produces no pollution, is renewable, can be used almost anywhere, and is an inexhaustible, abundant, and free fuel supply.

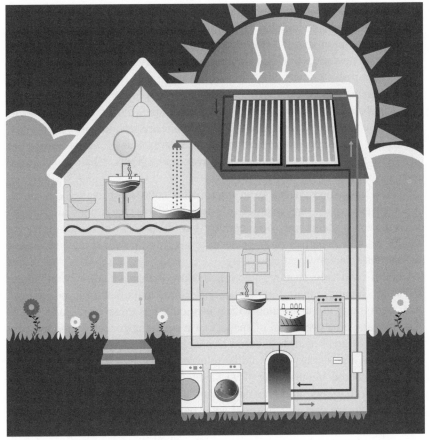

Figure 26.2. Solar panel electric inverter.
Source: Provided by the author.

In the home a solar water heating system will save approximately $500 over electricity in the first year of service and savings will improve due to increasing electricity rates. Solar systems are nearly maintenance-free, only have to be replaced every fifty years (unless you use storage batteries), and are usually guaranteed for twenty to thirty years. Furthermore, no moving parts are required so solar energy produces electricity very quietly. Thirty-five states allow homeowners to sell excess solar energy to utilities. A typical home installation array might generate about a 5 kWh daily, using about twenty-five panels.

A one-kilowatt system eliminates the burning of approximately 170 pounds of coal, it saves 300 pounds of carbon dioxide from being released into the atmosphere, and it also saves up to 105 gallons of water consumption monthly. Solar panels can mitigate the sun beating on the roof, inadvertently cooling roofs and lowering AC energy costs.

The ability to harness electricity in remote locations not linked to a national power grid is much more cost-effective than laying the required high voltage wires. Solar power generation is resilient against large-scale blackouts as well as acts of terror.

Solar technology is rapidly improving, especially in photovoltaic technology, which soon will utilize solar film on glass, paint, tiles, and other means that can be used on any surface. New solar energy technologies even allow for a more efficient energy production on overcast days. Many companies now offer low-cost lease options, and government grants, rebates, and incentives are available.

Solar Cons: Solar energy is an intermittent source not available at night, under clouds, or in bad weather, it's less available for immediate heating demand, and systems may only convert 1 to 40 percent of the sunlight that hits the panels. A battery or an alternative source of power is needed to have continuous solar-powered electricity.

Certain solar cells require materials that are expensive and rare in nature, and solar systems contain fragile materials. Some manufacturing processes of solar equipment are associated with greenhouse gas emissions. Solar panels can also take up a great deal of space, cause aesthetic concerns, and may not work well in areas with a polluted atmosphere. There is also a technology risk—a much better system could be released in the future.

Solar-powered photovoltaic (PV) panels are made of crystalline silicon, a plastics technology, and convert the sun's rays into electricity by exciting electrons that are captured in small solar panel wiring in silicon cells, using the photons of light from the sun, into a DC electrical current, the kind used by your car battery. An inverter changes the current to AC, or the power used by your house.

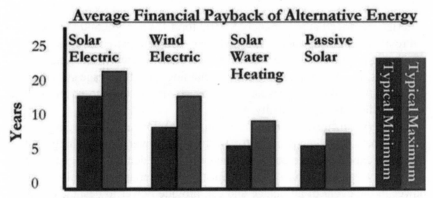

Average Financial Payback of Alternative Energy

Figure 26.3.   Percentage of energy efficiency converting fuel to electricity.
Source: www.wsj.com/news/us/.

HOME BATTERIES

Home batteries are meant for use to fill the power gap when the grid is down, or for partial power when the grid is at its peak cost, or when the sun is hiding out. Depending on home energy needs and the size of the battery, it can last between seven and forty hours. A battery is not intended for home peak use, like running loads of laundry while the AC, televisions, and computers are on.

The sun isn't always shining when you need power, and sometimes the sun is shining when you don't need power. To solve this obvious problem, people are using batteries to store energy. Basically, batteries have two sides. One is filled with electrons and the other side is empty; they are separated by a barrier. When the two sides are connected via a wire, a chemical reaction occurs which creates a flow of electrons or electricity. To recharge a battery the process, with the help of a substance called lithium, is reversed.

Although grid-tied systems can save money and earn their owners incentives while the sun is shining and the utility power grid is up, they must disconnect when the grid is down during an outage.

As an alternative to connecting the solar panels directly to the grid and "running the meter backwards" during the day (net metering), people can store their own electricity in home battery systems—thereby avoiding caps and special charges that may apply to net-metered systems.

These systems use lithium-ion batteries because they are capable of more charge-discharge cycles. A 7 kWh battery is about the size of a refrigerator. A 3 kWh battery can be wall mounted. The median manufacturers' suggested retail price of a complete AC-coupling system with sufficient battery storage is about $16,000—electronics-only packages run around $8,600, and Tesla batteries are priced approximately $3,500 for 7 kWh, or $3,500 for 3 kWh.

Pros: Although still more expensive than lead-acid batteries, volume manufacturing for the electric vehicle industry is spurring significant battery price reductions. In addition to new battery technology, home storage systems also employ advanced electronics and software control systems to further reduce costs and increase functionality.

A battery can provide financial savings to its owner by charging during low-rate periods (when demand for electricity is lower) and discharging during more expensive-rate periods (when electricity demand is higher). Thus, the battery can store surplus solar energy for later use. This also ensures power in the event of an outage and can provide power to designated appliances (i.e., refrigerator or server).

Manufacturers claim that the batteries are recycling-friendly. Boosters believe that 160 million battery packs could "transition" power usage in the United States to renewable energy, while 900 million battery packs could shift the entire world's energy needs.

Cons: There is the question of whether solar power coupled with home batteries is really a renewable, nonpolluting power—the batteries contain toxic materials and may be made via nonrenewable sources, and they may not be recycle-friendly.

As of right now, it makes little financial sense for the majority of people who go solar to also get a battery storage system and go off the grid, as it could cost up to $25,000. The payback period would be fifteen to thirty years, depending on your energy needs. Batteries also have complex installation systems and increase maintenance requirements. The average homeowner in the United States stays in their home for ten to fifteen years. Tesla's batteries are warrantied for only ten years.

Remember that first of all, houses run on AC current but the battery produces DC current. This means that you need to take the DC current and convert it to AC current, which means buying a converter. With a 7kWh battery you can get about 1 kWh, or maybe five hours of moderate use—so not everyone can crank up their fave toys and devices. This system will run your refrigerator, HVAC, and a couple of other important devices.

PASSIVE SOLAR WATER HEATING

With this system, glazed flat-plate collectors are insulated along with weatherproofed boxes that contain a dark absorber plate under one or more glass or plastic covers. Unglazed flat-plate collectors—typically used for solar pool heating—have a dark absorber plate, made of metal or polymer, without a cover or enclosure.

Integral collector-storage systems feature one or more black tanks or tubes in an insulated, glazed box. Cold water first passes through the solar collector, which preheats the water. The water then continues on to the conventional water heater, providing a reliable source of hot water. These systems should be installed only in mild-freeze climates because the outdoor pipes could freeze in severe weather.

Evacuated-tube solar collectors are parallel rows of transparent glass tubes. Each tube contains a glass outer tube and metal absorber tube attached to a fin. The fin's coating absorbs solar energy but inhibits radiative heat loss. These collectors are used more frequently for US commercial applications.

Direct circulation systems circulate household water through collectors and into the home. They work well in climates where it rarely freezes. Indirect circulation systems pump a nonfreezing, heat-transfer fluid through the collectors. This heats the water that then flows into the home's water system.

PHOTOVOLTAIC SOLAR

Simply put, a solar panel creates electricity by allowing photons, or particles of light, to knock electrons free from their atoms, generating a flow of electricity known as the photoelectric effect. Solar panels actually comprise many, smaller units called photovoltaic cells and small wires in the panels (photovoltaic simply means they convert sunlight into electricity).

By the way, Albert Einstein described the nature of light and the photoelectric effect, on which photovoltaic technology is based, for which he later won the Nobel Prize in Physics in 1921.

THINGS TO CHECK BEFORE GOING SOLAR

Make sure you understand your utility company's rates and have an accurate idea of the amount of energy your home uses each month. Unless you're building a self-contained home off the grid, don't worry about batteries.

Ideally, solar systems should be on the southwest area of your roof, but the direction is not as important as some people may insist. Even southeast, east, north, and northwest can give acceptable results. Adding a solar system will not cause a reassessment of property. In fact, you'll probably get a rebate from the state or federal government for going solar. Do cover your solar investment with proper insurance and know about solar warranties on parts and installation. Solar panels should last thirty years or more. Be sure to ask about maintenance.

Panels should not harm a roof, though the kind of roof you have makes a big difference in installation prices. It will definitely be costlier to install solar panels on Spanish tile than on plain old asphalt shingle roofs. The extra installation time can add 10 to 25 percent in additional expense to the job.

FUEL CELLS

A fuel cell is an electrochemical energy conversion that changes hydrogen and oxygen into water, and produces electricity in the process. Hydrogen is the most abundant element in the universe. When a hydrogen-rich fuel such as natural gas, renewable biogas, a fossil fuel (or even treated water) enters the fuel cell stack, it reacts electrochemically with air to strip off electrons that produce an electric current, heat, and water. The resulting electrochemical reactions in the fuel cell produce direct current (DC) power, which can be converted to alternating current (AC) power, depending on how the power is to be employed. DC current can be used for powering a vehicle.

Panasonic and Tokyo Gas are developing an "Ene-Farm" home fuel cell unit, which is the world's first commercialized fuel cell system targeted at household heating and electricity generation. The fuel cell can reduce primary energy consumption by 37 percent and cut CO_2 emissions by 49 percent. Some manufacturers claim their models achieve 95 percent combined heat and electrical efficiency and are exceptionally durable, while achieving greater than 60,000 hours of generation of electricity while cycling daily. The overall result is a reduction of as much as 50 percent in household CO_2 emissions and can save more than $650 yearly. The initial cost of a Panasonic system is about $17,280, with a predicted payback period of seven to ten years.

The Bloom Energy Box utilizes a solid oxide fuel cell (SOFC) that converts fossil fuels, such as gasoline, diesel, natural gas, propane, and methane to generate electricity through a clean electrochemical process. It's been reported that Bloom's fuel cells emit 884 pounds of CO_2 on average per megawatt-hour (mWh) of electricity produced. Compare that to 2,249 pounds for a coal-fired plant. However, it's not much less than the 1,135 pounds an existing natural gas plant emits. In 2010, the company announced plans for a smaller, home-sized Bloom server priced under $3,000. Bloom estimated the size of a home-sized server at 1 kW, although others recommended 5 kW. The price of 1 kW is about $3,000.

Pros: Fuel can be made to run from hydrogen, the most plentiful element on Earth. Hydrogen has been described as "the fuel of the future" because it is abundant and benign in terms of emissions; proponents say it holds tremendous promise. Fuel cell technology operates at half the cost of solar with a productivity rate eleven times greater. Furthermore, fuel cells are highly efficient, exhibiting maximum efficiency even at low-power levels. Fuel cells reduce greenhouse gas emissions, as their waste products are only heat and water.

The financial payback is fast, with many customers supposedly recouping costs within three to five years. Continued research will improve the technology and it may become a serious future player in the energy mix.

Cons: Some fuel cells run on hydrogen produced by fossil fuel. Due to technical barriers and resulting high costs, even ardent supporters do not see hydrogen power as a short-term solution for America's energy needs. Consequently, although some businesses are using this technology, at present it is still very expensive and not economically viable on a large scale or for homeowners. Reliability and durability of fuel cells, particularly at high temperatures, is still evolving. There are also safety concerns with combustible hydrogen (though it is far less dangerous than petro-based fuels).

GEOTHERMAL

Approximately 4,000 miles beneath the Earth's surface is a molten mass of superheated gas and magma cooking at roughly 7,200°F. The amount of thermal energy contained in the Earth's crust is enormous and can be tapped by simply drilling a hole, sending water down a pipe, and running the returned steam through a turbine to produce electricity. Geothermal energy is also used to heat and cool structures that use heat pumps, which derive their energy source several meters underground.

During the winter, a geothermal system absorbs extra heat from the Earth and transfers it into the home. During the summer, the system takes heat from indoors and moves it back underground. Today there are more than 1,000,000 geothermal installations in the United States, generating about 2 percent of the electricity in Utah, 6 percent of the electricity in California, and almost 10 percent of the electricity in northern Nevada.

Geothermal heat pumps (GHPs) are the HVAC system of choice for many Net Zero–use energy buildings. Cost can also depend on the expense and difficulties in building a plant. Costs of a geothermal plant are heavily weighted toward early expenses, rather than energy sources to keep them running.

Pros: Few facilities can produce electricity between 4.5 and 7.3 cents per kilowatt-hour, making geothermal competitive with conventional fossil fuel–fired power plants. Geothermal is almost entirely emission-free and has the smallest carbon and land footprint of any major power source. According to the EPA, replacing an ordinary HVAC system with geothermal is the environmental equivalent of planting 750 trees.

The geothermal process can scrub out sulfur that might have otherwise been released underground. No fuel mining or transportation is needed in a geothermal system, nor is it subject to the same fluctuations as solar, wind, or water power. Geothermal energy is not susceptible to price fluctuation like crude oil and the supply is limitless.

Properly sized and installed GHPs deliver more energy per unit consumed than conventional systems. For further savings, GHPs can be equipped with a device called a "desuperheater." In the summer cooling period, the heat that is taken from the house is used to heat the water for free. In the winter, water-heating costs are reduced by about half.

The geothermal system is inherently simple and reliable. Most of the infrastructure for GHPs could be built underground. Geothermal plants are small in size compared to atomic or fossil fuel plants, thus they have a smaller impact on the environment. Geothermal power plants also run continuously day and night with an uptime typically exceeding 95 percent. The power plants can have modular designs, so additional units can be installed in increments when needed to fit growing demand for electricity.

Geothermal units are stored indoors, so there are no outdoor units creating heat and noise. They are also protected from the elements. Surveys consistently show that more than 95 percent of all geothermal system owners would recommend it to a friend. The US government has offered tax credits for individuals who use the technology in their homes. On average, a typical home of 2,500 square feet, with a heating load of 60,000 Btus and a cooling load of 60,000 Btus, will cost between $20,000 to $25,000 to install with a payback period of approximately ten to twelve years.

Cons: Prime sites are very location-specific, often far from population centers, and some sites are better suited for geothermal than others. Geothermal energy uses more water than any other form of electricity generation, but development of new cooling technologies and advanced energy-conversion techniques will reduce this. Geothermal uses water in three stages: water used to extract the Earth's heat, degraded water to top up the geothermal fluid, and fresh water for cooling. Also, geothermal may emit sulfur dioxide and silica. Sometimes, the process of digging for geothermal energy, in extreme cases, may cause earthquakes.

Since geothermal energy is still a relatively new concept for private home use, it can be expensive to install and is often higher in cost than that of other heating and cooling systems. Extreme care and caution is needed as water that travels through the piping is superheated. Installing a geothermal energy system can require a lot of land to have it properly installed. Geothermal heat can't be "transported" to other generation sites, like nuclear and fossil fuel plants. Current technology does not yet allow the best exploitation of this energy resource.

HYDRO POWER: GOING WITH THE FLOW— DAMS, TIDES, AND WAVES

DAMS

The Federal Energy Regulatory commission (FERC) regulates approximately 2,540 hydroelectric-producing dams. Due to the Endangered Species Act and changing attitudes toward man-made dams, many are being dismantled. The only ecologically sound dams are created by beavers who are the only builders that will probably create any more dams in this country.

Only 3 percent of approximately more than 80,000 man-made dams in the United States are currently used to generate electrical power. Some small dams are being retrofitted to produce hydroelectric power, which is clean and sustainable.

Pros: Hydroelectricity is currently the largest producer of reliable, safe, renewable power in the United States. In 2010, hydroelectricity produced around 6.2 percent of the nation's total clean electricity, which totaled 60.2 percent of US renewable power. Once dams are built they are among the most efficient energy sources, with low operational and maintenance costs. Today's hydroelectric power plants have an efficiency of approximately 90 percent; only a small amount of energy gets wasted in the process of generating electricity. Hydropower plants are among the longest-lived power plants.

The lake that forms behind a dam can be also used for irrigation and recreational tourism in the form of water sports. And luckily, hydroelectric power plants have no toxic emissions or waste disposal issues. Hydroelectric plants do not require a lot of workers and maintenance costs are usually low.

Cons: Dams require suitable locations and can damage the environment. There are also high up-front costs, especially when building large hydroelectric power plants. In time of drought and seasonal fluctuations, hydroelectric power plants may not be able to produce electricity because there isn't enough water flow. Due to limited resources and changing attitudes, only one hydroelectric project has been started in the last two years, and accidents and failures can be extremely hazardous.

TIDE POWER

There are three ways to use the ocean's waves: high and low tides, movement of waves, and temperature differences in the water. Some of the types of energy from water movement include one that is called VIVACE (vortex induced vibrations for aquatic clean energy). This is a unique hydrokinetic energy system that relies on "vortex induced vibrations," a purely experimental system that draws energy from slow-moving water currents.

Tidal power, used primarily in Europe, converts the energy of tides into electricity. Two high and low tides each day produce a huge amount of moving water and harnessing it could provide a great deal of energy. California, for instance, has more than 745 miles (1,200 kilometers) of coastline, of which about 20 percent could be used for producing electricity. The state has plans for twelve plants.

Tides are more predictable, reliable, and plentiful than wind energy and solar power, however converting them into useful electrical power is not easy. Tidal energy systems typically involve erecting a dam across the opening of a bay. As the tide comes in and out, the flow of water is directed toward a series of turbines to generate electrical power. Wave or aquamarine power is created when a float or buoy generates electrical power by driving turbines that flow with the natural movement of the waves.

With most of the Earth's surface covered with water, a great amount of energy can be produced by placing turbines at strategic locations under strong (artificial or natural) currents and tides. Australia, Denmark, France, Canada, Spain, Portugal, the United Kingdom, and Israel are presently using wave power. A report by the US Department of Energy revealed that wave and other water power resources across the United States could potentially provide 15 percent of the nation's electricity by 2030.

Pros: Tidal energy is considered to be a renewable and predictable source of energy since it does not require any fuel and tidal plants can last up to 100 years. Maintenance for tidal and wave plants is low. There is minimal visual impact as most of the device is underwater.

Turbines can be anchored to the seabed or float to generate electricity from tidal currents, and have an efficiency rate of 80 percent in converting the potential energy of the water into electricity. Wave power makes no noise, is almost completely below the surface, is inexhaustible, and creates zero emissions. Energy analysts believe there is enough energy in the ocean waves to provide up to 2 terawatts of electricity—enough to power 180,000 homes for one hour.

Cons: At present tidal power plants need to be constructed close to land, which could reduce shipping and recreation areas. Strong ocean storms and saltwater corrosion can damage plant devices, and changes in tidal movement could substantially reduce efficiency.

Converting tidal power into useful electrical power is not easy and is expensive, considering tidal power can only be captured for a maximum of a 10-hour cycle per day. For these reasons, tidal energy systems are in their infancy in the United States and have not been considered economically feasible.

Tidal technology also has the disadvantage of affecting the surrounding ecosystem and wildlife in the area of the workings; fish mortality is from 20 to 80 percent around a tidal plant. Sea life could be harmed or disrupted by the blades in the turbines.

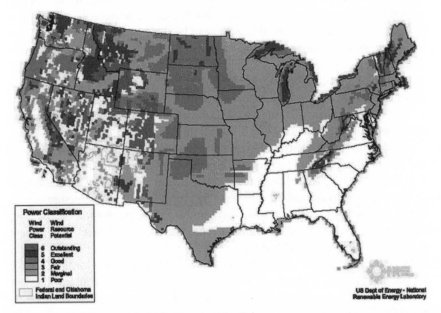

Figure 26.4.   U.S. map of wind resource potential.
Source: U.S. Department of Energy.

EOLIC POWER

Farmers once used windmills to pump water and grind their grains. Today, we use wind turbines to generate electricity by spinning "wind" blades that turn a shaft connected to a generator to create electricity. At present, wind power, the fastest growing alternative energy source, provides about 2.5 percent of energy in the United States. Between 2008 and 2012, wind power has provided 36.5 percent of all new generating capacity in the United States.

Wind power is expected to account for nearly 5 percent of total US electricity generation in 2015.

The American Wind Energy Association (AWEA) estimates that about 13 million US houses could employ small windmills. Systems cost about $40,000 to $50,000 to install a 5 kW system and take fifteen to twenty years to repay the investment. Zoning restrictions may apply.

Scientists at the California Institute of Technology (Caltech) have been conducting a field study and claim the power output of wind farms can be increased at least tenfold by optimizing the placement of turbines on a given plot of land. The average wind farm requires seventeen acres of land to produce one megawatt of electricity that can sustain 1,000 homes for one hour.

Turbines can be as tall as a twenty-story building and have three 200-foot-long (60-meter-long) blades. Winds have to be sustained at approximately ten to twelve miles per hour to produce electricity, which typically costs around five cents per kWh.

Pros: There's enough wind in the Unites States to power the country ten times over. According to the US DOE, all US electrical energy needs could be met by the wind in Texas and the Dakotas alone. One large wind turbine can power all the electricity needs of 350 to 500 homes.

Wind is very cost-efficient. Average turbine lifespan is 122 years. A wind turbine can lower your electricity bill by 50 to 90 percent. The actual space that a small turbine tower occupies is small, usually less than 100 square feet.

The fuel for a wind turbine is essentially free once the infrastructure is paid for and operational costs are low. Any excess power can be sold to the grid. Also, tax incentives may be available from the local or federal government for those who install wind turbines.

Wind turbines have a low lifecycle carbon footprint; they will not leave a toxic legacy. Wind causes no pollution; a one-megawatt wind turbine will annually displace emissions of 1,600 tons of carbon dioxide (as much as 900,000 trees), nine tons of sulfur dioxide and four tons of nitrous oxide, reducing smog, acid rain, and greenhouse gases. New turbines are even being made safer for wildlife. Some predict by 2050, the answer to one-third of the world's electricity needs will be found blowing in the wind.

Cons: The wind is inconsistent, unsteady, and unpredictable, so batteries are needed to store the energy produced by wind turbines. Wind power is also a fairly new resource, relying on government subsidies to remain competitive. Of course, not all geographical locations are suitable for wind turbines; check local wind speed averages. Turbines typically operate at only 30 percent capacity (but to put that in perspective, solar panels operate at only 15 percent efficiency).

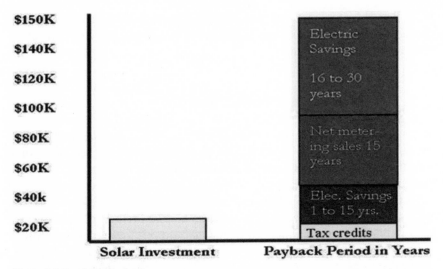

Figure 26.5.   Solar savings.
Source: Provided by the author.

Wind farms are considered by some people to be a noisy eyesore and they have a negative impact on wildlife as birds and bats have been sliced and diced. Turbines have been known to suffer from mechanical fatigue and can be damaged by storms and lightning, too.

BIOFUELS

Biofuels are quasi-renewable fuels derived from natural oils such as soybeans, fish processing, insects, plants, paper, vegetable oils, waste oils, or agricultural and light industrial waste. Because biofuels are made from plants, are not excavated from finite sources, and are biodegradable, many consider them to be sustainable.

But since they have to be cultivated, concerns come into play such as water management and erosion, soil health and monoculture (planting only one kind of crop), overuse of fertilizers, production of GHGs, social and economic standards, the value of the crops as food, and the value of land (new standards emphasize the use of marginal, degraded, or previously cleared terrain for growing biofuels). The impact and whether they are truly renewable is yet to be seen.

In a process called transesterification, the glycerin (a simple sugar compound) is separated from fat or vegetable oil. The sugars can be used to create ethanol, the fats to manufacture biodiesel.

Biogas or biofuel is a clean and renewable energy source that may be substituted for natural gas to cook, to heat water or power a furnace, to generate electricity, or to run engines.

BIODIESEL

It can be made from any plant oil or animal fat. Some examples include soybean, grapeseed, and palm kernel oils, as well as animal fat left over from meat processing or from recycled restaurant cooking oil, often called waste vegetable oil (WVO).

Although it has been promoted mostly as a fuel for diesel-powered vehicles, biodiesel—sometimes referred to as bioheat fuel—is perfectly suited as an additive or replacement fuel in a standard oil-fired furnace or boiler. Most types of biofuels are carbon-neutral. This means that the amount of carbon dioxide created by the burning of biofuels is equal to the CO_2 absorption capacity of the plants from which they are derived. Biodiesel has even been used in cleaning oil spills.

Pros: Particulate matter dropped by almost 50 percent when using B100 (100 percent biodiesel) and dropped by 12 percent when using B20 (20 percent biodiesel). Global warming impact from carbon dioxide dropped by almost 80 percent using B100. Hydrocarbons were reduced by nearly 70 percent using B100 and 21 percent using B20. Hydrocarbons include many different individual toxic compounds. Carbon monoxide decreased 48 percent with B100, 12 percent using B20.

Biodiesel is the only alternative fuel to have fully completed the health effects testing requirements of the Clean Air Act. Its use will reduce respiratory disease. Biodiesel is also safer to transport than diesel fuel because it has a higher ignition temperature.

Restaurants utilize approximately 1.4 million gallons of cooking oil each year. Biofuel can be produced gallon-for-gallon from used cooking oil that would otherwise be discarded in landfills or shipped to China for processing. This displaces millions of gallons of petro-based diesel fuel in the United States each year. It reduces our dependence on unstable and costly foreign sources of oil and is an additional cash crop for our farmers.

Biodiesel from soybeans costs an estimated $2 to $2.50 per gallon to produce. Biodiesel from yellow grease is about $1 a gallon cheaper than the soy product. Biodiesel can be made at home, saving 50 percent on fuel costs. Blends can be created with a mixture of biodiesel and regular diesel gasoline with reasonable results. Biodiesel is biodegradable and has a pleasant aroma (like popcorn) in comparison to the toxic smell of petroleum diesel fuel.

Cons: Current worldwide production of vegetable oil and animal fat is not sufficient to replace liquid fossil fuel use. Also, total cost-effective production for biodiesel technology is not yet proven.

Biofuels can be difficult to find and are not always cheaper than petrodiesel. The quality can vary greatly and a fluctuation of 1 to 2 percent lower fuel efficiency can occur. Some form of gelling and restrictive flow in very cold weather may be experienced. There is also a slight increase (2 to 4 percent depending on the blend) in nitrous oxide (or NOx) which can form a noxious emission.

Promoters of biofuels have created a false impression of an easy solution to energy needs, but the transition is not so simple. Replacing only 5 percent of the nation's diesel consumption with biodiesel would require diverting approximately 60 percent of today's soy crops to biodiesel production. Converting crops into biofuels will also mean less will be available to feed people and animals. Extensive biofuel production could invite extensive deforestation in tropical areas that grow sugar cane and soybeans, such as tropical rainforests, so other noninvasive methods and plants will be needed.

ETHANOL

It is one of man's oldest substances, dating back 9,000 years and is basically high-powered alcohol. Ethanol gained favor again in 1974 during the fuel shortage, but interest quickly declined when it was over. Ethanol fuel is widely used in Brazil and in the United States, and together both countries were responsible for 88 percent of the world's ethanol fuel production in 2009.

This fuel is an alcohol-based product made from corn, sorghum, potatoes, wheat, sugar cane, and even biomass such as cornstalks, some weeds, and vegetable waste. It is a quasi-renewable resource and is most often used as a biofuel additive for gasoline.

Ethanol production consumes close to 1.6 billion bushels of grain, and about 15 percent of total US corn production. Farmers planted almost 93 million acres of corn in 2007, a 19 percent increase over the previous year, and the highest figure since 1944 (when yields per acre were far lower). Ethanol is used in many products ranging from fireplace fuel to perfumes.

Pros: Overall, ethanol is considered to be better for the environment than gasoline as it displaces the use of toxic gasoline components such as benzene, a carcinogen. It is nontoxic, water soluble, and quickly biodegradable.

Ethanol is a renewable fuel that comes from agricultural feedstock and can be produced domestically, lessening dependence on foreign oil. Ethanol reduces the amount of GHGs by 13 to 50 percent, relative to gasoline. Production of carbon dioxide should be "net zero" as crops used to make ethanol absorb CO_2 from the atmosphere during their growth.

Sawgrass or switchgrass, a weed that can be cultivated on land considered non-farmable by some US farmers, does not need petro-based fertilizer and could result in 88 percent less greenhouse gas emissions than petro-fuel. Sawgrass in ethanol production is a hearty cellulosic material that uses 100 percent of the plant and produces ten times the energy as opposed to corn that uses only the protein kernel.

Cons: Most ethanol produced in the United States is corn-based. Some see this as a disadvantage because the crop is food for humans and livestock and when used to produce ethanol, it causes a spike in food prices. The challenge of growing enough crops to meet the large demands of ethanol production is significant and, some say, insurmountable. Clear-cutting land (such as rainforests) to plant crops to make ethanol is considered unsustainable and irresponsible.

Corn farming involves heavy inputs of nitrogen fertilizer (made with natural gas), applications of herbicides and other chemicals (made mostly from oil), heavy machinery (which runs on diesel), and transportation (diesel again).

Ethanol prices are not very stable and fluctuate, so ethanol is sometimes cheaper but sometimes more expensive than gasoline, by as much as forty cents per gallon. Distribution is very uneven and states located far from processing centers pay more for the fuel.

Ethanol has to be mixed with gasoline, which produces aldehydes, which are carcinogens. The blending of ethanol is not uniform, either, though there are test kits available to check ethanol content. Ethanol gasoline can cause problems by dissolving and hardening plastic and rubber components of fuel systems, and absorbs water that may cause rust and corrosion, especially in small engines, such as those in lawnmowers.

Producing ethanol is not economically feasible in the long run because it is not energy-efficient. It takes 1.3 gallons of ethanol to do the work of one gallon of gas.

METHANOL

Also known as wood alcohol or wood naphtha, methanol is a light, colorless, flammable liquid with a distinctive odor very similar to ethanol. Originally, the production of methanol came from coal. Today, it is produced from the methane component in natural gas, and can be mined as a mineral as huge deposits are on the ocean bed. Renewable methanol refers to any type of methanol produced from non-fossil fuels that come from municipal waste, industrial waste, biomass, and carbon dioxide. As much as 30 percent of landfill material in the United States is organic waste, creating methane—which is both good and bad.

Pros: Methanol can be produced from carbon dioxide culled from industries, preventing that gas from entering the atmosphere. Renewable methanol offers carbon- and GHG-reduction benefits ranging from 65 to 95 percent. It also displaces large amounts of gasoline and diesel, and reduces nitrogen oxides as well as volatile organic compounds that form ground-level ozone or smog. Methanol can be also created from natural gas or biogas, making it very flexible and versatile as an energy source.

Researchers at Sandia National Laboratories in New Mexico have found a way of using sunlight to recycle carbon dioxide and produce fuels such as methanol. Scientists at the National Aeronautics and Space Administration's Jet Propulsion Laboratory in Pasadena, California, have developed a direct methanol fuel cell technology that uses liquid methanol to produce electricity.

Methanol burns 75 percent more slowly than gasoline, and methanol fires release heat at 20 percent the rate of gasoline, making it far safer and cooler when it burns.

Cons: Plants for generation of methanol are expensive—approximately 1.8 times that of an equivalent energy output. Methanol can be dangerous since the liquid can be absorbed through the skin and toxic vapors through inhalation.

Methanol may be much less volatile than gasoline, but it only produces roughly 50 percent of the energy and delivers fewer miles per gallon than gasoline. At present there is a low demand in US production of methanol; however, demand is likely to increase over the next several years as a gasoline additive.

BURN, BABY, BURN

High-tech incineration is not simply about burning things to create heat, but is rather a high-tech way to use garbage to create energy. The heat produced by an incinerator is used to generate steam, which may then be used to drive a turbine in order to produce electricity. There is a debate whether incineration is a beneficial renewable energy, and whether or not it releases damaging GHG emissions.

A more accurate description for this high-tech incineration is "plasma gasification." The heat of ionized gas can range upward of 27,000°F, vaporizing garbage that passes through it. However, most run at 1,800°F. According to the EPA, 12.5 percent of solid waste in the United States was incinerated in 2012 for energy; the other 65 percent was dumped in landfills.

There are only eighty-seven trash-burning power plants in the United States, and almost all were built at least fifteen years ago. Twenty-four states and some federal laws have categorized waste-to-energy as a renewable resource eligible for subsidies. No new waste-to-energy plants are being planned or built in the United States, according to the EPA. There is an incinerator in Minneapolis that generates enough energy, via a steam turbine, to power 24,000 homes and heat a sports stadium. It produces no pollutants, combustion flames, or smoke, only minor toxic emissions or offensive odor, and meets all of the EPA's standards.

Pros: Many consider municipal waste a constant supply, categorizing incinerating it as a renewable resource. Waste-to-energy incinerators consume more garbage than a normal incinerator and produce less pollution, while producing almost as much power as a coal-fired power plant. However, the cost-efficiency of incineration does depend on keeping an expensive plant working constantly. A 2009 study by the EPA and North Carolina State University scientists favored waste-to-energy plants over landfills as the most environmentally friendly use for urban waste that cannot be recycled. With incineration, the volume of the uncompressed garbage at landfills can be reduced by approximately 70 percent.

Incineration also offers strong benefits for the treatment of certain waste types in niche areas such as clinical wastes and certain hazardous wastes where pathogens and toxins can be destroyed by high temperatures.

The Delaware Solid Waste Authority found that, for the same amount of energy, incineration plants emitted fewer particles, hydrocarbons, and other GHGs than coal-fired power plants, but more than natural gas–fired power plants. The EPA claims that embracing incineration technology could not only reduce toxic emissions (technologically improved filters can catch pollutants, from mercury to dioxin), but also yield copious amounts of electricity. The end products of the process are inorganic solids that can be used to make asphalt, concrete, and gypsum.

Cons: Many believe that more than 90 percent of materials currently disposed of in incinerators and landfills can be reused, recycled, and composted. Providing subsidies or incentives for incineration encourages local governments to destroy these materials, rather than investing in environmentally sound and energy-conserving practices like recycling and composting.

One of the reasons that waste-to-energy plants are not used in the United States is the relative abundance of cheap landfills. Landfills only charge municipalities an average of $35 per ton of trash, compared to disposing a ton of garbage at a plasma gasification plant at $172 per ton. Also, if there is not enough garbage to reach a power plant's maximum capacity, it won't produce maximum potential power, increasing cost.

Incineration plants are expensive to build, operate, and maintain, they produce moderate pollution, and they have the highest capital cost among the twenty-six different ways to generate electricity. Older incinerators emit varying levels of heavy metals such as vanadium, manganese, chromium, nickel, arsenic, mercury, lead, and cadmium, which can be toxic at very minute levels.

Harrisburg, Pennsylvania, has been flirting with bankruptcy because of a $300 million loan it took to reopen and refit an old public incinerator with new technology. In Maryland, the price tag for one 1,500-ton-per-day incinerator is more than $500 million, twenty-five times more than a similarly sized recycling facility.

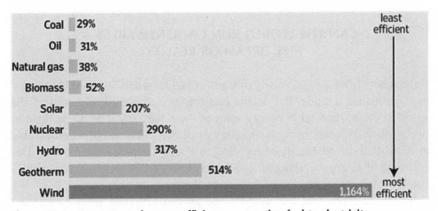

Figure 26.6 Percentage of energy efficiency converting fuel to electricity.
Source: blogswaj.gov

BUY RIGHT AND SAVE—YOUR RIGHT TO CHOOSE

The price of almost all kinds of fuel fluctuates over the course of the year. If you use heating fuels such as fuel oil and propane, purchasing them in the summer often means you'll pay less per gallon than you would if you waited until fall to fill up.

Most people believe that the local energy utilities have to provide power at non-negotiable rates. That changed in 1992 when Congress passed the National Energy Policy Act, opening the energy industry to competition. For years the utility companies had a monopoly and without much resistance they could charge what they wanted.

Deregulation, tax exemptions, and incentives offered by the government, along with sustainable or renewable resources, are encouraging people to take electricity matters into their own hands and effectively change their electrical resources. Companies that offer the power of choice and manage customers' customized energy needs will aid in searching for the best, cleanest, most inexpensive source of energy.

An increasing number of power companies are offering the choice of an independent contractor or an energy service company that constantly shops for the best wholesale prices to keep your costs down, using an alternative form of energy. Your local utility owns the power lines that carry electricity and they will continue to bill you for the delivery of the electricity source of choice, but they cannot add extra fees, and will remain responsible for the safety, reliability, and delivery of electricity, and will be governed by the state regulatory commissions.

CAN THE WORLD RUN ON RENEWABLES— PIPE DREAM OR REALITY?

Researchers from the University of California, Davis and Stanford University have published a study that details one scenario to completely convert the world to clean, renewable energy sources—and they say it could be done in twenty to forty years using technology available today at costs comparable to fossil fuel–based energy. According to a recent report posted by the Department of Energy's National Renewable Energy Lab (NREL), renewables could contribute 80 percent of American electricity by the year 2050.

Scientists claim that the world's energy can originate from 50 percent wind, 40 percent solar, 4 percent geothermal, 4 percent hydroelectric, and 2 percent wave and tidal power. Your choice may change the way power is produced, bought, and sustained in the future.

27

The Grid

The Arteries of Energy

Energy is the largest industry on Earth, powering the world's unquenchable need for power. Catastrophic and unpredictable weather events, terrorism, resource shortages, shifting economic centers, and a decrepit power grid are events that interfere with energy and its delivery. Think back to the gas shortages of 1979 and the power brownouts and blackouts of the 1990s that caused billions in economic damage, and then were forgotten about a short time later.

FACTS AND FIGURES

Reliable and inexpensive electricity is a basic building block of modern society. You can live without your television, your computer, and even your cell phone for days (but try to find a coin-operated phone booth). For most of us being cut off from electricity would be like living in the Stone Age.

For many generations, there has been a kind of social compact with power companies and their customers. It boiled down to a single phrase: "Pay your bill and when you hit the switch, the power will be there." For several generations, that compact worked well. But the arteries of that compact are suffering a serious case of arteriosclerosis.

The US national power grid is a Frankenstein-like creation, grafted and sutured together on an outdated electrical framework, assembled via early twentieth-century engineering technology, fueled by the need for power during and after WWII with many sections depending on one another and sometimes failing in a cascading manner. This system has kept us out of the dark for some time, but it's succumbing to senescence, decay, and overload; there is no light at the end of the tunnel and retrofitting, replacement, and repair could cost as much as $2 trillion. Those estimates do not include the costs of building new and expanded high-voltage transmission systems, including 160 million wooden power poles. That would tack on another $100 billion. Building a new power grid could create nearly two million jobs during tough economic times.

The power grid is our interstate highway of energy, an interconnecting road-map of high-voltage wires delivering electricity from power plants to users that functions by two primary systems: power plants and the distribution system. It is a complex network of independently owned and operated power plants and transmission lines regulated and monitored by the nonprofit North American Electric Reliability Corporation (NERC). Under NERC's jurisdiction are the users, owners, and operators of the bulk power system (BPS), which serves more than 334 million people from Canada to Baja California, Mexico.

Electrical energy is regulated in terms of demand, the system powering up when one region peaks and lowering when demand is lessened. In this way, electricity can be maintained at a steady level across many districts. This aids petroleum-based power plants, enabling them to be more efficient and to operate at constant production levels. Other types of intermittent alternative energy can be stored via various methods (such as stored water to run a hydroelectric plant, and wind turbine or solar charged batteries) for future use. These natural energy sources are by nature unpredictable, depending heavily on factors such as water, wind, weather, and available sunlight.

In addition, the country's copper-based electric grid is estimated to leak electricity at 7 percent and in some instances it can be as much as 60 percent of the electricity that is transmitted in the United States annually. Today, the US power grid has been given a grade of "D" by the American Society of Civil Engineers (ASCE). Power grids can lose up to 40 percent of the power they generate at a cost of approximately $20 billion a year. The Electric Power Research Institute (EPRI) estimates that electricity disruptions cost the economy upward of $150 billion each year in damages and lost business. With power plants usually located far from where the electricity is used, this adds up to a lot of wasted power.

The number of minutes without power in the country from 2002 to 2011 has risen from 97 to 112 annually, while cost for such loss has risen from $163 to $232 per customer.

An interconnected grid can work well as a distribution system because it allows for sharing, a double-edged sword. If one power company needs to take a power plant or a transmission tower offline for maintenance, the other parts of the grid can pick up the slack and power can be diverted to wherever it's needed. However there are times, particularly at peak demand, that the nature of the patchwork grid makes the entire system vulnerable to collapse.

The US power grid is the largest business investment by man in history. The National Academy of Engineering (NAE) named the early United States power grid the most impressive, largest engineering and construction project undertaken by man.

Most of the nearly 500,000 miles of transmission lines were built fifty or more years ago. In the last decade, demand for electricity increased by about 25 percent, the construction of transmission facilities decreased about 30 percent, and blackouts and brownouts have doubled in that time; it's been estimated that we will need another 30 percent more power in the next two-and-a-half decades.

American citizens will experience 214 minutes of blackout each year. The US power grid fails more often and for longer than its counterparts in Europe and Japan. Deerfield, Illinois, has the dubious honor of being the blackout capital of the United States. It has suffered more than 1,400 blackouts since the turn of the century, of which 83 percent are due to infrastructure failures.

Fifty-five million people in a nine-state area in the northeastern United States and Canada in 2003 were without electricity due to infrastructure failure caused by a sagging power line. It shorted out on a tree, causing a "cascade effect," taking out electricity for people in eight states and parts of Canada and causing $6 billion in damages.

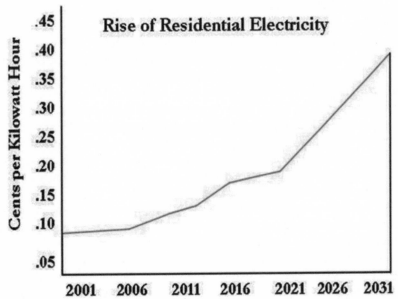

Figure 27.1.   Rise of residential electricity use.
Source: Provided by the author.

Most utility companies hear about power failures when they get calls from their customers. A smart grid will alleviate that. But without major expenditures we may face power rationing in the next couple of decades. Climate change affecting weather patterns and increasing demand are only going to exacerbate the problems. A smart grid will enable better control, will give us the ability to lower the energy used by our smart electronic devices, and will allow our appliances and home energy systems to feed energy back into the system during peak use or emergencies.

Congress is never in the political mood for the kinds of expenditures required to reprocess our grid. However, expanding and securing our national power grid is not a question of "if," but of "when." The United States without power is an America literally in the dark.

HOLD-UPS IN CONSTRUCTION

The power grid in the US infrastructure has not been appreciably upscaled or renovated for decades and has broken down in the recent past; it needs to be replaced in the near future. The grid is a highly complicated mechanism with approximately 3,500 utilities, 14,000 substations, half-a-million miles of lines, thousands of power plants, and tens of thousands of transformers. It is exposed to the weather, the landscape, and is under constant stress, deteriorating a little bit every day.

Many factors have forced a slowdown in the construction of new US power plants. Coal is seen as both friend and foe. Fear of nuclear power, especially after the 2011 Japanese tsunami, has been revived in many people. In addition, the NIMBYs (Not In My Back Yard) and the BANANAs (Build Absolutely Nothing Anywhere Near Anything) have issues about eco-problems such as noise, GHG emissions, transmission lines, increased traffic, transportation of hazardous substances, terrorism, and ruining property views. Against this backdrop are the escalating needs of an energy-hungry public and conservationists who are trying to reduce the vast amount of power wasted in Americans' homes and offices.

The national power grid, the most important segment of our energy infrastructure, is not properly protected against terrorism, either physical or computer-directed. A carefully planned attack on the grid could deny large regions of the country access to bulk power for weeks or even months, according to *Forbes* magazine and could also result in hundreds or even thousands of deaths due to heat stress or extended exposure to extreme cold, or doing without necessary power. It would cause billions of dollars of damage especially if combined with extreme weather.

A new grid would do a far better job of connecting users to sources of energy utilizing "smart" technology, including a far more efficient real-time metering system of energy "stockpiling" that would help prevent power outages and aid in averting security threats.

Researchers have made a pivotal breakthrough using cable made up of nanotubes, cylinders made up of atomic particles of different materials whose diameter is around one to a few billionths of a meter, as they can carry electricity over long distances with negligible loss.

Another answer is to "get smart" with the construction of a digital, information-age technology system that connects everyone to reliable, efficient, abundant, affordable, clean, and secure electric power anytime, anywhere. An intelligent answer can be realized through a "smart grid" which integrates advanced digital computing functions into the nation's electrical power network while contributing to the goal of reducing carbon emissions.

28

The Change

Petroleum Penance and the Price of Fossil Fuels

FACTS AND FIGURES

Love it or loathe it, the carbon atom has given people, especially Americans, a very abundant, cheap source of energy and the world's best lifestyle. However, burning so much petro-fuel has left us with consequences which we ignored and didn't plan for—the fallouts of pollution, attendant health problems, and the possibility of accelerating us toward a new ice age.

Climate change is not a new thing, it's been happening for hundreds of millions of years; it's part of our planet's biological clock. Sometimes the change is immense, other times it's minor on a geologic timeline. In addition, the key to the thermostat of the Earth is carbon dioxide. When the Earth and the atmosphere are flooded with CO_2, it causes anoxia, an extreme form of "low oxygen," which warms the planet. It is believed anoxic events are strongly linked to the slowing of ocean circulation, climatic warming, and elevated levels of greenhouse gases caused in the past by volcanic action and the release of CO_2 as the "central external trigger for euxinia" (the loss of oxygen).

In our primeval past, it caused catastrophic and colossal climate change when the Earth was a gigantic green hothouse, melting the ice caps, rising sea levels, and making the oceans and both poles tropic, but not livable. The last colossal warming episode of about 100,000 years ago lasted about 250,000 years and is called an interglacial age or the greenhouse end effect.

An example of what can happen when too much greenhouse gas enters the atmosphere happened as recently as 1275 when there was massive volcanic action, which triggered a chain reaction affecting sea ice and ocean currents in a way that lowered temperatures for centuries. The volcanic ash would

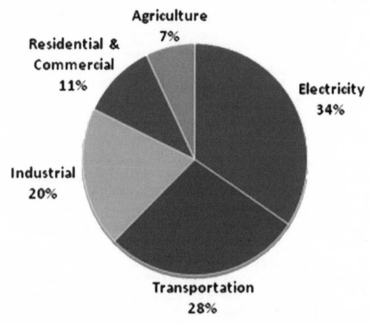

Figure 28.1. Activity generation of greenhouse gases.
Source: U.S. Environmental Protection Agency.

have darkened the atmosphere causing temperatures to drop. In fact, there was snow in Europe and people were ice skating on the River Thames in July.

Although this happened in the past as part of a natural phenomenon, the amount of carbon dioxide in the atmosphere at present is increasing at a rate exponentially faster than ever before and has doubled since the industrial revolution. If it doubles again within the next one hundred years, some scientists believe we may face the tipping point of causing irreversible climate change. And we still have more than enough fossil fuel to discharge sufficient carbon dioxide into the air to make that change a fait accompli.

Water vapor, which occurs almost 100 percent naturally, constitutes Earth's most significant greenhouse gas, accounting for the majority of Earth's greenhouse effect. Interestingly, many "facts and figures" regarding global warming completely ignore the powerful effects of water vapor in the greenhouse system, carelessly overstating human impacts on the environment as much as twentyfold.

However, Andrew Dessler and colleagues from Texas A&M University believe that the heat-amplifying effect of water vapor is potent enough to double the climate warming caused by increased levels of greenhouse gases the atmosphere. When you add carbon dioxide to the atmosphere, warming will result.

Table 28.1.   Growth in Residential Carbon Dioxide Emissions

Pollutant	Natural Gas	Oil	Coal
Carbon Dioxide	117,000	164,000	208,000
Carbon Monoxide	40	33	208
Nitrogen Oxides	92	448	457
Sulfur Dioxide	1	1,122	2,591
Particulates	7	84	2,744

Source: US Energy Information Administration

The answer to this problem may seem obvious—simply slow down the use of fossil fuels—but it's not that easy. The dilemma is with countries like China and India that are becoming industrialized giants creating escalating appetites for first-world affluence: guzzling gas in petro-driven vehicles, constructing hyper highways leading to a glut of suburban and urban spread, and building scores of new fossil fuel–burning power plants to feed this growth, reflecting their escalating addiction to energy.

In any case, the debate rages on about which data is right and what outcome is real. No one knows for certain what's going to happen in the next century, but it's a good bet that we have to do two simple things: support and push for alternative energy sources and practice conservation of our resources. We hope this book will help educate and offer some simple, but significant, solutions and suggestions for a more sustainable life on Earth.

FACTS AND FIGURES

- Industry, electric power generation, agriculture, and transportation are the four top sources of greenhouse gases.
- The main greenhouse gases contributing to global warming are those consisting of water vapor, carbon dioxide (CO_2), methane (CH_4), nitrous oxide (N_2O), and miscellaneous other gases.
- China is now the largest producer of greenhouse gases in the world. In 1990, China and India together accounted for 13 percent of world carbon dioxide emissions. In 2007, China and India's combined share of GHGs had risen to 26 percent, largely because of their strong economic growth fueled by their increasing use of coal.
- In 2035, it's predicted that carbon dioxide emissions from China will account for 31 percent of the world total.
- China, the United States, and India have announced CO_2 reduction targets from 25 to 40 percent by 2020.

- It's predicted that world energy-related carbon dioxide emissions will grow from 29.7 billion metric tons in 2007 to 33.8 billion metric tons in 2020 and 42.4 billion metric tons in 2035, almost a 13 percent increase in twenty-two years.
- At the present rate, coal's share of world carbon dioxide emissions, which grew from 39 percent in 1990 to 42 percent in 2007, will increase to almost 46 percent by 2035.
- Between 1990 and 2004, US emissions of carbon dioxide increased 15.8 percent.
- Topping off the warmest decade in history, 2010 experienced a global average temperature of 58.3 degrees Fahrenheit (14.63 degrees Celsius), tying 2005 as the hottest year in 131 years of recordkeeping.
- The fourteen hottest years on record have all happened in the last fifteen years. Average temperatures in the northern hemisphere in the last fifty years were higher than in any other such period in the last 500 to 1,300 years.
- The multinational Arctic Climate Impact Assessment (ACIA) report concludes that in Alaska, western Canada, and eastern Russia, average temperatures have increased as much as 4 to 7 degrees Fahrenheit (3 to 4 degrees Celsius) in the past fifty years.

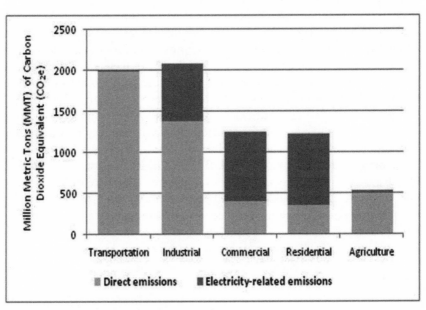

Figure 28.2.   US Fossil Fuel Emission Levels.

- The concentration of carbon dioxide in the atmosphere has risen from 290 parts per million in 1900 to nearly 400 ppm today.
- Carbon dioxide has a very long lifetime. It remains in the atmosphere for several thousand years. Currently, CO_2 emissions contribute 64 percent of the total greenhouse gas emissions and are rising.
- The rate of sea level rising from 1993 to 2003 was 42 percent faster than the rate from 1961 to 2003.
- Experts forecast higher prices for agricultural commodities due to potential factors such as climate change, price of gas, and increasing scarcity of water.

RESIDENTIAL AND COMMERCIAL OPPORTUNITIES TO REDUCE POLLUTION

Landfill waste, and the pollution it causes when decomposing, can be reduced and exploited as an energy source by capturing greenhouse gases and preventing them from being released into the atmosphere. We can lower emissions by choosing lower-carbon options such as using local products that don't have to be transported, materials that impound carbon, and materials manufactured at "green" industrial facilities.

Improving building design and construction by using natural light, shade, and ventilation reduces the need for light fixtures and HVAC appliances. Additionally, we can go on "energy diets," improve and adopt energy efficiency via the use of efficient appliances, and employ other techniques to minimize energy consumption and the associated greenhouse gas emissions from electricity produced by fossil fuels. Adhering to conservation guidelines, reducing the use of appliances, artificial lighting, and HVAC equipment, selecting smaller residential and commercial spaces, and reducing the energy required for building construction and operation will all help to lower pollution levels.

Importantly, refuse to be doomed. We have heard naysayers before. And we have overcome enormous problems in the past. The pace of things, most importantly regarding our attitudes about how and when productive and redemptive change is going to take place, is quickening. Let's keep a positive attitude and hope that those in generations to come might pick up this book and benignly smile about past problems that have already been overcome.

29

Pools, Hot Tubs, and Spas

Pooling Your Resources

During summer it gets blazing hot in most towns. The most popular kid on the block during summer isn't a good athlete, terribly smart, or overly attractive. But his family has the only pool in the neighborhood. Much to the consternation of his mother, their backyard becomes a kind of meeting place when the sun is high in the sky and the days are scorchers.

Children will stay in the pool late into the day, ignoring parents' protestations until their flesh is pruned, limbs become numb with exertion, jaws involuntarily start chattering, eyes become bloodshot with chlorine, and lips turn ice-blue from the chill water. They love it.

Of course kids don't have to clean the pool, chlorinate the water, change the filters, or pay the water and power bills, that's for the grown-ups. Perhaps this chapter will offer hints and secrets about how to lower the costs of a family pool, spa, or hot tub, making them just as enjoyable and more economical.

Millions of people, and even monkeys in Japan in winter, look forward to a hot dip and a simmer that will remove physical cricks from a body, turning it from kinked and cable-like into warm pasta. But it takes some intelligence and care to ensure a safe and economical soak.

FACTS AND FIGURES

It's estimated that close to 10 percent of all residences in the United States have swimming pools. In many homes during the summer, pools are the largest consumers of water and energy. Heating water is the overwhelming single-largest source of energy use for pools and is a significant and largely

247

untapped energy savings opportunity. Heating, pumping, and filtration are responsible for 70 percent of the energy used to operate a typical pool.

In California, pools consume the energy output of one medium-sized power plant, and heated pool water could cover the city of San Francisco by seven feet and uses twice the amount of energy as Chicago in summer.

Water evaporation and "splash out" during the summer accounts for more than 70 percent of total energy lost in both outdoor and indoor pools and can average 80 to 200 gallons per week, or about 2 to 5 percent volume of a typical medium-sized pool.

The American Red Cross recommends 78°F as the water temperature for competitive swimming. However, this may be too cool for young children and the elderly, who may require 80° to 84°F to be comfortable. Almost all of a pool's heat loss—about 95 percent—occurs at the surface. Raising the water temperature just 1°F can cost an additional 10 to 30 percent of energy annually to run a pool depending on location. It costs three times as much energy to run a pool heater as a home furnace.

On average, an energy-efficient pump will use 30 to 45 percent less energy than a older pump. If 100,000 swimming pools had more energy-efficient filtration systems, global demand for electricity would be reduced by 102,000 megawatts per year, enough to power roughly 800,000 homes each day.

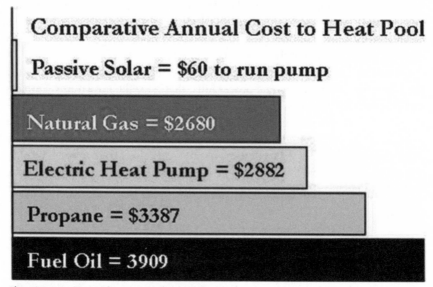

Comparative Annual Cost to Heat Pool

Passive Solar = $60 to run pump

Natural Gas = $2680

Electric Heat Pump = $2882

Propane = $3387

Fuel Oil = 3909

Figure 29.1.   Annual cost to a heat pool.
Source: Provided by the author.

MAINTENANCE

Maintenance costs for a pool are far less expensive if you do it yourself. Up-keep costs should run about $300 to $1,000 per year depending on the size of the pool. Pool maintenance companies will suggest they come from once a week to twice a month, depending on the season and the use of the pool, which can run from $75 to $165 per month.

Probably the most widely used chemical for sanitization in pools is chlorine. It destroys algae, bacteria, and any other unhealthy organic matter in the water. An inexpensive chemical kit should be used to test the water when adding chlorine or adjusting pH levels. Chlorine comes in granular, tablet, and liquid form, and is used in about a 15 percent solution.

Use a grease pencil to mark the water level of your pool at the skimmer. Examine the mark 24 hours later to check for leaks, keeping in mind evaporation and "splash out" water, which can account for up to three-quarters of an inch. When back-flushing the pool, use the water for landscaping. There should be no effect on plants and animals, which can tolerate the concentrations that are recommended for pool water. Saltwater from pools will not adversely affect plants.

A solar-powered heating system can cut pool energy usage by 5 to 10 percent and has very low operating costs. Solar heating systems can also raise pool water temperatures 10° to 20°F inexpensively. Passive solar heating systems start at around $3,000, but price depends on use, size of the pool, and other factors. Pool heaters can prove to be a source of wasted energy, but an energy-efficient pool heater could save 50 to 80 percent of the pool's heating expenses.

Turn down the pool heater when the pool is not in use. Keep a thermometer in the water and set your thermostat to the lowest temperature that still maintains a comfortable swimming setting. Mark the "comfort setting" on the thermostat dial to avoid accidental or careless overheating. Lower the thermostat setting to 70°F when the pool is to be unused for three or four days. For longer periods, shut the pool heater off. Get your pool heater tuned up annually as a properly tuned pool heater will operate more efficiently.

Make use of the sun by locating your pool in the sunniest part of the yard avoiding overhead plants and trees. If possible, screen it from the cooling, prevailing wind with existing structures such as the house or garage, or add a solidly built fence as a windbreak, as even modest winds increase evaporation rates. A mere 7 mph wind on the pool surface can increase energy consumption by 300 percent.

PUMPS AND FILTERS

The swimming pool pump is one of the biggest energy consumers for the home. A two-speed pump can cut energy use by 50 percent. Make sure your swimming pools, fountains, and ponds are equipped with recirculating pumps or you are going to waste a lot of water. Use a timer on your pump—many pumps waste energy by running too much or all day.

In the United States, the average cost of electricity is about $60 to $90 per month for a residential pool. By reducing filtering hours to four hours per day (which uses 196 kWh monthly), a pool owner realizes a monthly savings of 392 kWh, or about $40 per month.

POOL COVERS

The single-most inexpensive and effective means of reducing the pool costs is simply using a pool cover, which can save energy and can keep the water in the pool an average of 10°F warmer, cutting summertime pool heating costs by up to 90 percent. Pool covers only cost between $85 and $250 for most residential pools. However, a well-built security cover can cost up to $3,000 and last up to fifteen years. A cover also reduces water and chemical evaporation by up to 70 percent, saving nearly 1,000 gallons of water per month. A cover will help keep pools clean, which means less filter pump use, less maintenance, and more money saved.

SALTWATER VERSUS CHLORINE (FOR POOLS AND SPAS)

Just as in pools, salt in the spa water is converted into natural chlorine sanitizing the water. It doesn't need much salt—as low as one-thirtieth the salinity of the ocean—or somewhere between tap water and what's in a typical contact lens saline solution. In fact, you won't even taste it. And most saltwater systems will require the salt system to be checked only once a month.

A chlorine generator is a filtering system that eliminates buying chlorine. First, the pool water must be converted from a freshwater to what is called a "saltwater pool." Converting from a chlorine to a saltwater pool calls for the installation of an in-line salt chlorine generator. It generally has two parts: the power unit that supplies DC power for electrolysis and the in-line electrolytic cell which converts diluted saltwater to chlorine. The parts can cost from $400 to $2,000 depending on the size of the pool and any extra accessories. If you're handy, it can be a fairly easy DIY project. If not, it might cost from $250 to $500 to have a salt unit installed. Twenty pounds of salt per 1,000 gallons of fresh water is added. A chlorine generator produces chlorine automatically using the pool water itself.

Salt Pros: In the ocean the salt concentration is between 20,000 to 35,000 parts per million, in a saltwater pool, it's just 3,000 to 6,000. Salt kills algae and germs, creates no chemical smell, and takes less time to maintain than a chlorine-maintained pool. Pool water from a saltwater pool is safer for family and pets, and is less harsh on your skin and hair. A salt pool also saves maintenance time.

Saltwater pools are becoming more popular than chlorine pools as the system is more energy-efficient. A 40-pound bag of salt costs $6 to $9 and needs to be replaced roughly once a month. The costs of maintaining a saltwater pool are less than chlorine, and they are easier to care for.

Salt Cons: There is a higher initial cost when installing or switching to a salt system. It costs from $1,000 to $3,000 to retrofit an existing pool from chlorine to saltwater. Saltwater is more expensive when installed, but afterwards it saves the cost of chlorine, which adds up to about $200 per summer.

Saltwater pools take longer than chlorinated pools to balance if bacteria are present. The salt in the water is corrosive to cement, which constitutes the surface of the pool. It should be checked yearly for pitting. Pool components and equipment will become damaged slightly faster with regular exposure to saltwater as well. The generator needed to maintain a saltwater pool system also requires electricity. The increased cost based on electricity should be taken into account when considering a conversion.

Chlorine Pros: There is a smaller up-front cost to install a chlorine system and the system is easy to operate—just add chlorine tablets to pump or floating device. Chlorine systems will clear the water up faster than a saltwater system if bacteria are present and chlorine pool water will not damage pool surfaces or decking.

Chlorine Cons: Chlorine has a strong odor and has to be maintained carefully in order to avoid sickness, bloodshot eyes, hair turning green, and stained clothing or irritated skin when using it. A balance of all chemicals is important in a chlorine-based pool. Every week a pH test should be conducted before chlorine is added. Chlorinated pools also have higher monthly pool chemical and maintenance costs. Some physicians claim that chlorine in pools is akin to secondhand smoke, especially in children. Chlorine byproducts are not healthy for those with allergies and asthma.

POOL SAFETY, LISTEN UP!

Approximately 260 children under the age of five drown in residential swimming pools and spas in the United States every year. Another 3,000 under the age of five are treated in hospital emergency rooms following pool accidents.

Think insurance; pools are considered an attractive nuisance. Locked pool fences are one of the more common means to ensure safety. Pool safety nets over the water provide a safe, secure barrier. A swimming pool net can typically be removed and replaced in about ten minutes. Safety covers, saving energy as well as lives, are anchored to a deck with straps that pull the cover tightly over the pool.

One of the latest safety features that can be added during a pool remodel is anti-entrapment equipment. Anti-entrapment equipment prevents hair, limbs, or other body parts from being sucked and pulled toward a pool drain.

A swimming pool can also be remodeled to include equipment to accommodate the injured, disabled, or elderly persons so that everyone can enjoy the curative powers of water therapy. Whenever young or elderly people are in the pool, a lifeguard should be present. Teach your children to swim as soon as possible. Many children are taught to swim before they can walk. Check the experience and ability of all children before going into the pool and always have an adult present whenever children are around.

HOT TUBS AND SPAS

The term "hot tub" originally referred to the wooden, barrel-shaped tubs, which became popular in the late 1960s, especially in California. When the industry began building tubs of molded fiberglass or with filters, thermoplastic shells, and high-speed jets, they were given the tag "spa" to differentiate them from their wooden cousins. Although hot tub is a generic term, Jacuzzi is a brand name, so all Jacuzzis are spas, but not all spas are Jacuzzis.

If your hot tub does not have an updated digital control system, upgrade it. Newer control systems can be quite affordable and will pay for themselves quickly.

HEATING AND PUMPING

Most tubs and spas come with electric heaters. A modern, well-insulated spa/hot tub with a quality insulated cover will cost, on average, only about a dollar to two dollars a day to operate, depending on heating source and power costs. An advantage of gas heating, besides rapid heating, is the lower cost of day-to-day operation since gas generally costs less than electricity to use.

There is no significant cost difference in heating with a 110-volt system versus a 220-volt system. For a truly "portable" installation, 110-volt is generally more practical, but a 220-volt system offers the advantage of faster heating, more power available to operate multiple motors, jets, lights, etc., and a properly hard-wired 220-volt system has no exterior cords to trip over or become unplugged. If your hot tub has a low-wattage, continuous circulation pump, leave it alone. It's designed to run all the time.

PUMP POWER

The more jets, the more horsepower required from the pumps, the higher the operating costs. An average-sized energy-efficient hot tub consumes 5 to 7 kWh per day, while a poorly insulated, inefficient hot tub may use 12 to 18 kWh per day. Depending on where you live, spas cost anywhere from $50 to $100 a month to operate, including chemicals.

To comply with certain energy-efficiency standards, the California Energy Commission (CEC) created Title 20. Not all hot tubs are made equally and not all are compliant with these energy standards, so do some research before making a purchase.

Circulation pumps use a smaller amount of electricity than jet pumps, so they will assist in lower monthly operating costs. They are also quieter to run than models that do not have circulation pumps, which may be nice if the spa is sitting outside the bedroom or on a deck. Models with circulation pumps usually cost more.

MAINTENANCE

CALCIUM HARDNESS (FOR SPAS AND POOLS)

Agents called flocculants are used in water treatment processes to improve the settling and filtering of particles to the bottom. It hardens the water, preventing it from slowly eating away and breaking down your hot tub's shell, pipes, and other parts. This chemical is inexpensive, can be easily located, and needs to be added at the beginning of every fresh refill.

The proper level for calcium hardness is 100 to 250 ppm.

THE WATER PH

To keep your sanitizer at the right level and working efficiently, you need to keep your water's pH balanced. This is a measurement of whether the water is too acidic (which could be corrosive) or too basic to interact with other chemicals. The pH is a measure of the acid or base of a solution. If your water has low pH, then your water will be acidic, like vinegar. If you water has high pH it will be dry, like baby powder.

Municipal water is chemically treated and has characteristics designed for the type of components found in household water systems, so it needs a little adjustment for the types of plumbing, pumps, heaters, and shells of a spa.

Use test strips for spa water (a typical bottle has fifty of them) by dipping it into the water and examining the color. Compare it to the color on the side of the bottle. The test strips will reveal whether you need to increase or decrease acidity or alkalinity. The correct pH will help extend the life of your spa. Keep a log and test the spa water two to four times per week. Make adjustments as needed to keep your levels in the proper ranges.

The proper pH Level should be between 7.4 and 7.6.

ALKALINITY

Alkalinity is a pH stabilizer which helps keeps your pH from changing drastically. First, adjust your alkalinity to the correct level, and then fine-tune your pH levels if needed. If both your pH and alkalinity levels are low, just adding alkalinity will increase both, but make sure to adjust the pH if the alkalinity doesn't bring it up to the correct level.

If both your pH and alkalinity levels are high, use pH decreaser to drop it back to the right level. These two chemicals are inexpensive but extremely important—especially in a hot tub. Because a hot tub has such a small body of water, the pH and alkalinity have a tendency to fluctuate a lot. It's important to keep a close eye on these levels by testing frequently.

A low pH and alkalinity will cause damage to your hot tub, especially your heater, because of the acidity of the water. High pH and alkalinity will cause scaling which leaves a milky residue around anything the water flows through, including the filter. The heater is at risk both ways. Acid will eat away at the heater element and the high pH will cause a scale around it, which will make it work harder to heat your hot tub.

The ideal level is 80 to 120 ppm.

SANITIZERS

Sanitizers are chemicals added to the water to kill standing bacteria and other germs and to ensure clean, clear water. Chlorine, bromine, baquanine, and mineral-based purifiers are all common water purification chemicals.

There are only four sanitizers approved by the EPA—chlorine, bromine, biguanide, and mineral sanitizers. Select only one. Once you pick one, there are several ways to get an appropriate amount in your spa. Here are some of the most popular options available.

Bromine

Up to 85 percent chlorine, bromine comes in tablets and powders that dissolve in the water. It's a little less irritating to people with sensitive skin than chlorine. Using a dispenser regulates the amount of bromine that is used. It's an easy system to understand. Tablets can reduce how many times per week you need to check your water. When using the powdered form, levels need frequent checking.

It's more effective at killing certain types of algae and bacteria and works well in a wide range of pH. However, the sun's UV rays eat up bromine very fast, and there is no additional chemical to help stabilize it like there is for chlorine. Consequently, it shouldn't be used in spas with direct sunlight.

The proper level for sanitation using tablets is 2 to 4 ppm; for sanitation (powder), it's 3 to 6 ppm.

Baqua Spa: The alternative sanitizer

A biguanide sanitizer is a liquid nonchlorinating product that kills bacteria much like chlorine and bromine do. It will make the water look "sparkly" and feel smoother. It calls for less frequent additions than chlorine and bromine and doesn't produce an odor.

It costs more than bromine and chlorine, and it may be hard to find. Not all pool and spa dealers carry these products. Check with your hot tub manufacturer before using it because biguanides are known to deteriorate some parts in your hot tub, including rubber gaskets and certain plastics.

The proper level for sanitation is 30 to 50 ppm.

Biguanide

Biguanide is a hydrogen peroxide–based system. Those who are sensitive to chlorine or bromine should try biguanide. It's typically less harsh and odorous than chlorine or bromine and most spas can use it.

It needs frequent manual testing that can be puzzling for some people. It's incompatible with other sanitizers, so users have to stay with the same brand of biguanide due to proprietary formulations, and the entire product line must be used, including biguanide formulated filter cleaners, stain and scale controllers, etc. It's also more expensive than its chlorine counterpart. To change to a different sanitizer, a spa must be drained, cleaned, and refilled.

Chlorine

It is probably the most commonly used sanitizer in spas and hot tubs as a destroyer of algae and bacteria. Chlorine comes in liquid or powdered form. Test strips designed for a spa using a chlorine sanitizer will show you if there is too much, not enough, or just the right amount. If the chlorine level is correct, there is very little noticeable odor.

It's fairly simple to use and to understand. However, it needs to be frequently checked, and small amounts have to be added repeatedly. High chlorine levels from manually added chlorine can irritate some people. Chlorine sometimes has an unpleasant odor, and undiluted liquid chlorine can burn skin and bleach fabric white. It's cost-effective, easy to manage and apply, and is a very aggressive bacteria killer.

The proper sanitation level is 1 to 3 ppm.

Mineral systems

This uses copper, silver, and other minerals to kill bacteria in the water, but it's slow and not as aggressive as chlorine. Along with using a mineral purifier in your tub, you will need to add a little bit of chlorine as a backup. It also helps to give the water a fresh smell. Without chlorine, the water would smell stale.

It's cost-effective, easy to manage, and uses a small amount of chlorine.

Mineral sanitizers area pellet-sized ceramic beads coated with silver. The container is placed in the water, within a filter or specially designed holder. The silver inhibits bacteria growth and usually lasts about four months and allows minimum use of chlorine. However, they can't be used with bromine.

The proper sanitation level is .05 ppm of chlorine.

MAINTENANCE

Use a mild, nonabrasive, non-sudsing cleaner and a soft rag or nylon scrubber to remove dirt build-up. Use common baking soda to clean small surface areas. A full cleaning of the waterline and surfaces can be done when the spa is drained. Just be sure not to use any old household cleaner or soap. Floating debris can be removed with a skimmer net. There are also spa vacuums available for the obsessive spa cleaners. Keep the spa clean, and drain and refill every two to four months.

On a once-weekly basis you will need to shock your hot tub by adding two to three tablespoons of shock oxidizers to get rid of accumulated chlorine compounds. Add this with the jets running and wait fifteen minutes. Test the water for bromine, pH, and alkalinity levels with your test kit or test strips. In general, you want your bromine level at 3 to 5 ppm. Right after you shock it, you may see a higher number, but it will settle.

COVER

The most significant energy-saving option is the hot tub cover, so make sure the tub or spa cover fits snugly. Use the straps to latch the cover when the hot tub is not in use; this will reduce heat leakage and provide a safety measure to keep children out.

Keeping a cover in good condition is essential because most heat loss will be through the surface of the water. Replace the cover if the interior foam is broken or water-soaked, which will increase energy consumption from heat loss.

Hot tub covers have different insulation values, but the basic rule of thumb is the denser the core of the cover and the thicker the cover, the better the heat retention. Standard hard covers are from two to four inches thick and have an insulating value of approximately R-12.

Hot tub spa covers cost around $300 to $500 dollars and usually only last about three years. About every two to four months, take the spa cover off and unzip the panels to let the foam dry and breathe. Use a cleaner such as Lysol to help cut down on the moldy smell the cover can produce.

First, remove the cover and spray it lightly with a garden hose to loosen any dirt or debris. Using a mild soap solution (one teaspoon of dishwashing liquid or two to three tablespoons of baking soda to two gallons of water), scrub the vinyl in a circular motion with a large sponge and rinse with a garden hose. Rinse the bottom of the cover without using soap, and wipe it clean with a dry rag. To condition the cover after cleaning, apply a vinyl protective coating on the top only so the cleaner's chemical agents don't get into the hot tub and affect the water's chemistry. To clean the underside of the cover, use a nonabrasive sponge for persistent dirt or stains. Let it air-dry on a warm or sunny day.

EXTERIOR

The acrylic shells on most hot tubs are simple to clean. They are nonporous surfaces, which means dirt and germs cannot penetrate them. Still, just like anything else that sits outdoors, the shell can get dusty. Wiping it down with a damp cloth periodically will keep your hot tub looking as nice as the day you bought it.

REPLACING YOUR SPA WATER

Soaps and detergents can build up in your spa to cause residue. Follow the instructions in your owner's manual and drain and refill the water in your spa to clear detergent and soap residue that may have accumulated over time.

USE A PRE-FILTER

When using a pre-filter, attach it to an ordinary garden hose to remove organic contaminants, metals like copper and iron, and tannins from your new water.

CLEANING/REPLACING THE SPA FILTER

Water needs to be able to flow easily through the filter in order for it to be heated and cleaned. The spa filter can be located under the skimmer basket and accessed from inside the spa, or it can be a small tank that is opened up underneath the spa to clean or replace the filter. If underneath the spa, you may have a valve that can be shut to prevent water from rushing out when you open the filter. Loosening a large nut or just turning the filter body counterclockwise is the usual method to access the filter cartridge.

Because mineral particles or calcification from hard water can clog any water filtration system, following these light cleaning tips each month to keep your spa's water flowing properly. Spray each cartridge with a garden hose, rotating while spraying to thoroughly remove any debris between filters, and keep them clean and in good operating condition. Replace your filters every three years.

Every six months, spa filters should soak overnight in a muriatic acid solution or a filter degreaser. Soak the filters overnight with one part acid to three parts water. Use a standard filter cleaner or degreaser, but be sure to rinse the filter until all of the cleaner is eliminated. Not rinsing the filters well will make the water foam.

If your spa filter has a pressure gauge attached to it, the cartridge needs cleaning when the pressure rises eight to ten pounds, or when flow is noticeably reduced. If you have no gauge on your filter, you should clean the filter on a regular schedule or every four to eight weeks, depending on how often the spa is used. Replace your spa filter every twelve to twenty-four months, again depending on usage, or change it every ten to fifteen cleanings, because that's what really breaks down a cartridge.

WINTERIZING YOUR SPA

Help keep the spa hot year-round, even in areas with freezing temperatures, by purchasing a vinyl-covered, fiberglass-insulated blanket for inside of the equipment compartment door. This is also an additional precaution against partial freezing of some of your spa's components while maximizing energy efficiency. Regularly brush snow off of your spa cover and splash warm water on ice rather than prying it off.

ON VACATION

Before you go, adjust the pH according to the owner's manual and sanitize the water. Lock the light and jets and spa cover to prevent access. When you return, balance the pH and sanitize the water prior to using. Keep your spa water clean from algae, bacteria, and other unwanted impurities by maintaining a safe amount of sanitizer. Be careful—too much sanitizer in your spa water may irritate your lungs, skin, and eyes.

Drain older, non-energy-efficient hot tubs when not in use over long periods of time. Hot tub water can freeze, which can cause damage to equipment. Repair any leaks and adjust jets so as not to send streams of water out of the tub. Hot tubs that are heavily used should be drained every three to four months. Use that water for plant irrigation.

ENERGY USE AND ECONOMY

To enhance heat retention, insulate the underside of the shell with high density foam. Some manufacturers also use lower-density foam, resulting in a less energy-efficient hot tub. If a kWh costs about $0.12 from your electric company, your energy cost for heating that much water in the winter is about $6.25 for a one-time use.

Turn on the tub in the morning for use that evening. If you're using the tub more than six or seven times a month, you may want to consider running it all the time and investing in a very high R-value cover for the hot tub. Set the hot tub heater thermostat to maintain 102°F, which is the temperature recommended by most health departments for adults and children. Heat water during off-peak times and reduce peak load cost. Program the tub timer to "off" during peak hours.

Set normal filtration cycles for single- and two-speed pumps for four hours, twice per day. Based on your usage pattern, reduce the filtration cycles to three hours twice a day—during off-peak hours so you can maintain clear, clean, and safe water.

Remember that a spa is an attractive nuisance, keep it closed off or tightly closed. Privacy panels, landscaping, or fencing can all be effective windbreaks; cutting wind exposure reduces the amount of energy needed to heat the spa.

30

The Garden and the Yard

Saving Gold in Your Greenery

AN OLD, ODD, AND IRONIC STORY

For eons nature was in balance and bountiful with trees, wildflowers, milk-weeds, and all green things were plentiful on Earth. They grew in any type of soil, withstood drought and floods, and multiplied with abandon. They shaded and held the land, and fed a multiplicity of animals; nectar from fragrant blos-soms attracted butterflies, honeybees, flocks of songbirds, and created a vast palette of natural colors and edibles, and everything acted in harmony.

Then people, who had also flourished, created towns and tried to tame na-ture. They labeled the natural plant life "weeds" and went to great lengths to annihilate and replace them with monochromatic grass and engineered plants that didn't attract and nourish animals and other creatures.

Lawns, for instance, are not very hardy, efficient, or in harmony with na-ture. They are vulnerable to climate and need prescribed amounts of water, plant food, and fertilizer. They require lots of attention and resources and fill a questionable need, except for those who insist on playing golf or croquet.

People go to great pains to grow their turf and shrubbery and keep them green. The ritual begins each spring with reseeding, fertilizing, and applying herbicides (many of which are toxic), and poisoning any plants or animals that breach the yard. The planned plants have to be mowed and cropped con-stantly. It's not a cash crop you can sell—but it costs a lot of cash to keep the garden growing and green. People rake up the clippings, put them in bags, and pay money to throw them away.

Then in the summer when rain diminishes and the heat increases, they pay more money to water so they can continue to mow and pay to get rid of the trimmings. When they need to "feed the foliage," they buy their clippings

261

back—now a part of what is called compost, fertilizer, or plant food—to help keep their gardens lush, and they use more chemicals to rid themselves of the animals that "nature" once fed. This keeps their property values high and neighborly status secure.

They also pay to have their trees and leaves removed. The same people later buy it back in a new form called mulch and spread it around to keep their plants healthy, in place of the leaves and bark from their trees that they threw away that kept their plants healthy. Many of these same people claim that they wish to protect and be in harmony with nature, because that is what is called "being environmental."

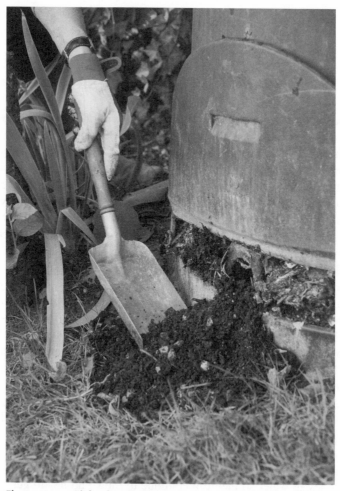

Figure 30.1.   Rich, clean compost.

FACTS AND FIGURES

Keep in mind the weather zone in which you live. For example, when living in an arid zone, it's best to use natural plants, which are going to be drought-resistant. You should expect to pay anywhere from 5 to 15 percent of your home's value on landscaping. Using the national median value of a home at about $215,000, this will translate to somewhere around $10,000 to $20,000.

By 2012, total estimated revenue of lawn and garden products in the United States was about $30 billion and the average spent was $350 annually per household. Last year the nationwide average spent on lawn and garden activities was $449, which was down from $457 the previous year and $466 the year before that. Of all the home outdoor water use (from 30 to 40 percent), half is used for lawns.

Think about garden to table. Building a raised bed (8' × 4') and filling it with compost and soil will run about $80. Buying veggies to put in the raised bed will cost you another $15 or $20. The average family with a vegetable garden spends just $70 a year on it and grows an estimated $600 worth of vegetables.

Just 48 percent of homeowners did their own lawn care last year, and even fewer (36 percent) have a flower garden or a vegetable garden (22 percent)—the lowest numbers in the last five years. Eleven million fewer households participated in gardening in 2010 than participated in 2005. However, the share of the nation's gardening time and budget spent by those over age fifty-five is actually increasing. In 2010, a whopping 70 percent of the nation's gardening time came from homes without children.

WATERING YOUR PLANTS AND VEGGIES

A good general garden guideline is an inch of water per week and twice that much in very hot climates. Plant in blocks instead of rows to create shade for the root systems and reduce evaporation. Group plants with similar water and plant needs. Check the soil for moisture before you water and do not water until the soil has dried out to a depth of at least four inches. Don't water wet soil. Get on your knees and weed. They compete with "planned plants" for water.

Inappropriate watering causes most of the root system to "drop off." The symptoms of a drowning plant are burnt leaf margins, leaf shedding, and terminal decline—oddly enough very much like the symptoms of drought stress. Drought-resistant plants only need to be watered once or twice a month with a minimum of four to five gallons each time.

PESTICIDES, HERBICIDES, AND FERTILIZERS

Approximately 4.4 billion pesticide treatments are made each year to US gardens and yards, adding up to 350 million pounds per year, some of which gets into the water table. Even though elevated levels of heavy metals are found in some inorganic fertilizers, the EPA has concluded that the hazardous materials in inorganic fertilizers generally do not pose risks to public health or the environment.

However, the Food Quality Protection Act (1996) recognizes that many of the chemicals used present unacceptably high health risks, particularly to infants and children. According to the Environmental Protection Agency, 60 percent of herbicides, 90 percent of fungicides, and 30 percent of insecticides are carcinogenic. They claim that only 1 percent reduces pests effectively.

The number and concentrations of pesticides found in household dust exceed those found in food, water, or air. Pesticide contamination in the home can persist for years, particularly in carpets, due to the lack of sun, rain, and other factors that help break down pesticides outdoors.

Earthworms are important for soil health, but where pesticides are used, 60 to 90 percent are killed. For flowerbeds, gardeners often use herbicides that prevent the germination of weed seeds, but will not affect any established plant and follow up immediately with mulch. But some of the preemergent herbicides are considered health and environmental hazards.

Corn gluten is a nontoxic byproduct of corn processing and kills weed seedlings within days of application. It also adds nitrogen to your soil. Just one application, before weeds emerge, reduces weed survival by 60 percent and increases garden growth.

Use a minimum amount of organic or slow-release fertilizer to promote a healthy and drought-tolerant landscape. Organic fertilizers have been known to improve the biodiversity of soil life and long-term productivity of soil, and may prove a large depository for excess carbon dioxide. Using organic nutrients (compost) increases the abundance of soil organisms by providing organic matter and micronutrients for organisms, which aid plants and can drastically reduce the need for energy, pesticides, and fertilizers, and increases water-holding capacity of the soil.

Organic pesticides are inexpensive and easy to make:

- Mix one teaspoon of liquid dishwashing detergent with one cup of vegetable oil. Shake vigorously to emulsify and add to a quart of tap water. Steep three tablespoons of dry, crushed hot pepper or hot sauce in one-half cup hot water (covered) for half an hour. Strain out the particles of peppers, and then mix with the solution.

- Use at ten-day intervals as an all-purpose spray for insects.
- Placing fist-size nylon bags of Milorganite organic fertilizer on 24-inch stakes camouflaged in the plants feeds them while keeping deer away.

Organic herbicides are also inexpensive to make:

- Try spraying vinegar directly on weeds, as this is a natural and safe alternative to chemicals. Take care not to spray any other plants, as the vinegar can harm them just as it does the weeds. Try one gallon white vinegar, one cup salt, one tablespoon dish soap. Use a spray bottle and make sure that every weed is coated with the mixture.
- Pouring boiling water over the weeds is also an option.
- Killing perennial weeds with any of these methods will take repeated applications to exhaust the nutrients stored in the root.

THE IMPORTANCE OF BEING MULCHED

Mulching reduces evaporation from the soil surface and reduces irrigation needs by approximately 50 percent. Organic mulch can be made from many materials, including rock, pumice, wood, newspaper, cardboard, straw, plant and tree material, and landscape fabric. For general landscape applications, use spun or woven permeable landscape fabrics rather than solid sheet plastics. Black or dark-colored plastic mulch conserves moisture and increases soil temperature in vegetable gardens.

Use organic material such as coconut coir (fiber), peat moss, or even plain old compost around plants. Mulch absorbs several times its own weight in water, thus retaining moisture that plants can use during dry spells. Use organic mulch to a depth of approximately four inches, depending upon the particle size of the mulching material.

Mulching aids in prevention and weed control and helps stop soil erosion. It protects roots from fluctuating and extreme temperatures. Grass clippings can be used as mulch in the vegetable garden. Do not use clippings from lawns treated with herbicides or other pesticides.

RESOURCEFUL X-LANDSCAPING

Think xeriscape—a landscaping philosophy that uses as many native, drought-resistant plants as possible and arranges them in efficient, water-saving ways. The next time you add or replace a flower or shrub, choose a drought-tolerant type. It could save up to 550 gallons of water each year. Converting to a water-efficient landscape through proper choice of plants and careful design can reduce outdoor water use by 20 to 50 percent, and improve the look of your landscape.

Five thousand square feet of bluegrass will require approximately 18,500 gallons a month, while Buffalo grass needs 3,000 gallons a month. Drought-resistant plants need only a few gallons a month. High-water-use plants will use much less water if they are located in a shady area with protection from wind.

Water plants deeply but less frequently to encourage deep root growth and drought tolerance. To decrease water from being wasted on sloping lawns, apply water top to bottom for five minutes and repeat two to three times. Water only when necessary. More plants die from overwatering than from underwatering. Adjust your watering schedule each month to match seasonal weather conditions and landscape requirements.

Choose shrubs and groundcovers instead of turf for hard-to-water areas such as steep slopes and isolated strips. Think small and plan big when buying plants. Smaller plants are far less expensive and will grow into your expectations. Use bricks and stones in place of lawn and plants.

Get into full-scale landscape design by doing it yourself. A landscape architect can cost a couple of hundred to thousands of dollars. Draw your own plan, and if need be, hire a landscape designer only to review it, lowering your cost for professional help. Save money by doing as much grunt work as possible yourself. A three-gallon bush may cost $20, but the price skyrockets to $40 or $50 when it's planted by a landscaping professional.

Segregating Plants by Use

Consult with your local nursery person for information on plant selection and placement for optimum outdoor water savings. Trees can be used as windbreaks and can reduce HVAC costs in winter and summer. Leave lower branches on trees and shrubs and allow leaf litter to accumulate on the soil. This keeps the soil cooler and reduces evaporation.

COMPOSTING: FROM SCRAPS TO SOIL

Composting doesn't have to be hard, smelly, dirty, or foul. Mother Nature is composting constantly and the finished product is dark, rich, earthy, clean, and sweet-smelling soil. Why pay premium prices that can cost $30 a yard or more (plus delivery) at the nursery or home improvement store? You have all the ingredients at home. Many American towns and cities are beginning to compost their green waste and offer it free to their citizens—call your city works department to see what they have to offer.

Yard and food discards make up approximately 30 percent of the waste stream in the country. And with a little effort, you can save money, help conserve energy, reuse resources, lighten the load of your local landfill, keep inorganic fertilizers out of your yard, and make plants happy and productive by feeding them, and therefore yourself, well.

Composting involves mixing yard and household organic waste (no meat products) in a pile or bin and providing conditions that encourage decomposition. It's a process fueled by millions of microbes that continuously recycle waste by producing a rich organic soil and fertilizer that will improve your garden's health and make it more resistant to infestations by pests or decimation by drought.

All you need to compost is a basic understanding of a few simple principles, and a little bit of elbow grease. Nature does the rest.

Ideally, start your composting in spring. Anything plant-based that was living at one time is great for compost bins, but too much of any one material will slow down the composting process. Compost all yard wastes, except for diseased plants or any plants that have been exposed to pesticides. Pay attention to the compost "heap" and keep it moving and damp.

A GARBAGE CAN = A HOMEMADE COMPOST BIN

Many ready-made kits are available on the Internet and in hardware stores and home improvement centers. But if you have a plastic garbage can (a 20-gallon can is priced around $15), it will work nicely. Along with the can you'll need an 8-penny or large nail and a hammer to poke enough holes in the garbage can to ensure complete circulation, as oxygen is critical to compost successfully, and two bricks or something that will prop the can off the ground. Place the can on top of the prop-ups and follow directions for getting started.

THE COMPOST DIET

The compost needs a balanced diet of nitrogen (green material) and carbon (brown material). A ratio that contains equal portions by weight (not volume) of both works best. An overload of any single type of material can throw off the balance of the pile and will compact it, slowing down the process and causing it to stink. Chop the materials as best you can as organic waste will turn into compost faster if it's in small pieces.

Carbon is aged manure, cottonseed meal, alfalfa meal, blood meal, shredded newspaper, cardboard (torn or shredded), straw, wood chips, and sawdust. These help jumpstart the microbes responsible for breaking down organic matter into compost.

Nitrogen comes from food scraps; eggshells, coffee grounds, fruit and vegetable scraps, and plant clippings are all outstanding materials. Adding kitchen scraps that are typically high in nitrogen helps heat up the compost pile and speeds up the composting process.

If you want a fast turnaround, create a "hot" compost pile by adding more nitrogen and moisture, and turning the heap regularly to improve the air circulation. If adding ashes to your compost bin, do it sparingly. They are alkaline and affect the pH of the pile. In contrast, add acidic materials including pine needles and oak leaves. Algae and seaweed make excellent additions to your compost pile. Be sure to rinse off any salt before using.

Even urine is acceptable; it's sterile and contains large amounts of urea, an excellent source of nitrogen for plants and also a good source of phosphorus and potassium, and is widely considered as good as or better than commercially available chemical fertilizers. You'll have to dilute—ten to fifteen parts water to one part urine.

GETTING STARTED

The first levels of compost piles can be placed in thin layers of alternating greens and browns; later they can all be thrown in together and mixed well. Place the more woody material at the bottom and between layers to help with air circulation. The green material is the next layer, about six inches thick. Top this with a six-inch layer of brown material.

Keep adding to the initial pile at regular intervals. When the can, heap, or bin is full, it will start to heat up as the decomposition process gets underway.

THE CRAFTING OF A COMPOST PILE

The perfect size for a compost pile is at least 3 feet × 3 feet × 3 feet. It's a manageable size to turn, and perfect for retaining heat while still allowing airflow. If composting with a pile, not a container, bigger is often better. Heat builds up with a big pile. Keep your compost pile in direct sunlight to continue the composting process through the winter. Hay bales can be used to further insulate the pile.

If composting with a tumbler, make sure to turn it when adding new materials. If composting with a pile, or in a static (nontumbling) compost bin, be sure to mix up the contents so that the pile gets oxygen and can break down effectively.

High temperatures are essential for destruction of pathogenic organisms and undesirable weed seeds. The optimum temperature range is 135° to 160°F for the composting process. Worms (found at nurseries) are great for compost piles, as they do a lot of the work for you. But give them some time to get accustomed to a new environment.

Sprinkle with water, but don't keep your compost too wet so that it gets soggy and starts to stink. Don't let the compost completely dry out. A compost pile needs moisture to keep the composting process active. Repeat steps until your layers reach about a three-foot thick compost pile. When the heap begins to cool down slightly, add water if it is drying out, turn to introduce oxygen and undecomposed material into the center, and to regenerate heating. The composting process is complete when mixing no longer produces heat in the pile, or generally about two to four months.

Soak finished compost in water to "brew" compost "tea," a nutrient-rich liquid that can be used for foliar feeding (technique of feeding plants by applying liquid fertilizer directly to their leaves), for starter plants, or to enrich basic watering.

Finished compost is usually less than half the volume of the materials you started with, but it's much denser. When finished it should look, feel, and smell like rich, dark soil. You should not be able to recognize or smell any of the items you used for compost. Apply finished compost to your garden about two to four weeks before you plant, giving the compost time to integrate and stabilize within the soil.

TURF WARES/TURF WARS: FACTS AND FIGURES

Americans spend $25 billion on lawns annually. According to the *Environmental Magazine*, the total area of lawn in America is about 40 million acres (about the size of Pennsylvania). The total area of lawn in America is increasing in size by roughly 2.1 million acres every year with an average lawn of about 5,000 square feet. It's unlikely lawns will be eliminated altogether, but you can reduce the area of your lawn through use of groundcovers, decks, patios, ornamental grasses, flowers, and shrubs. Some places, Los Angeles, for example, are actually paying residents to eliminate lawns because of water shortages.

When selecting a turf species, choose one that matches your climate and site conditions. "Eco-lawn" grass is a drought-resistant blend of grasses that requires little or no mowing and no fertilizer. To switch to this kind of lawn, simply cut your existing lawn as short as possible and overseed with eco-lawn seed.

Most lawns that are kept green all summer will need extra nitrogen. Nearly 50 percent of this can be supplied by leaving clippings on the lawn. The best time to apply the other 50 percent is mid- to late October. Instead of raking leaves, use a mulching lawn mower to shred the leaves and leave them on the lawn. By spring they will have decomposed, adding nutrients and organic matter to the soil.

Lawn aeration brings microorganisms to the surface that will eat most of the thatch (effluvia that gathers on the surface), allowing the roots to get deeper in the soil and fostering thicker grass which naturally kills weeds.

LAWN PROS AND CONS

Pros: Lawns can be stately and beautiful. A healthy lawn increases soil stability through its deep and expansive root structure, which reduces land degradation and erosion from wind and water. Soil health and stability are greatly reduced in the absence of root systems and organic matter from grass and other vegetation.

According to a Mississippi State University study, a healthy lawn has the same cooling effect as an 8.5-ton air conditioning compressor. About half of the heat energy directed to a grassy area is eliminated by evapotranspiration (moisture transferred from the land to the atmosphere by evaporation).

Nonvegetative surfaces (such as rock, artificial turf, cement) do not have the same cooling effect and in some cases, can actually create a mini "heat-island" effect, increasing the ground-level temperature.

Lawns act as carbon sinks, taking up carbon dioxide from the atmosphere, thereby playing a small role in managing climate change. The 40 million acres of lawns in the United States take up between 6 and 17 teragrams (a teragram is equal to one trillion grams) of carbon each year depending on how they are managed, according to NASA. Also, leaving grass clippings on the lawn increases carbon uptake.

Lawns act as natural filters taking up dust, pollutants, and particulate matter from the air and water (up to 12 million tons per year). Lawns also significantly reduce noise pollution, particularly in urban areas.

Cons: The average suburban lawn receives ten times as much chemical pesticide per acre as farmland. The chemically dependent lawn is more prone to disease and less able to handle stresses from drought, heat, and insects. The US EPA estimates that about 80 million US households dump nearly 90 million pounds of herbicides and pesticides on lawns each year.

The 2 percent of the US land surface that is covered in lawns accounts for only about 5 percent of the carbon dioxide absorbed by all plants (18 percent of municipal solid waste is composed of yard waste). The typical American lawn sucks up 10,000 gallons of supplemental water (nonrainwater) annually. Mowing the lawn actually reduces the plant's leaves, cutting down its ability to use photosynthesis.

Researchers in Seattle found a correlation between the pesticides polluting sampled streams and the use of lawn and garden chemicals. Of the thirty most commonly used lawn pesticides, sixteen pose serious hazards to birds, twenty-four are toxic to fish and aquatic organisms, and eleven have adverse effects on bees. Researchers reporting in the *Journal of the National Cancer Institute* found that exposure to garden pesticides can increase the risk of childhood leukemia almost sevenfold.

Like small children, pets can't read the "Keep Off—Pesticide Application" signs. A study revealed that exposure to lawns treated with herbicides four or more times a year doubled a dog's risk of canine lymphoma, while the *Journal of the American Veterinary Medical Association* reported that, when exposed to chemically treated lawns, some breeds of dogs were four to seven times more likely to suffer from bladder cancer.

WATERING THE TURF

If walking on the lawn leaves a footprint behind, or if it is an off color, that's a sign the grass needs water. The average American family uses 320 gallons of water per day for lawns during the growing season, much more water than the same size area planted with shrubs or groundcover. Don't sprinkle grass lightly; deep-soak it. Light watering can't get water down deep into the soil and encourages the grass to develop shallower roots making it less drought-resistant and more prone to winterkill and insect damage.

Lawns need an inch or two of water per week to thrive depending upon the climate and soil conditions. In dry areas, a regular watering at least once a week is important to maintain good plant health. First, water dry spots instead of the entire lawn. It's not necessary to water grass every day. Delay regular lawn-watering during the first cool weeks of spring. This encourages deep rooting and makes the lawn healthier for the rest of the summer. It also delays the first time you have to mow the grass.

During drought or times of restricted landscape watering, most lawns, including bluegrass will withstand reduced watering demands by going dormant and only need to be to be watered every three weeks. Use sprinklers for large areas of grass and adjust sprinklers to water the lawn, not the house, sidewalk, or street.

Set a kitchen timer when watering the lawn or garden to remind you when to stop. Don't water the lawn on windy days when most of the water blows away or evaporates, and water either early in the morning or late in the afternoon when the temperature is cooler. You could also install a rain sensor on an irrigation controller so the system won't run when it's raining. Aerate the lawn at least once a year so water can reach the roots rather than run off the surface.

MOWING THE MEADOW

Don't give your grass a Marine buzz cut. Most turf grass species are healthiest when kept between 2.5 and 3.5 inches tall. A taller lawn shades roots and holds soil moisture better.

When mowing, wear proper clothing and ear protection. Check the level of the oil and gas in the lawn mower. Before mowing, check the lawn for any toys, big sticks, and/or rocks and remove them.

Try to cut the lawn every four to seven days and mow in alternate directions—this allows the grass to be cut evenly with the proper height. The best time to cut is after the sun is down—it puts less stress on the grass and the mower. Mulching-type mowers allow you to leave grass clippings on the lawn.

Sharpen mower blades once a year. If you're a little handy you can do this yourself:

- Disconnect the spark plug wire to prevent the lawn mower from accidentally starting.
- Drain the gas from the lawn mower.
- Tip the mower on its side. Use a wrench or socket to remove the mounting nut or bolt to remove the blade from the lawn mower.
- Clamp the blade in a vise.
- Run a metal file along the factory-beveled edge of the lawn mower blade. Keep the file at an angle to the bevel of the blade, in many cases a 40- or 45-degree angle.
- If there is extensive damage to the blade, sharpen the blade using a bench grinder. Move the blade back and forth against the wheel of the grinder at the same angle.
- Check the balance of the blade using a balancer. A blade that is not balanced can cause damage to the lawn mower. Balancers and instructions can be found at gardening centers or hardware stores.
- Reinstall the cleaned and sharpened blade on the lawn mower.

Every twelve to eighteen months you might notice the mower is not cutting well. This means it is time for you to adjust the blades with a gauge that determines the optimal distance between the bed knife (the stationary blade) and the rotating blades. If you don't have one, a home improvement center will.

Yale University has estimated that the United States uses more than 600 million gallons of gas to mow and trim lawns each year—about two gallons of gas for every man, woman, and child. Mowers also consume engine oil in their crankcases and two-stroke mowers consume oil in their fuel and exhaust it as carbon dioxide. If you have an old mower, consider replacing it for a cleaner-running machine. Each year, more than 17 million gallons of fuel are spilled during the refueling of power lawn and garden equipment. That fuel seeps into our soil.

Per hour of operation, a gas lawn mower emits ten to twelve times as much hydrocarbon as a typical automobile. A gasoline-powered weed eater emits twenty-one times more and a leaf blower thirty-four times more hydrocarbon than a lawn mower.

Gas mowers also contribute to noise pollution. A typical gas-powered mower creates 85 to 90 decibels, technically a noise violation in most towns. If you are using an average gas-powered mower, unless you can finish the job in fifteen minutes you should be wearing earplugs.

Using the Environmental Protection Agency's Nonroad Emissions Model, a gas mower used for twenty-five hours or to cut one-third acre of lawn will emit the following each year:

- 87 pounds of carbon dioxide.
- 48 pounds of carbon monoxide.
- 5.6 pounds of volatile organic compounds.
- 0.25 pounds of nitrogen oxides.
- 0.02 pounds of sulfur dioxide.
- 0.02 pounds of particulate matter.

A gas mower will also:

- Apply the equivalent of seven gallons of emissions due to creating and transporting fertilizer.
- Burn up to five gallons of gas for energy used for water treatment plants.
- Consume an additional gallon of gas for cleanup.

USING ETHANOL IN GARDENING MACHINES

Use a fuel additive to reduce cost and wear and tear on your internal engine, fuel parts, and rubber or plastic fuel delivery parts and gaskets. Ethanol condenses water when stored too long, so stock enough for one month, and store fuel in a dry place. Test kits are available to analyze ethanol content in gasoline. Too much ethanol is hard on an engine. Use only 10 percent ethanol, or pure gasoline.

Clean tanks if equipment is not used for more than one month. If an engine has been idle for more than a month, drain fuel and replace with new fuel.

ELECTRIC ALTERNATIVE

Think about an electric mower. They're less expensive to operate (about 3 cents of electricity per kWh), and they significantly reduce toxic emissions. An electric mower maintaining one-third of an acre for a season costs about $3 of electricity on average. Electric mowers are 75 percent quieter than gas mowers. Push mowers consume no fuel and make little noise, are good exercise and will eliminate 80 pounds of noxious emissions a year, and a couple of pounds around the waist.

Save fuel by using traditional hand rakes and brooms instead of power ones while also reducing air and noise pollution. Trim down grass clippings by mixing 5 percent clover into your lawn seed.

IMITATE THE TURF

Pros: Artificial turf is pesticide-free, doesn't require treatment with fertilizers, and is much more durable than grass; because playability is much higher, it allows broader access. Turf can be played on all the time and gives youth sports organizations practice space they might not otherwise have in times of scarce fields. There is no problem of spring and fall rains resulting in cancellation of numerous games and practices—one match on a muddy field can ruin or reduce field use for the rest of the season.

Durability and an even playing surface means fewer injuries, unlike grass that gets torn up by rough play and eventually turns into vast patches of slippery mud, an uneven playing surface, or rough patches and potholes that can cause injuries.

An average grass playing field uses about 50,000 gallons of water per week during the growing season. Artificial turf does not need water, fertilizers, or the high maintenance required by grass.

Cons: Artificial turf is made from petroleum-based materials which are resource-intensive to manufacture and transport. Some artificial turf is painted with lead paint, creating an unsafe recreation area for children and animals.

Artificial turf has also been shown to leach zinc, inorganic compounds, and other chemicals, particularly from inorganic fill. Some questions exist as to whether artificial turf is as financially friendly as touted, citing the need for repairs, vacuuming, refilling, and even some watering, suggesting that the fields may not last as long as advertised and raising the thorny problem of "clean and green" disposal.

The heat-absorbing properties of an artificial field make it uncomfortable to play on in hot warm weather, and it can be 37°F hotter than the surrounding air temperature.

Athletes who use synthetic turf are seven times more likely to receive turf burns than those who play on natural grass. These open lesions are often the source of contracting and spreading dangerous infections. Medical experts have found that staphylococci and other bacteria can survive on polyethylene plastic, the compound used to make synthetic turf blades, for more than ninety days. Blood, sweat, skin cells, and other materials can remain on the synthetic turf because the fields are not washed or cleaned. Breathing in dust of ground-up tires and sports shoes (fill) could exacerbate breathing problems for asthmatics.

Once a community goes with artificial turf, it has no choice but to install another artificial turf field when the first one needs to be replaced because after plastic replaces natural grass, it kills any living organisms in the subsoil making it impossible to grow anything on that surface without years of intervention and rehabilitation for the soil.

31

Irrigation Systems
Watering without Waste

My grandmother always had a wondrous garden, where everything bloomed and grew in vivid colors and wafting fragrances of fabulous ripeness. It seemed that all she had to do was smile at plants and they would burst into bloom. She also spoke to them, claiming it helped them grow, and told me to be careful because it's easy to kill plants with water and over fertilization.

I had always been envious of her green thumb, as mine was purple. When I mumbled at my plants, it seemed to stunt their growth and dwarf their beauty and bounty, and I was always too generous with water and plant food. But I persevered, determined to get a ripe tomato or two for my layout of cash, calories, and resources. I persisted, followed grandma's advice, and now every year I look forward to a largess of fruits and vegetables for my table. My girlfriend is cursed with the purple thumb, and has a knack of knocking off almost every plant she buys by the flat. Now it's my turn to transform her thumb to green. Here are some hints to get yours to do the same.

FACTS AND FIGURES

Almost one-third of the water your family uses during the summer—more than 100 gallons a day on average—ends up on your yard and garden. Landscape irrigation in the United States is estimated to account for more than 7 billion gallons per day during the summer. A 10,000-square-foot yard, about one-fourth of an acre, will use 6,234 gallons of water to get a one-inch coverage. Between 50 and 60 percent of landscape water goes to waste due to poor planning, evaporation, or runoff caused by overwatering.

On average, people squander ten to fifteen minutes' worth of water when using a hose, which adds up to at least 50 to 100 or more gallons of wasted water. A garden hose on full can pour out 530 gallons of water in an hour. Almost 13,000 gallons of water will flow from a garden hose nonstop for nearly a whole day–enough to fill a 24-foot pool. An irrigation system with pressure set at 60 pounds per square inch with a leak of only ⅟₃₂ of an inch in diameter (about the thickness of a dime) can waste about 6,300 gallons of water per month.

Consider what types of plants your system will water, where they will be planted, and how much water those plants will need. You may need more than one system to meet the needs of various plants. Not all plants have the same water requirements, and soil conditions in various parts of your yard may vary.

There are several types of basic irrigation systems:

• The oldest is simply hand watering.
• The sprinkler systems we all used to enjoy running through as kids.
• Gaining ground is the drip system that is far more controlled.
• Soaker hoses are popular.
• A current technique is called the slotted pipe system.
• Any single method, depending on several factors, can be the best system.

Your local water utility company or nursery is a great place for free advice concerning water conservation in the garden.

PRACTICAL SUGGESTIONS FOR WATERING

Watering is going to vary depending on where you live, what kind of plants you have, and what kind of watering system you use. To obtain a more sophisticated and accurate measurement, check the Internet for water calculators such as those found at www.bewaterwise.com.

Hiring professionals to perform regular maintenance in each yard could reduce irrigation water by 15 percent or about 9,000 gallons annually, but it can be expensive and you can do it yourself.

The key to properly watering plants is all about paying attention because there are no hard or fast rules. You could save as much as 1,000 gallons a month by watering your plants only as much as they need. Use a trowel, shovel, or soil probe to examine soil moisture depth. If the top two to three inches of soil are dry, it's time to water.

The best time is to water is early in the day or in the evening because this gives the plants time to dry out. It's much more difficult for plant diseases to get a foothold when the foliage is dry. Watering to excess in the evenings can lead to turf and plant disease and rot problems because the water sits on the plants all night, especially in humid climates. During the day, water can cause plants to burn from the magnified reflection of the sun on the water. Water also evaporates faster in the afternoon.

Plant in the fall when conditions are cooler and rainfall is more plentiful. Water less in the spring and fall and more during hot summer months.

Grassy areas on sunny southern sides of buildings or on slopes and areas near sidewalks and driveways need to be watered more often. Shady areas and northern exposures need water less frequently.

Create little walls around individual plants or groups of plants to hold water in place so it can soak in deeply. Water small patches by hand to avoid waste. Self-watering plant containers have a water reservoir at the bottom of the container which will keep plants well-watered for a few days.

Soil moisture sensors determine the amount of water in the ground available to plants which, when properly installed and maintained, can save a household more than 11,000 gallons of water annually in large gardens.

PLAN AHEAD

Pull out your ruler and rough out a sketch of the area to be watered. This will give you an idea of how much area you have to cover and the amount of material you'll need. Note the location of your faucets and the different needs of your various plants and trees.

The water pressure for your line should be at least about 40 psi. We have talked about testing water pressure with a gauge, but the easiest way is to call your water company and ask them. You should also know what that means in gallons per minute.

Another way to figure is to use a five-gallon bucket under your spigot running at full blast and time how long it takes to fill. Divide five (gallons) by the number of seconds it took to fill the bucket, and then multiply by 60 seconds. This gives you the number of gallons of water per minute. For example: If you measured 36 seconds to fill the five-gallon bucket, your equation is: $5 \div 36 = 0.14$. Next, $0.14 \times 60 = 8.4$ gallons per minute.

Estimate how the system(s) you choose will fulfill your needs. Consider the diameter of a sprinkler spray, placement of devices to ensure a good watering pattern, and the various amounts of equipment you'll need to assemble your system.

SPRINKLER SYSTEMS

Different systems deliver water in various ways, from a portable device hooked up to a hose to sophisticated underground systems that work on time schedules with flow regulators.

Spray-type sprinklers (often simply called "spray heads" or "sprays") are the sprinklers that create a fixed fan-shaped pattern, somewhat like a shower nozzle spray. Rotor-type sprinklers (called "rotors") are the sprinklers that have one or more streams of water that rotate over the landscape. A valve circuit or valve zone is a group of sprinklers that are all turned on and off by the same valve.

When installing, make sure tall grass, groundcovers, or shrubs are not blocking or deflecting water spouting from sprinklers. Use sprinkler heads with a pop-up height of four inches or more, unless in a lawn where you must be careful to ensure than a mower won't strike the sprinkler head. Keep in mind that water can spray into the side of the shrubs, especially if the shrubs are six feet or more from the sprinkler and will grow out to where the water is. Shrubs can be planted twelve inches from the edge, especially mature plants.

If you irrigate with automatic sprinklers, program your irrigation timer so that it waters in two or three short cycles rather than one long period of time. Place sprinklers so that they are between four to six inches from the edge of sidewalks, curbs, and patios so as not to waste water. Make sure sprinklers turn completely off. Water flowing when the system is off may encourage mold or algae to grow on the cement or ground. Look for low-head drainage, which occurs when the sprinkler system has been installed on a sloped area. Water left in the pipes puts a lot of stress on the sprinklers and drains, exploding through the sprinkler when the water is turned on.

A smart controller does the work of periodically adjusting the sprinkler operating times to reflect the current water needs of the plants. Install a rain switch sensor that detects measurable rainfall and will turn off the automatic valves.

Sprinkler Pros: Portable sprinklers can be anywhere in the yard and are only limited by the length of a hose. Sprinklers are about 50 to 70 percent efficient and do not require surface shaping or leveling and can be applied to large surfaces and areas of variable topography. Flexibility is possible with sprinklers because their heads are available in a wide range of discharge capacities. Chemical and fertilizer applications are easily used via sprinkler systems.

Sprinkler Cons: In high wind or dry and hot conditions, sprinkler systems have poor uniformity in distribution and application efficiency, which can cause evaporation and water loss. Clean water is also necessary in order to prevent clogging of the sprinkler nozzles. The unavoidable wetting of plant leaves could result in increased sensitivity to diseases, and fertilizers and pesticides are often flushed out of a sprinkler system.

DRIP IRRIGATION

Drip irrigation systems consist of a network of plastic pipes to carry a low flow of water under low pressure to drippers, micro sprinklers, micro sprayers, dripper lines, drip tape, or soaker hoses that emit beads of water directly to a plant's roots, lessening waste and soaking the soil before water can evaporate or run off or puddle. The basic elements of a drip or trickle system consist of the head, the tubing, and the emitters.

Emitters deliver small amounts of water to the plants and small sprinkler emitters can be installed to provide a spray pattern similar to a lawn sprinkler. Depending on the design, emitters can either be attached directly to a pipe or attached via a "spaghetti tube," a very small flexible tube that can be placed next to plants or in pots.

The size and pattern of the emitter will determine the amount of water delivered and some are adjustable to deliver different flow rates of water, varying in the amount of water delivered and area covered via various spray patterns per hour. Some distribute as little as one-half gallon of water per hour while others deliver up to ten gallons per hour. Remember that well-mulched vegetable gardens high in organic matter or shady flower gardens will require shorter watering times than gardens with sandy soils or those in full sun. Stake the drip tubes to the ground about every three feet. Cut-up metal coat hangers (bent in a U shape) work well and are cheap.

In a drip irrigation system, soil erosion and weed growth is minimized. After the initial set-up, drip irrigation or soaker hoses do the work of watering for you. For a little extra nutrient try a liquid soaker hose fertilizer that until recently was only available for commercial use.

Pros: Drip irrigation is more than 90 percent efficient because it applies water directly to the plant's root zone, uses between 20 to 50 percent less water than conventional in-ground sprinkler systems, and provides an even distribution of water.

Going from sprinklers to drip irrigation can cut lawn water use up to 50 percent, saving about $70 off the average annual household water bill. Drip irrigation systems are more efficient as no water is lost to wind, runoff, and evaporation. Drip works well with narrow and odd-shaped areas. It is easy to install, easily expandable, reasonably inexpensive, and is the most efficient method of irrigating.

Fertilizer and nutrient loss is minimized with drip irrigation due to localized application and reduced leaching.

Cons: If emitters are placed too far apart or are too few in number, root development may be restricted by the limited soil area wetted. Water seeping at ground level is hard to see and makes it difficult to know if the system is working properly. An indicator device that raises and lowers a flag to show when water is flowing is available to overcome this issue.

Regular maintenance inspections are needed to maintain system effectiveness. Clogs are much less likely with filtered water and proper pressure regulation used in combination with self-cleaning emitters. The sun can affect the tubes used for drip irrigation, shortening their usable life. Also, PVC pipes often suffer from rodent damage, requiring replacement of tubes that increases expenses.

Drip tubing can be a trip hazard, especially for dogs and children, but is less problematic if covered with mulch and fastened with wire anchor pins every two to three feet. Be careful not to cut them during garden maintenance.

Drip irrigation might be unsatisfactory if herbicides or top-dressed fertilizers need sprinkler irrigation for activation. In lighter soils, subsurface drip may be unable to wet the soil surface for germination.

SOAKER HOSES

Use soaker hoses throughout the garden to provide water directly on plant roots. They are made of water-permeable fabrics, perforated recycled rubber, or other porous materials. When attached to a hose with the water turned on low or medium, moisture droplets seep out along the length of the hose at a rate no faster than the ground can absorb it. When using soaker hoses, make sure the holes face down to avoid evaporation. While drip irrigation is more precise and versatile than a soaker hose, it is more expensive and requires a bit more work to install.

Pros: Soaker hoses provide an efficient way to water plants without waste. The hoses also conserve water, adding it to the soil slowly enough that it soaks in instead of standing on the surface or drying out too quickly, which improves the look of your garden and further reduces water loss. Nor do they waste water in areas that don't need a drink. Plants don't need their leaves watered; they need their roots watered.

A soaker hose in good condition disturbs the soil very little, and therefore conserves soil and will not wash away soil, seeds, or seedlings. Turning on a soaker hose also conserves time as it is much quicker, more efficient, and easier than watering by hand. While the hose drips away, you can bring in the harvest. They are inexpensive and easy to install, just roll them out over the area you wish to irrigate and cover them with mulch.

Cons: Soaker hoses have a short lifespan and tend to deteriorate quickly. As they age, their pores fill up with sediment and they lose their ability to seep water. Furthermore, soaker hoses are very fragile. Crimping or stepping on a hose almost guarantees a leak, and this problem will only worsen with age. Always be careful when working around a soaker hose; it is very easy to slice one in half with garden tools.

The primary advantage of soaker hoses—water conservation—can also be a disadvantage if your plants are not growing in conventional rows. Remember, soaker hoses have limited coverage and can only deliver water to the ground directly beneath them. Your garden layout is a key consideration in the soaker hose question. That soaker hoses can be buried out of sight is both an advantage and disadvantage—if out of sight they're also out of mind.

SLOTTED PIPE

This system consists of a series of pipes that are custom-perforated on one side where water is released through small tubes. The slotted pipe system needs planning, but is not difficult to install. In most cases, no special tools or skills are needed.

If you intend to water a vegetable garden, you may want one pipe next to every row or one pipe between every two rows. You will need a length of solid pipe the width of your garden. You will need lengths of perforated pipe the length of your rows (the laterals) times the number of rows. Measure the distances between laterals and cut the solid pipe to the proper lengths. Place T-connectors between the pieces of solid pipe. Approximately in the center of the solid pipe, place a T-connector to which a hose connector will be fitted.

The plastic pipe is punched with an inexpensive tube punch that ensures the proper hole size. Emitters or spaghetti tubes snap into the hole. No gluing or soldering is required. Cut perforated pipe to the length of the rows and attach perforated pipe to the T-connectors. Attach so that the perforations are facing downward. Cap the end of the pipe. Connect garden hose to hose connector on solid pipe. Adjust water from the spigot until water slowly emerges from each of the laterals and check emitters to make sure they are working properly as they can become clogged. Timing systems are available at hardware or home improvement centers at reasonable prices.

Pros: Some systems come with preassembled emitters at regular intervals. Pipes can be easily customized to fit special needs; they conserve water since it only goes where it is needed. The method won't disturb soil. In most cases, no special tools or skills are needed for assembly.

Cons: Because the holes are small, they have to be kept clean to avoid clogging and they can also easily be plugged if you put them in the wrong places. Lifespan is short compared to other systems. Slotted pipes should not be buried.

CONTROLLING THE FLOW

Buy a flow timer, also called a water timer. They measure the actual water flow and are calibrated. It can be set to give you the water needed for the square footage covered by the sprinkler, drip irrigation, or soaker.

Reset automatic controllers according to the seasonal needs of plants and be sure to inspect controls at least once a month to adjust run times. Winter watering will minimize stress to trees, shrubs, flowers, and turf in areas of drought or minimal rain. Set to water once a month during dry winter periods.

ONCE INSTALLED BE ON GUARD

Look around for wet spots that indicate there might be a leak in irrigation pipes. Simple shut-off devices are installed or built into many sprinkler heads. These are often called geyser preventers, a reference to the geyser-like spray of water that occurs when a sprinkler head or nozzle is broken off. Turn on each section or valve, one at a time, and carefully inspect your irrigation system. Automated emergency shut-off devices save water by automatically shutting off the water when something breaks in the irrigation system.

Plastic tubing is used to get the water from the source to the garden. This comes in many sizes. A variety of fittings are available to go around corners and to connect pieces. Check with a supplier for the maximum length of tubing that can be run in any one direction. A general recommendation is a 400-foot maximum for ½-inch tubing. The length of a drip hose tube should not exceed 200 feet from the beginning to the end of the tube, and the total length of any laterals should not be more than 150 feet.

The head is the part of the system that connects to your water supply. The major components of this may include a pressure regulator, a filter, an anti-siphon valve, and an automatic timer. While this may sound complicated and expensive, it is not. Installation of these components will create a better operating system. Some sprinkler head models have built-in pressure regulators. The pressure regulators save water by reducing the water pressure at the sprinkler head nozzle.

Many drip systems are designed to be used with low water pressure, under 25 psi. Normal city water pressure is about 55 psi. Therefore, a pressure regulator should be installed. Use pressure or turbulent emitters if you have an elevation difference of more than five feet. Never bury emitters underground; roots will grow into them and clog them. Don't bury drip tubes; rodents will chew them up.

Consider installing a backflow preventer. This is a valve that prevents the accidental backflow of water in the system getting into a main water line. This may be required by ordinances in some municipalities. Considering the minor cost, it is probably a wise investment for anyone considering an irrigation system.

A timing device can be added to automatically turn the system on and off. This can be as simple as a battery-operated attachment or a more permanent timer that is wired into the electrical system.

BE A WATER MISER

Reroute graywater (the relatively clean waste water from baths, sinks, washing machines, and other kitchen appliances) to trees and gardens rather than letting it run into the sewer line. Check city codes, and if it isn't allowed in your area, start a movement to get that changed. Look for alternate sources of water: creeks, ponds, and shallow wells are all examples. Keep a bucket in the shower to catch water as it warms up or runs off. Use this water to flush toilets or water plants.

Consider buying multiple rain barrels or cisterns to catch water from your gutter system to use on plants. A plastic garbage can that holds about thirty gallons—and includes a child-proof lid—costs about $30. More expensive barrels have a spigot for easy dispensing on plants.

If you accidentally drop ice cubes when filling your glass, don't throw them in the sink. Drop them on a houseplant instead. When you have ice left in your cup from a take-out restaurant, don't throw it in the trash; dump it on a plant. Collect the water from rinsing fruits and vegetables and reuse it to water houseplants. When cleaning out fish tanks, give the nutrient-rich water to houseplants. This is the idea behind aquaponics.

Don't install or use fountains or other water ornaments unless they use recycled water. Trickling or cascading fountains lose less water to evaporation than those spraying water into the air. Avoid water toys that need a constant stream of water. When the kids want to cool off, use the sprinkler in an area that needs watering the most.

MAINTENANCE

Learn how to shut off your automatic watering system in case it malfunctions or you get unexpected rain. Know where your master water shut-off valve is located both on the street and for your house. In case of emergency, this could save water, money, and prevent damage to your pipes, and home.

Continually check for leaks in all pipes and plumbing connections indoors and outdoors. Use filters. Most valve and sprinkler malfunctions result from contaminants, small grains of sand, pipe scale, or even small snails. Periodically check controller batteries, clean rotor-type sprinklers, and clean and adjust spray-type sprinklers. Replace any broken or malfunctioning sprinklers.

You can't mix different sprinkler models on the same valve circuit. Also never mix spray-type heads and rotor-type sprinklers on the same valve zone.

If your irrigation system is located in an area where hard frosts occur, make sure you properly winterize each season by installing frost-free sillcocks (simple outdoor water faucets that are located and attached to the exterior of a house) on outdoor water faucets or purchase inexpensive insulated covers for spigots.

In winter, turn off the water to the irrigation system, especially for temperatures below freezing. Set the automatic irrigation controller to the "rain" setting. Turn on each of the valves to release pressure in the pipes. Empty hoses before a freeze and drain all of the water out of any irrigation components that might freeze.

Some water providers will conduct an irrigation audit, either for free or at minimal cost. You can also look for a certified landscape irrigation auditor (CLIA) using the Irrigation Association's Web site.

32

Plant a Tree

For You and Me

I think that I shall never see
A poem lovely as a tree. . . .
Poems are made by fools like me,
But only God can make a tree.

—Apologies to Joyce Kilmer

Although just about everyone has been entranced or filled with wonder by a tree, surprisingly, most of us take them for granted.

Not Wangari Maathai. She won the Nobel Peace Prize in 2004 for "her contribution to sustainable development, democracy and peace." Her grassroots campaign to counter deforestation by encouraging women to plant trees locally resulted in the planting of over thirty million trees in Kenya and other African countries, and helped to create income, provide sustenance, and husband the environment improving the lives of millions of people. In its "Reforesting the Earth" paper, the Worldwatch Institute estimated that our planet needs at least 321 million acres (an area almost twice the size of Texas) replanted just to restore and maintain the productivity of soil and water resources, meet industrial and wood fuel needs in the Third World, and annually remove roughly 780 million tons of carbon from the atmosphere.

You don't have to have one to fall on you to understand the implication and the importance of trees. Besides inspiring poetry, they absorb carbon dioxide and release oxygen. They comprise one of the world's most sustainable products and offer comforts that all animals appreciate, especially poets and dogs.

FACTS AND FIGURES

Trees offer charm, beauty, grace, and serenity that cannot be measured in volts, watts, amperage, and Btus. Trees provide background to hide, soften, complement, or enhance architecture. They provide edibles, cooling shade and privacy, frame and emphasize beautiful vistas, screen out objectionable views, reduce glare and reflection, and offer a counterbalance for man-made environments. Trees aid in our well-being, make life more enjoyable and peaceful, and offer a rich and continuing inheritance for future generations.

Tree-lined streets and green spaces have been shown to have positive physical and psychological benefits including lowering rates of stress, mental illness, violence, and crime. Hospital patients who have a view of trees heal faster, use fewer pain medications, and leave the hospital an average of one week sooner than other patients.

Trees have tremendous symbolic value; they humanize cities, acknowledge our affinity for the natural world, and provide a focus for community participation in landscaping the urban environment.

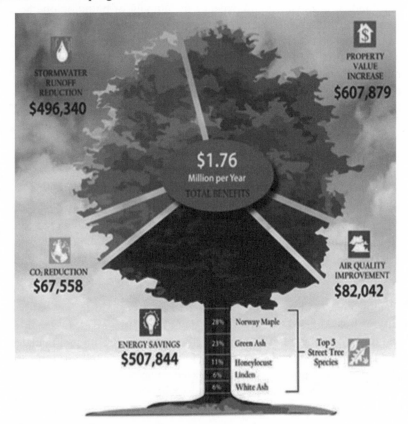

Figure 32.1. The economy of a tree.

ENVIRONMENTAL BENEFIT

America has 749 million acres of forestland at present. In 1920, there were 735 million acres of forest, and although not virgin, the United States has 14 million more acres of forest than it did ninety years ago, even though the population of the United States is three times as large. An average-sized tree produces enough breathable oxygen in one year for a family of four. It also helps reduce air pollution, controls storm water runoff, reduces the need for air conditioning in hot weather, offers wind breaks in winter, requires less attention than most plants, adds thousands of dollars to a property's value, and can save up to 15 percent of household energy costs if properly planted. Attractiveness and comfort ratings are about 80 percent higher for a tree-lined sidewalk compared to a non-shaded street. Quality-of-products ratings were 30 percent higher in districts having trees over those with barren sidewalks.

Trees also reduce the greenhouse and heat island effects by shading homes and office buildings. This reduces air conditioning needs up to 30 percent. There is up to a 60 percent reduction in street level particulates with trees. Three hundred trees can counterbalance the amount of pollution one person produces in a lifetime. If every American family planted just one tree, the amount of carbon dioxide in the atmosphere would be reduced by one billion pounds annually. This is almost 5 percent of the amount that human activity pumps into the atmosphere each year, and 300,000 trees can offset the pollution produced to power 250,000 homes for one week.

Reductions in energy use resulting from shade trees can save up to 2.4 tons of CO_2 emissions per year. The US Forest Service estimates that all the forests in the United States combined sequestered approximately 309 million tons of carbon per year from 1952 to 1992, offsetting approximately 25 percent of US human-caused emissions of carbon during that period. Trees reach their most productive stage of carbon storage at about ten years old.

Depending on their type, location, and health, trees can live from 100 to 1,000 years. Each tree also directly absorbs about 25 to 50 pounds of carbon dioxide from the air annually. For every ton of new tree wood that grows, about 1.5 tons of carbon dioxide are removed from the air and 1.07 tons of oxygen are produced. An acre of trees absorbs enough CO_2 over one year to equal the amount produced by driving a car 26,000 miles.

Planting trees and expanding parklands has noticeably improved the air quality of Los Angeles County. In one day in one urban park (averaging 86 acres) tree cover was found to remove 48 pounds of airborne particulates, 9 pounds of nitrogen dioxide, 6 pounds of sulfur dioxide, 2 pounds of carbon monoxide, and 100 pounds of carbon. Based on pollution control technology, this "removal service" would equal almost $50,000 per year.

Trees prevent and/or reduce soil erosion and water pollution. They also prevent harmful land pollutants contained in the soil from getting into our waterways and slow down water run-off and ensure that our groundwater supplies are continually being replenished. For every 5 percent of tree cover added to a community, storm water runoff is reduced by approximately 2 percent.

Trees shade rivers, streams, and lakes, which reduces water temperatures and provides protection for fish. A typical shade tree intercepts 760 gallons of rainfall in its crown each year, thereby reducing runoff of polluted storm water and flooding. Wind speed and direction can be affected and deflected by trees.

Tree leaves and twigs provide excellent mulch for flowerbeds and gardens. Trees can enhance community economic stability by attracting businesses and tourists. People love to linger and shop longer along tree-lined streets. Apartments and offices in wooded areas rent more quickly and have higher occupancy rates. Businesses leasing office spaces in areas with trees find their workers are more productive and absenteeism is reduced. A US Department of Energy study reports that trees reduce noise pollution by acting as a buffer and absorbing 50 percent of urban noise.

Windbreaks on farms reduce loss of topsoil, cooling and heating bills, and help with snow entrapment, wind reduction, aesthetics, and wildlife habitat. Trees shelter livestock, effectively reducing weight losses during cold winter months and providing shade for moderating summer heat. Trees hold snow away from roads, help keep them open, and reduce road maintenance costs.

ECONOMIC BENEFITS

Over a fifty-year lifetime, one tree generates $31,250 worth of oxygen, provides $50,000 worth of air pollution control, recycles $37,500 worth of water, and controls $31,250 worth of soil erosion, or $162,000 in total value per tree. One tree cleans 330 pounds of CO_2 from the atmosphere through direct capture in the tree's wood.

The maximum potential annual savings from energy conserving landscapes around a typical residence ranged from 13 percent in Madison, Wisconsin, to 38 percent in Miami, Florida. Projections suggest that 100 million additional mature trees in US cities (three trees for every unshaded single family home) could save over $2 billion in energy costs per year.

Three trees planted in the right place around buildings can cut air conditioning and heating costs from 15 to 35 percent in a one-fifth-acre house lot with 30 percent vegetation cover. One large front yard tree saves $30 in summertime air conditioning by shading the building and cooling the air, cutting energy use by about 250 kWh, which saves about 9 percent of total annual air conditioning cost. In the winter, trees around the home act as shields against wind and snow, and heating costs can be reduced by as much as 30 percent.

Structures surrounded by trees sell for 18 to 25 percent higher than those with no trees. One tree adds about 1 percent to the sales price of a property, or about $25 each year when annualized over a forty-year period.

In San Diego County, a developer found he could increase the sale price of his houses by 25 percent by scaling back his development by 15 percent and adding natural open space corridors with plants and trees visible from every home. A study of housing values near Philadelphia's Pennypack Park found that the park accounted for 33 percent of the land value for lots abutting the park and its economic influence was felt up to 2,500 feet away. The park directly contributed to a net increase of $3.4 million in real estate value.

Heat sinks are 6° to 19°F warmer than their surroundings with trees. Trees reduce heat in cities by giving off water vapor and shading various surfaces. The asphalt paving on streets contains stone aggregate in an oil binder. Without tree shade, the oil heats up and changes into a greenhouse gas, and leaves the aggregate unprotected; with trees, street life is extended by up to twenty-five years.

CARETAKING

You might think that trees pretty much take care of themselves, but giving your trees the right care from day one is essential for long and healthy life. Proper tree care begins with selecting the right tree and planting it in the right place. In some cities, such as Seattle, groups of neighbors can request ten to forty trees from the city in exchange for planting and maintaining them.

When planting trees and trimming them, be sure they will stay clear (by at least 15 feet) of electric lines and utilities, including light standards. Newly planted trees do best when exposed to moderate temperature and rainfall and they need time to root and acclimatize before the onset of the heat and dryness of summer or the freezing temperatures of winter. New trees should be watered immediately and generously after planting them. During the first couple of growing seasons, newly planted trees expend a lot of energy trying to get their roots established in the soil. Deep watering can help speed the root establishment and consists of keeping the soil moist to a depth that includes all the roots. After two seasons a tree's roots will have been established.

The most common mistake when planting a tree is a digging hole that is too deep and too narrow. Too deep and the roots don't have access to sufficient oxygen to ensure proper growth. Too narrow and the root structure can't expand sufficiently to nourish and properly anchor the tree. Overwatering is another common tree-care mistake. Please note that moist is different than soggy, and you can judge this by feel. A damp soil that dries for a short period will allow adequate oxygen to permeate the soil.

Water should be applied to established trees once a month during the winter and as often as once a week during the heat of the summer. Trees, especially those that have been in the ground less than three years, need 25 gallons of water, equivalent to approximately a 1.5-inch rainfall event, a week to become established and thrive. To get an idea of how much or how long you should water, try sticking a thin metal rod into the ground soon after you irrigate. The rod should slide easily through the wet soil and become harder to push further when it reaches dry soil or when your soil probe won't penetrate the ground more than 3 to 6 inches. Commercial watering gauges are available at a home improvement center or nursery and, keep in mind, trees adapted to drier climates need far less irrigation than other species.

Mycorrhizal fungi are an extremely beneficial additive for newly planted trees. Add these all-natural, symbiotic fungi to the soil to promote the growth of the root system and discourage damaging fungi that could hinder the tree's development. Think about position when planting a tree in terms of sunlight and general direction of the wind. And don't forget to mulch your trees! Bare root, container-held, root-balled, and burlapped trees should be planted a little differently. Ask your nursery or dig around the Internet for sage advice. The Arbor Day Foundation has information on planting and provides trees. And maybe make a poem about a tree.

33

Chores Wars
Using Your Personal Energy Efficiently

For most of us, chores are the things you have to do to be able to do the things you like to do. Here are some suggestions to trim some time off those tasks each week to find more time and energy in your life to do the things you'd rather be doing. You might even save some money too.

Planning is the first best use of time, especially if you have a family. Doing the household chores together can cut the time it takes to complete them alone. Sharing in each other's daily tasks can create family harmony and is a great way to spend time together. Undesirable chores should be rotated by time or by person. Dividing household chores equally amongst the family, as well as rotating tasks, will keep everyone in agreement and ensure feelings of fairness.

FACTS AND FIGURES

An average person spends more than twenty hours per week on household chores. Ninety-eight percent of people feel good about themselves when their house is clean, and 97 percent of people believe their families appreciate a clean home.

PRACTICAL SUGGESTIONS

Housecleaning can be a very time-consuming job and a bit overwhelming when you think you have to tackle the whole job at once. Look at it in a series of small jobs rather than one huge whole.

There are several software programs and applications that can help if you ask yourself these questions:

- Do I often need to remind people to do their fair share?
- Do my roommate, children, spouse, and I argue about doing chores?
- Do I sometimes forget what needs doing until it is too late?
- Do I feel flustered and like I don't have enough time to organize?
- How often do I, family, and roommates put off, find excuses, or ignore doing chores?

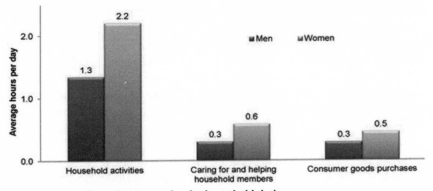

Figure 33.1.   Average hours per day for household duties.
Source: Bureau of Labor Statistics.

Create schedules and rules via some software programs and phone apps that will automatically generate a schedule of chores and e-mail them daily or weekly. Better yet, have everyone help to create a schedule from scratch so everyone gets to contribute and collaborate. If really pressed for time, outsource chores if the time saved is worth it to you.

For do-it-yourselfers, make, organize, and prioritize a list of your duties, get them on autopilot, and after a while they'll get done in less time. Ten minutes a day speed-cleaning your kitchen is better than an hour on the weekend when you have play time planned.

There will always be reasons to procrastinate, but getting something done is better than the energy expended worrying or putting it off. Consolidating tasks saves time and energy. It's multitasking, which should simplify and speed up the process and produce pleasant byproducts. Catch up on your reading while waiting for things to be dried, wipe down the kitchen counters while waiting for the coffee machine, and fold laundry while watching your favorite TV show. Talk to the kids when doing dishes together—with two people working together, things seem to get done quicker. Call a friend or relative and chat while working; what really makes the time pass is conversation. Whether carpooling or shopping for a friend, division of labor can save time and energy, and lower greenhouse gases.

Many tasks are better left for the evening or, better yet, for when no one else is home. Cooking, drying clothes, and using the dishwasher can heat up the kitchen, so schedule those tasks properly. Use microwave ovens and crockpots, which produce much less heat and require less supervision and energy than stoves for cooking. One-pot cooking also lessens dishes to be washed. Taking on labor-intensive tasks can also make you feel uncomfortable during the hottest or coldest times of the day and create a need to run the furnace or air conditioning. If possible, do chores and errands when the temperature and weather are not so contrary.

Avoid activities in the afternoon that require a great deal of traveling through the doors of your home, which allows cool air to escape and hot air to enter the home. When possible, spread heavy and light tasks throughout the day. Always schedule rest periods and take this time to relax muscles and the mind.

Plan meals in advance. Also try to prepare or cook more than one meal at a time. With a large enough freezer, a single day's cooking can yield a week's worth of time and cost-effective meals.

Try to be cheerful about chores, not matter how unpleasant. It will set an example for the next person and should reduce grumbling. Do the best you can. No one likes a sloppy job. And finally, reward yourself for a job well done and on time.

DON'T FORGET THE KIDS

If you have kids that you can bribe or motivate to pitch in, it's a good way to teach family responsibility and cooperation. No matter what age your kids are, there is something they can do and it's best to start their responsibilities early.

Be clear about the task and write directions if need be. With each job assigned to them, give them a demonstration, demands, and penalties—that way no one can claim they didn't understand the rules and their consequences.

Motivate the kids. When a job is finished, use praise, cash allowances, or both. Go easy on criticism that will turn them off to the process.

Create a chore chart and have everyone sign it. This will vary depending on your family's needs and size, but will help the kids know what they are responsible for and it will help keep them on track. Everything becomes boring after a time and kids can lose interest quickly, so rotate tasks. Chores can even become a fun family affair when everyone works together.

34

Energy Assists

More Power to Power More People

This book is as much about saving green as doing green. By now you know that energy efficiency, being green, and saving money isn't about hugging trees. Besides conservation, it's about paying attention to rebates, incentives, free programs, and tax breaks to upgrade your home's alternative and efficient energy systems and devices. Many of these aids and incentives are not necessarily attached to your income or age, but to your desire to do the right thing. And always shop and negotiate for deals.

Energy assistance programs can save you hundreds of dollars, maybe thousands, a year on water and power bills, new purchases, and upgrades. Keeping more money in your wallet—where it belongs—will help to make your home a more pleasant and sustainable one in which to live. It's a win-win for you, for the environment, and for the planet, with a little leg-up from Uncle Sam and associates.

FACTS AND FIGURES

Your local power companies, county, state, and federal agencies are rich sources of energy information and economic assistance. For example, in California, Pacific Gas and Electric has an Energy Partners Program that offers free basic home energy audits, educational and information programs, and some complimentary products and services that aid in conserving energy. Call your local utility company so they can inform you of the programs they offer.

While states identify renewable technologies differently, most include choices for creating electricity from wind, geothermal, biomass, biogas, low impact hydroelectricity, and fuel cells. Look for similar state and federal programs (EPA/DOE/EIA) on the Internet that might be offered via your local power companies. Alternative programs are listed by state to assist low-income customers, the disabled, and senior citizens.

A taxpayer may claim a federal credit of 30 percent of a qualified energy saving expenditure for a home that is owned and used as a primary residence. Senate Bill 1254 of 2010 created a tax credit for electricity produced by certain renewable resources. Qualified renewable energy systems installed on or after December 31, 2010, may be eligible for the tax credit based on the amount of electricity produced annually for a ten-year period. Expenditures for equipment are counted when the installation is completed. Costs include labor for on-site preparation, assembly or original system installation, and for piping or wiring to interconnect a system to the home. To keep up with the latest info, check with your state and local Internal Revenue Service office and the DOE.

Local elected officials are another resource. Call or write their offices; they have staff that should be able and willing to assist you.

POSSIBLE INCENTIVES

Federal energy tax credits, state assistance programs, and county assistance for low-income families are available for many types of home improvements. Tax credits can help offset the initial investment of some of the larger energy-efficient home improvement projects you may be considering. Check your local, state, and federal agencies to see if you qualify.

Federal and state Low-Income Home Energy Assistance Programs (LI-HEAPs) and Weatherization Assistance Programs (WAPs) may cover:

• Caulking and weatherization.
• Insulation.
• Exterior door replacement.
• Faucet aerators.
• Glass and window replacement.
• Combustion air ventilation.
• Natural gas appliance testing, repair and/or replacement.
• CFLs (free compact fluorescent bulbs): five per home and ceiling, torchiere, and porch light fixtures.
• Refrigerator replacement.
• Occupancy sensors.
• Low-flow showerheads.

- Duct testing and sealing.
- Switch and outlet gaskets.
- Exhaust venting, duct repair and replacement.
- Water heater repair and replacement.
- Blower door testing.
- Smoke detectors.
- Rebates and installation of doors, windows.
- Basic health and safety repairs and additional minor home repairs.

The City of Tallahassee, Florida, offers a rebate of $1 per square foot (up to $2,000) for EnergyStar-qualified new homes, which include single-family detached, single-family attached, low-rise multi-family, and existing-home renovations. For state assistance, Google or call your state public utilities commission for energy assistance or the DOE home page and look for the "In Your State" section.

Look for assistance with weatherizing and in obtaining new energy-saving appliances. For example, state governments will often pay for a significant portion of the bill for you to install a solar system in your home.

The DOE's Office of Energy Efficiency and Renewable Energy Network offers a wealth of energy-efficiency information (www.eren.doe.gov). This information is also available toll-free at 1-800-363-3732, or at http://www. energy.gov/ using search terms such as energy assistance, assistance with energy bills, rebates, tax credits, and/or by checking out the "Quick Clicks" on their home page.

Assistance is also available for paying utility bills and weatherizing homes. Sources of assistance include: The Salvation Army at 800-933-9677, the Federal Low Income Home Energy Assistance Program at 800-433-4327, county offices (energy assistance programs), and your local power company. In California PG&E customers can help assist other needy bill payers by adding $1 to $10 monthly to their bill in the REACH program.

The Weatherization Assistance Program (WAP), through the DOE, enables low-income families to permanently reduce their energy bills by making their homes more energy efficient.

Some fire departments will even supply and install free smoke detectors for the elderly, disabled, or needy.

There are now at least eight states that assist with adding a solar system to your home, which supplies electricity at a lower rate than your utility company. The four companies that have stepped up to offer these $0-down options (some offer free installation) are: SolarCity (OR, CA, TX), Sunrun (CA, AZ, CO, NJ, MA), groSolar (PA, CA), and Sungevity (CA). Check about your state with the DOE: http://www.energy.gov/.

Once a solar system is installed on your roof, you either make lease payments or pay monthly for electricity by the kilowatt-hour (net metering), the same way you pay your current electric utility, but far cheaper. You must own the home, have a good roof with enough sun access, and not be in foreclosure or behind on mortgage payments. Someone with a $500-a-month bill could save around $100,000 over ten years.

STATE INCENTIVES

Another great resource is the Database of State Incentives for Renewables and Efficiency (DSIRE), the most comprehensive source of information on incentives and policies that support renewables and energy efficiency in the United States. DSIRE is funded by the US Department of Energy. This allows you to view rebates, loan and grant programs, financing options, and tax credits offered in your region. Check out their Web site at http://www.dsireusa.org/ for an unofficial overview of financial incentives and other policies (listed by state).

Advanced Home Energy in California offers up to $5,000 in cash for energy upgrades—check your state for similar offers. Ask utility companies and county offices for various benefits including a free energy loss analysis and for possible grants and tax rebates.

MORE RESOURCES

Homeowners can still receive a federal tax credit for 30 percent of the cost of energy-efficient products (up to a total credit of $1,500). This includes the purchase of central air conditioning systems, electric heat pumps, furnaces and boilers, and whole-house ventilation fans (both the product and installation). Visit the US DOE Energy Saver Web site for more information at http://energy.gov/energysaver/energy-saver.

The only products that are eligible for vacation or second homes for the tax credit are:

- Geothermal heat pumps.
- Solar panels.
- Solar water heaters.
- Small wind energy systems.

ALSO CHECK OUT

- The Office of Community Services—Low Income Home Energy Assistance: www.acf.hhs.gov/programs/liheap/.
- Mortgages for Home Buyers: www.usa.gov/Citizen/Topics/Benefits.shtml.
- Home Improvements/US Department of Housing and Urban Development: https://portal.hud.gov/hudportal/HUD?src=/topics/home_improvements.
- Special energy-efficient offers such as cash rebates, low-interest loans, or other incentive programs are used to encourage buyers to purchase energy-efficient appliances. To find rebates in your area, use the EnergyStar Rebate Locator Web site: https://www.energystar.gov/index.cfm?fuseaction=rebate.rebate_locator.
- Go to the DOE EnergyStar page for information about products for home and office: http://www.energystar.gov/index.cfm?c=products.pr_find_es_products.
- Household Energy Efficiency—Learn more about HUD's Open Government Initiative: hud.gov/improvements/.
- Utility Bill Assistance programs: www.utilitybillassistance.com/.

35

"Safe" Yourself
What to Do After the Electricity Fails

There is a great story about how the birthrate jumped nine months after the great New York blackout of 2003, called "From Here to Maternity." It wasn't true. The birthrate nine months after the blackout did not show a statistically significant difference from the rate of birth recorded during the same period in any of the five previous years. If and when another blackout or brownout happens, and odds are that it will, it's best to be prepared, hope for the best, and plan for the worst. Of course, it won't hurt to cuddle up in the dark and tempt fate.

PLANNING FOR THE POWER GOING OUT

As our power grid becomes elderly and senescent and can no longer handle the demands of a growing society, your best bet is to be prepared, especially in a crisis. For a few bucks you can easily and competently plan for an emergency. And when that happens, you'll feel good that you planned ahead—and so will the people around you.

WHEN THE GRID GOES DOWN

Unplug everything. As the grid sputters back to life, it may create power surges that can destroy electronics. Leave one light switched on so you know when power has returned. Flashlights produce more light than candles and don't start fires, especially since you might not be able to contact the fire department. But keep candles handy for backup. Bring any outdoor solar powered lights inside for light, but be sure they get sunshine during the day. Power via backup generators will probably be on at the hospitals, but they'll also be packed with stooges who took stupid chances and got injured. Think about a personal generator if you are either in a distant place or where a lot of blackouts occur. They are irreplaceable if the power is out for days, and can be bought for anywhere from around one hundred to thousands of dollars depending on the amount of power you require.

ALTERNATIVE AUTO POWER

Your car can generate power for your house. A power inverter, which turns 12-volt DC current from your car into 120-volt AC current for your home, might be the only source of juice available during a blackout. Inexpensive inverters are available from small units that can power your computer, up to more expensive models that can run power tools and appliances. Check out the amperages for your home appliances and then match that with an inverter to suit your needs. Make sure you have a good supply of gas in the car because when the electricity stops, so do the pumps at the gas station.

ABOUT BATTERIES

A battery does not really store electricity; it is a chemical reaction waiting to happen. When a battery is placed inside an electrical circuit, the chemical reaction transforms chemical energy into electrical energy via the transfer of electrons. Until recently, batteries only offered a small capacity for power.

Americans use an average of about eight batteries a year per person to power everything from flashlights to computers. Instead of throwing dead batteries in the trash, take them to a toxic waste disposal area. Batteries that are thrown away produce most of the toxic heavy metals—dangerous substances like lead, arsenic, zinc, cadmium, copper, and mercury—that are found in household trash, and consequently in landfills, and can seep into the ground water and, eventually, into the food chain.

Non-rechargeable batteries have a longer shelf life, but rechargeable batteries last longer over all. Non-rechargeable batteries are cheaper, but rechargeable batteries are more cost-efficient. Americans throw out approximately 179,000 tons of batteries a year, of which about 14,000 tons are rechargeable. All batteries, including rechargeable, eventually die. This is because the chemicals inside the battery degrade over time and with usage. Charge rechargeable batteries hours before you intend to use them. You should also avoid leaving rechargeable batteries discharged for long periods of time, because the batteries will degrade more quickly when left discharged for six months or more.

One NiCad mobile phone or power tool battery is enough to pollute 158,503 gallons of water. That's equivalent to a third of an Olympic-sized swimming pool. New technology in lithium-ion batteries can start or power cars and can store energy from windmill turbines and solar systems. However, production of the new lithium batteries creates large amounts of toxic waste that is difficult to recycle. A Texas company claims it will soon produce a new ultracapacitor power system to replace the electrochemical batteries in everything from cars to laptops. Although not sustainable, they still use toxic chemicals that are far more green and environmentally friendly then lead batteries. Solid state rechargeable batteries (SSB) are created using semiconductor processing techniques on silicon wafers. They are completely different from traditional batteries and supercapacitors that contain dangerous chemicals and have toxic waste disposal issues.

HOME BATTERIES

(See Renewable Power chapter.)

LANTERNS AND FLASHLIGHTS

They are not going to do you any good with dead or dying batteries. LED flashlights and lanterns have a big benefit over incandescent models because batteries last as much as six to ten times longer. If you use lanterns with fossil fuels, be watchful of proper air circulation and with the operation of flammable material. Watch for marketing hype like "Heavy Duty." These are often the least powerful batteries you can buy. And, of course, turn off the devices that use batteries when you are not playing with them.

REMEMBER TRANSISTOR RADIOS?

In an emergency, if you don't have access to a car radio, a portable and inexpensive battery-powered radio may be your only source of weather and emergency information.

WATER, WATER, WATER

Disasters, small or large, have a cascading effect. When the electricity fails, the Internet and water system may soon follow. The largest source of available water is the water heater, then the toilet tank. If you can, fill up your tub and any buckets and bottles for washing and flushing. Drinking water should be kept separate from the impotable sources. Remember to secure the tub drain with waterproof tape, as plugs are not completely tight, and it won't take long for your wet stash to drain out.

When the light goes out, so does the refrigerator. Try keeping a few bags of ice available as long as you can by filling a few zippered plastic bags beforehand. They might come in handy for water or to ice-down minor injuries and to keep stuff in the freezer colder longer. Keep a few of the "blue" frozen bags in the refrigerator also.

MONEY, MONEY, MONEY

When the power goes out and credit cards don't work, cash will, so keep a few bucks ($50 to $100) in a safe place for emergencies.

DON'T FORGET THE BBQ

If you have a gas barbecue, keep the tank topped, or the charcoal scuttle full. Again, when the grid fails you won't have to do without a hot meal. Besides kind of being fun in an unfunny situation, barbecues might help make points with your neighbors by sharing your grill, and giving you the opportunity to finally enjoy your frozen food.

CO_2 IS HAZARDOUS

In emergencies one of the first things people do is make a fire; it produces light and heat, and is a means for cooking and comfort. People fire up fireplaces, gas stoves, and all types of heaters that can also mean cranking up the carbon dioxide and carbon monoxide content of the house, as well as increasing the probability of fire after a disaster. And those gases and accidental fires kill people every year. A good, inexpensive investment is a CO detector, and multiple fire extinguishers.

PLANS AND BACKUP PLANS

Before something happens, make sure that everyone in the family agrees on a meeting place in and out of the house, and on a plan and secondary plan for everyone to exit the house if necessary. Agree on a neighborhood meeting place—a nearby school, park, friend's house, or building to rendezvous if the situation calls for it.

Plan beforehand to notify members of the family, friends, and neighbors, especially those out of the affected area, in the event that a blackout or emergency lasts long or you have to evacuate. Make just-in-case arrangements with friends or relatives who are willing take you in, be a communication link, especially those who are out-of-towners. Your people are going to worry about you during a crisis and the longer you wait, the more difficult it might be to get a phone call through.

36

The New Rs
Redoing, Rethinking, Reusing

- Recycle—reprocess materials.
- Rescue—salvage.
- Reduce—what you buy and how it's packaged.
- Reclaim and Renew—fix and restore.
- Reuse—more than once.
- Reinvent and Repurpose—find and imagine new uses.
- Rethink—new life resolutions.
- Repair—things can be revitalized.

AN OLDER SHADE OF GREEN

The parents of the Boomer generation paraphrase an old Sanskrit phrase saying, "There is nothing new under the sun, and what is old is new again." For one, my mother pointed out that recycling is nothing new to her generation. "During the Depression," she would say, "nothing was left to waste that could be reused. And during World War II, we all pulled together to conserve and recycle our resources for the war effort. Nothing was thrown away."

They didn't call it being green back in those days. They returned their milk bottles, soda bottles, and beer bottles to the store. The store sent them back to the plant to be washed, sterilized, and refilled, and the same bottles would be used over and over. They walked up stairs, because they didn't have an escalator or elevator in every store and office building. They walked to the grocery store and didn't climb into a car every time they had to go two blocks because gas was expensive or rationed. They washed baby diapers because they didn't have the throwaway kind. Their clothes dryer was the wind and the sun, not energy-gobbling machines. Kids wore "pre-owned" clothes handed down from their brothers or sisters. They had one phone, a radio, or a single TV in the house—not in every room or pocket.

A TV screen was the size of a large dinner plate, not the dimensions of a ping pong table, it had to be turned off manually, and did not guzzle standby energy. In the kitchen, they blended and stirred by hand. When they packaged a fragile item to send in the mail, they used wadded up newspaper to cushion it, not Styrofoam peanuts or plastic bubble wrap.

To cut the lawn they pushed a mower that ran on human power not fossil fuel. They didn't need to go to a health club to run on electricity-operated treadmills, they walked. When thirsty, they drank from a fountain or tap instead of buying water in a plastic bottle. They refilled pens with ink instead of buying new ones. They replaced razor blades instead of throwing the whole razor away.

Back then, people took streetcars, and kids rode their bikes to school or rode the school bus instead of being a single kid chauffeured by a parent in an SUV. They had one electrical outlet in a room, not an entire bank of sockets to power a dozen appliances. They didn't need a computerized gadget receiving a signal beamed from satellites 2,000 miles out in space to order a pizza or to figure out what was on TV. They used a phone book and called with a heavy, hard-plastic phone that lasted forever.

The above decreased pollution, enhanced resources in a number of ways, reduced the use of energy to make new material, saved money, protected wildlife and habitats, and lessened the pressure on the environment and dumpsites. Maybe some old lifestyles can be recycled too.

Unfortunately, they were also the first throwaway generation and they taught their children well by example.

FACTS AND FIGURES: WASTE

Believe it or not, trash is the country's largest export by volume. China used to be the largest purchaser of our detritus. They would use it as raw material and recycle it to manufacture goods that we bought back. Talk about a deal. Add to that the environmental impact of long-distance round–tripping those goods. But those days look like they're over, which has panicked some of our industries, which are not geared up for getting their refuse bought or recycled. By the way, fifteen of the largest cargo ships (which partly transport recycled stuff) produce more sulfur oxide pollutants than the world's 760 million cars.

Americans represent 5 percent of the world's population, use more than a quarter of its energy, and generate 30 percent of the world's garbage. About 200 million tons of total waste is produced annually in the United States. In 2008, the average amount of waste generated by each person in America per day was 4.5 pounds. In total, 25 percent of waste is recycled, 9 percent is composted, and 67 percent is sent to a landfill or incinerated. If all the trash Americans generate in one year were buried, it would be 100 miles deep. The line of trucks delivering that trash would be 125,000 miles long, or halfway to the moon.

It's estimated that each year more than 7 billion tons of rubbish makes its way into the sea. The Ocean Dumping Ban Act prohibits all dumping of sewage, sludge, and industrial waste into the oceans, without exception, aside from certain fish waste and dredged materials. There is no part of our largest ocean, the Pacific, which does not have plastic or refuse in it. Scientific research from the Scripps Institution of Oceanography in California indicates that 5 to 10 percent of the fish caught in the Pacific contain small pieces of plastic.

An ocean gyre is a large system of circular ocean currents. With the movement of these currents, small items of plastic and other refuse are sucked into the middle of a swirling soup of flotsam, jetsam, and garbage. This "trash vortex" is known as the Pacific Gyre, the Great Plastic Vortex, the Pacific Plastic Island, or the Great Pacific Garbage Patch and it is the largest plastic dump in the world.

In 2008, a report found that 82 percent of surveyed landfill was leaking toxic or semi-toxic materials. But by far the largest polluters in the United States are the 6,700 coal-fired power plants and heavy industries that are responsible for 80 percent of all emissions in the United States.

Each year more than 18 billion "disposable" diapers are thrown away that consume 100,000 tons of plastic and 800,000 of tree pulp. It costs about $350 million to dump them, and they'll be with us in the landfill 3,000 years from now. Even the final frontier, space, isn't safe: There are more than 100,000 pieces of space litter in orbit.

ON A TYPICAL DAY, HUMANS:

- Produce about 2.3 pounds of CO_2 each.
- Generate 4.5 pounds of waste per person, of which 24.3 percent is recycled, 8.9 percent composted, and 66.8 percent sent to a landfill or incinerated.
- Add 2,700 tons of CFCs to the stratosphere.

- Pass from 1 to 3 pints of methane (by breaking wind, etc.) each.
- Add 15 million tons of carbon to the atmosphere.
- Destroy 115 square miles of tropical rainforest.
- Create 72 square miles of desert.
- Eliminate between 40 and 100 species.
- Erode 71 million tons of topsoil.
- Increase our population by 263,000.

FACTS AND FIGURES: RECYCLING

There are thousands of ways to conserve, recycle, reinvent, or reuse. Do some research and discover ways that suit you and your family. Recycling creates 1.1 million US jobs, $236 billion in gross annual sales, and $37 billion in annual payrolls. Recycling and composting prevented 82 million tons of material from being disposed of in 2009.

The closed-loop recycling process represents recycling at its finest—remanufacturing a product back into the same product—like an empty aluminum can, which can be recycled endlessly into more containers.

Open-loop recycling is the conversion of material from one or more products into a new product, such as recycling plastic bottles into plastic drainage pipes. This is sometimes called down-cycling or reprocessing. If the United States were to recycle 75 percent of the resources that it currently burns or dumps into landfills, we could create more than 1.5 million new jobs.

For every pound of waste you eliminate or recycle, you save energy and reduce emissions of carbon dioxide by at least one pound. By recycling just half of your household waste, you can save 2,400 pounds of carbon dioxide annually. This can be accomplished by paying attention to packaging, composting, thoughtful recycling, BYOB (bringing your own bag to stores), and being creative and reusing products for different purposes. Paper bags can biodegrade in a matter of weeks, and can also go into compost bins, yard waste piles, or the recycling bin.

A single quart of motor oil, if disposed of improperly, can contaminate up to 2,000,000 gallons of fresh water. Motor oil never wears out; it just gets dirtier. Oil can be recycled, re-refined, and used again, reducing our reliance on imported oil.

A typical family consumes 182 gallons of soda, 29 gallons of juice, 104 gallons of milk, and 26 gallons of bottled water a year. That's a lot of containers—make sure yours are recycled. The beverage industry used 46 percent less packaging in 2006 than in 1990, even with a 24 percent increase in beverage sales.

A growth industry in the future will be mining our waste disposal sites for the resources we've buried. Reusing items means energy, time, and fuel saved, and fewer emissions produced.

Contribute to and check out consignment stores. There is a surplus of reusable stuff, and it is much cheaper than new goods. Donate old sneakers to Nike's shoe recycling program. If only half of the 25.5 million tons of durable goods (such as used appliances, furniture, clothing, and machinery) now discarded in the United States were reused, more than 110,000 new jobs could be created.

Try to buy things that don't have packaging that require a lot material and energy (including petroleum) to produce and dispose of. About 33 percent of what we throw away is packaging. Avoid products with several layers of packaging when only one is sufficient. Use rechargeable batteries and properly dispose of used ones.

Remove yourself from any junk mailing lists you're on by calling the 800-number on catalogs and asking to be removed from their list. Contact Mail Preference Service at http://www.recycleplease.org and tell them to remove your name from mailing lists. If every American recycled their newspaper just one day a week, we would save about 36 million trees a year. It takes half as much energy to make recycled newspaper as it takes to make fresh newsprint from trees. However, most paper used presently is either recycled or made from sustainable forestry. When building with wood, check out sites for used wood, or make sure that it comes from a certified sustainable forest (http://www.sfiprogram.org/find-sfi-certified-forests-companies-products/).

DIMINISH DEBRIS IN OCEANS AND WATERWAYS

Volunteer for a state beach cleanup every September.

Most marine debris starts out on land. Put trash in a secure, lidded receptacle and dispose of cigarette butts in ashtrays, not on streets, sidewalks, or beaches that drain out to sea.

When boating, picnicking, or camping, bring a trash bag and be sure to handle waste properly. Bring along your own permanent food containers for picnics instead of using disposables.

Start conversations that inform and inspire your friends and coworkers to help stop marine debris at the source, which may mean your town's drainage system. Write to companies or visit local shops and restaurants and encourage them to reuse, recycle, and generate less packaging. Write to your elected officials and encourage them to support policies that protect our ocean.

GUIDELINES FOR RECYCLING APPLIANCES

Make sure that old appliances can't be fixed or are not energy-efficient before you throw them out.

Freecycle is a national message board that calls itself a "gifting" network, meaning you post items you have to give away. These items stay out of landfills and go to people who can use them. Sites such as yourenew.com and gazelle. com will pay for your used phones and other electronics. If you'd rather give your appliance to charity but aren't sure where to begin, Excess Access (https:// excessaccess.org) is a charity-matching Web site service. You pay a small fee ($5) to list your item, and they match you with a local charity that needs that item. Use Craigslist to sell or give away your working appliances. If your local charity doesn't accept old appliances, there may be someone in your neighborhood or community willing to take it off your hands. Be sure to check the rules and regulations regarding appliance recycling in your local community.

If you're buying a new appliance, check to see if your manufacturer or store will accept and recycle your old one in exchange. The EPA has a list of participating vendors (https://www.epa.gov/sites/production/files/2015-10/ documents/vendors.pdf).

Many appliance dealers will pick up your old appliance when they deliver a new item. But be sure to ask whether they have an appliance recycling program (you don't want them sending it to the landfill).

Your city or town may have an appliance round-up day or a location where you can drop off used appliances. Some recycling companies charge a fee to pick up and recycle your appliances; others will do it for free. Call around. Check out Earth911's (earth911.com) directory of companies and recycling facilities near you that accept "Non-Reusable Large Appliances."

If you plan to dump appliances yourself, prep for recycling according to local regulations, like removing the doors from old appliances to prevent curious children or animals from climbing inside and getting stuck.

REFRIGERATORS

All the refrigerators bought in one week would tower eighty miles high, according to greenecoservices.com. Luckily, Americans recycle almost all of their old refrigerators.

After your refrigerator is deposited, almost all of it can be recycled. The average ten-year-or-older refrigerator contains more than 120 pounds of recyclable steel. The energy saved by recycling that refrigerator is enough energy to run a new EnergyStar-qualified refrigerator for eight months. The US Environmental Protection Agency (EPA) requires that refrigerants be recovered. If you need extra assistance finding someone to recover your refrigerator for you, or if you see someone improperly disposing of one, please contact the Stratospheric Ozone Hotline at 1-800-296-1996.

ALUMINUM

At one time aluminum was more valuable than gold, now it's one of the most abundant materials on Earth. The 36 billion aluminum cans in landfills in 2013 had a scrap value of more than $600 million. Almost 63 billion or 63.5 percent of aluminum cans produced are recycled annually. More than 1,500 aluminum cans are recycled every second in the United States.

A used aluminum can is recycled and back on the grocery shelf as a new can in as little as sixty days. Used aluminum beverage cans are the most recycled item in the United States, but other types of aluminum, such as siding, gutters, car components, storm window frames, and lawn furniture can also be recycled. Recycling aluminum saves 95 percent of the energy used to make the material from scratch.

There is no limit to the amount of times aluminum can be recycled. Recycling one aluminum can saves enough energy to run a 100-watt bulb for twenty hours, a computer for three hours, a TV for two hours, or the equivalent of a half-a-gallon of gasoline. Energy saved from recycling one ton of aluminum is equal to the amount of electricity the average home uses over ten years.

The amount of aluminum currently recycled in one year is enough to rebuild the entire US commercial airplane fleet every six months. An estimated 80,000,000 Hershey's Kisses are wrapped each day, using enough aluminum foil to cover an area of over fifty acres—that's almost forty football fields. All that foil is recyclable. If we recycled all of our aluminum cans for one year, we could save enough energy to light Washington, DC, for 3.7 years.

GLASS

It never wears out—it can be recycled forever. A modern glass bottle would take 4,000 years or more to decompose, and even longer if it's in the landfill. We toss away enough glass bottles to fill two 1,400-foot skyscrapers twice a week.

In 2010, only 23.1 percent of glass, or more than 11 million tons, was recycled and most bottles and jars contain at least 25 percent recycled glass. When a new bottle is made from recycled material, it also causes 20 percent less air pollution and 50 percent less water pollution than making a new one. States with bottle deposit laws have 35 to 40 percent less litter by volume.

Most colored glass won't be recycled because of its various chemical components. As a result, waste colored glass is now being stockpiled in some locations, waiting for a use. Thanks to research conducted at the University of Greenwich, however, that glass may soon be used for filtering pollutants out of ground water. Much of the colored glass is used for purposes such as landfill, roadbeds, and weighing down refuse at municipal dumps.

If recycled glass is substituted for half of the raw materials for new product, waste is cut by more than 80 percent. Mining and transporting raw materials for glass produces about 385 pounds of waste for every ton of glass that is made. Even the mercury in fluorescent tubes can be recycled.

We save 1.2 tons of resources for every ton of glass recycled—1,330 pounds of sand, 433 pounds of soda ash, 433 pounds of limestone, 151 pounds of feldspar, and 860 kilowatt-hours of electricity—or 18 percent of the energy needed to form new glass.

OIL

More than 500 million oil filters are disposed of each year and the EPA estimates that more than 200 million gallons of oil wind up in landfills or down the drain every year. Recycling the 200 million gallons recoverable motor oil thrown away each year would produce enough energy to power 360,000 homes annually. If the 1.3 billion gallons of oil wasted each year by the United States were re-refined, it would save 1.3 million barrels of oil a day. Approximately 750 million gallons of used oil are reprocessed every year. When you get the oil changed in your car, asked for recycled oil.

Drained oil filters still hold about ½ cup of motor oil, enough to pollute 125,000 gallons of water. It takes 42 gallons of virgin crude oil to make 2.5 quarts of refined oil, but it only takes one gallon of used oil to make the same 2.5 quarts.

By the way, don't put any oil used for cooking down the drain. It causes arteriosclerosis in city sewers costing millions of dollars to clean them out every year.

PLASTICS

Ubiquitous should be a synonym for this boon and boondoggle to mankind. It's the greatest symbol of use, waste, and excess. Its many forms are useful and versatile from a product standpoint, but they aren't organic or biodegradable, and the materials and energy used to create them are petrochemically based, hence polluting air and water, and creating incredible amounts of solid waste. Consequently, they are not the best choice for the environment, so their overall merit will always be debated.

Which plastics can and cannot be recycled—or, more accurately, recomposed or reprocessed—has always confounded consumers. Different types of plastic can be recycled, a few cannot, and some need more difficult processing to be reformulated. Recycling regulations may vary from state to state—check with your local recycling or municipal waste management department.

Some recycling centers accept all types of plastic for recycling, while others only accept containers with coded numbers stamped on their bottoms. This is the Plastic Identification Code (PIC) created by the Society of the Plastics Industry to identify different types of plastic resins used in manufacturing. Those numbers are single digits from 1 to 7 surrounded by a triangle of arrows, used to clue consumers in as to how to distinguish the different types of plastics.

Recycling opportunities for other plastic products, including plastic foam cups and plastic cutlery, are expanding. Some yogurt and other small food containers are also recyclable. Check the numbers, manufacturers, or your local recycling center for your local regulations.

The amount of plastic produced from 2000 to 2010 exceeds the amount produced during the entire last century. Thirty-two million tons of plastic wastes were generated in 2011, representing 12.7 percent of total municipal solid waste (MSW). There are enough plastic water bottles on Earth to circle it more than 200 times. Every year Americans throw away enough paper and plastic cups, forks, and spoons to circle the equator 300 times and enough polystyrene foam cups to do it 436 times. Single-use plastic utensils, like the ones in cheese-and-crackers packages, are an incredible waste of resources and energy. Every year the United States makes enough plastic film to shrink-wrap Texas.

If every American household recycled just one out of every ten high-density polyethylene (HDPE) bottles they used, we'd keep 200 million pounds of the plastic out of landfills every year. Plastic bottle recycling grew by 97 million pounds in 2014 (increasing 3.3 percent) to more than 3 billion pounds for the year.

If all the nonrecycled plastics discarded in the United States annually were diverted to modern waste-to-energy facilities, they could produce 52 million megawatt-hours of electricity, enough to power 5.2 million households a year. This year more than 30 million tons of plastic will be recycled in the United States, but only about 25 percent of what is produced is recycled.

And, by the way, bubble wrap was originally invented as 3-D wallpaper. It is 100 percent recyclable.

PET

Polyethylene terephthalate (PET, PETE). Clarity, strength, toughness, barrier to gas and moisture. Soft drink, water and salad dressing bottles; peanut butter and jam jars

PE-HD

High-density polyethylene (HDPE). Stiffness, strength, toughness, resistance to moisture, permeability to gas. Water pipes, hula hoop rings, five gallon buckets, milk, juice and water bottles; the occasional shampoo / toiletry bottle.

PVC

Polyvinyl chloride (PVC) Versatility, ease of blending, strength, toughness. Blister packaging for non-food items; cling films for non-food use. Not used for food packaging as the plastics are needed to make natively rigid PVC flexible are usually toxic. Non-packaging uses are electrical cable insulation; rigid piping; vinyl records.

PE-LD

Low-density polyethylene (LDPE). Ease of processing, strength, toughness, flexibility, ease of sealing, barrier to moisture. Frozen food bags; squeezable bottles, e.g. honey, mustard; cling films; flexible container lids.

PP

Polypropylene (PP). Strength, toughness, resistance to heat, chemicals, grease and oil, versatile, barrier to moisture. Reusable microwaveable ware; kitchenware; yogurt containers; margarine tubs; microwaveable disposable take-away containers; disposable cups; plates.

PS

Polystyrene (PS). Versatility, clarity, easily formed   Egg cartons; packing peanuts; disposable cups, plates, trays and cutlery; disposable take-away containers;

O

Other (often polycarbonate or ABS). Dependent on polymers or combination of polymers   Beverage bottles; baby milk bottles. Non-packaging uses for polycarbonate: compact discs; "unbreakable" glazing; electronic apparatus housings; lenses including sunglasses, prescription glasses, automotive headlamps, riot shields, instrument panels.
Courtesy of Wikipedia

Figure 36.1.   Plastic types.
Source: wikipedia.org/plastictypes.

PLASTIC BAGS MADE FROM PET

Most plastic bags, an estimated 500 billion to one trillion used worldwide every year, are made from a type of plastic called polyethylene. Eighty percent of polyethylene is produced from natural gas. A great number of plastic bags and bottles made from "recyclable" PET (polyethylene terephthalate) material wind up buried in landfills and don't get recycled. They can remain there anywhere from 10 to 500 years, and the granules of the bags do find their way into the environment, then into wildlife.

During the 2009 International Coastal Cleanup, and the Ocean Conservancy noted that plastic bags were the second most common kind of waste found in the seas and on the beaches. It's also estimated that each year more than 100 million tons of plastic are produced, of which about 10 percent ends up in the sea.

A United Nations survey claims that an estimated 100,000 marine mammals and up to one million sea birds die every year after ingesting or being tangled in plastic marine litter. On land, many cows, goats, and other animals suffer a similar fate when they accidentally ingest plastic bags while foraging for food.

Plastic bags can be burned in power plants but, unless filtered, this will produce greenhouse gases. Recycling them saves twice as much energy as it produces in an incinerator. Once bags are recycled, they are made into lumber, trashcan liners, or more plastic bags. Recycling one ton of plastic bags costs around $4,000. Unfortunately, the recycled product sells for about $32. Guess who makes up the difference?

Estimates range from 100 to almost 400 billion plastic bags a year used in the United States and the average American uses between 300 and 700 plastic bags annually. The Irish use 27. If just 25 percent of US families used ten fewer plastic bags a month, we would save over 2.5 billion bags a year. Sources vary, but only about 1 to 12 percent of the bags are recycled. The rest enter the waste stream. In the United States alone, an estimated 12,000,000 barrels of oil are required to produce 100 billion plastic bags used annually.

Many cities have banned or are planning to ban or tax plastic bags to help stem the tide of plastic waste. Ask for compostable plastic bags now available that are derived from agricultural waste and formed into a fully biodegradable faux-plastic with a consistency similar to polyethylene bags.

PRACTICAL SUGGESTIONS: PLASTIC BAGS

Reusable bags hold far more than disposable bags, which means fewer trips back and forth from the car. Each time you use your own bag, you may get a small credit from grocery stores or you won't have to pay for paper bags. By reusing your own bags, you'll have less clutter and create less trash.

Send a green message to your children when they see you reusing plastic bags, or bringing your own bags to the store—they'll take notice and want to do the same. One of the most popular ways to reuse plastic bags is to use them as trash bags. Place them in small trash barrels in the bathroom, bedrooms, cellar, as doggy poop bags, and near the cat's litter box. Keep a plastic bag in your car to contain all of the trash that accumulates in your car. You can also reuse plastic bags as packaging for mailed articles. Use plastic bags as wrap for messy household and kitchen items. Donate your plastic bags to a local thrift store or charity. This prevents them from having to buy brand new bags. Post an ad on Craigslist for your bags. A local business or thrift can use them.

CRV—CALIFORNIA REDEMPTION VALUE

In some states, like in the old days, consumers pay a redemption value when they purchase beverages from a retailer, and receive refunds when they redeem the containers. Aluminum, glass, plastic, and bimetal containers are eligible for CRV. Notable container exceptions are milk, wine, and distilled spirits.

PVC PLASTIC

Chlorine production for polyvinyl chloride (PVC) uses almost as much energy as the annual output of eight medium-sized nuclear power plants each year. Creating a ton of PET plastic bottles produces three tons of carbon, adding 2.5 million tons of carbon dioxide emissions into the atmosphere. Although all of the thermoplastics are technically recyclable, many of them are not being collected for recycling because it is not economically viable to recycle them. Tell the manufacturers how you feel about this.

Over 14 billion pounds of PVC are currently produced per year in North America, and 7 billion pounds are thrown away in the United States, a waste as PVC compounds are 100 percent recyclable physically and chemically. Only 18 million pounds of PVC—between 1 and 3 percent—is recycled, according to the Association of Postconsumer Plastics Recyclers.

The Vinyl Institute claims that manufacturers' take-back programs, such as those for end-of-life vinyl-backed carpeting, wall coverings, and roofing, have been very successful and projects that more than 50 million pounds are recycled every year. And over 2.3 trillion gallons of treated water could be saved every year in the USA by using noncorrosive PVC pipes.

STYROFOAM/POLYSTYRENE (#6)

Although most forms of Styrofoam are recyclable, the problem is where to take it, and unfortunately recycling may not be realistic for small quantities. All you can do is reuse it, give it away, or hoard it if it becomes valuable. Each year, Americans throw away 25 billion Styrofoam cups, enough to circle the Earth 436 times. Seattle, Washington; Portland, Oregon; West-chester, New York; and Berkeley and Malibu, California, have all banned Styrofoam food ware. Laguna Beach and Santa Monica have banned all polystyrene (#6) food ware.

STEEL

Steel takes up to 100 years to fully degrade in a landfill. Approximately 131 billion cans are produced each year in the United States. All steel cans are 100 percent recyclable. Each new steel product is made in part from postconsumer recycled scrap metal and two-thirds of all cans on supermarket shelves are made of steel.

About 70 percent of all steel packaging is recycled, as is about 63 percent of all steel cans. Recycling seven steel cans saves enough energy to power a 60-watt light bulb for 26 hours. The steel industry's annual recycling saves enough energy to electrically power about 18 million households for a year. Recycling steel and tin cans saves 74 percent of the energy used to originally produce them. Steel recycling saves an average of 4,300 kilowatt hours per ton or 47 percent of the energy required to process steel from raw materials. Recycling steel takes 25 percent less energy and creates only 25 percent of the water and air pollution required to produce steel from raw materials. A steel mill using recycled scrap reduces related water pollution, air pollution, and mining wastes by about 70 percent. The recycling of steel saves enough energy to heat and light 18,000,000 homes.

If Americans only recycled one-tenth of the cans we now throw away, we'd save about 3.2 billion of them every year. The average American throws out about 61 pounds of tin cans every month (tin cans are 99 percent steel with a thin layer of tin). Americans throw out enough iron and steel to supply all the nation's automakers on a continuous basis.

Recycling more than 7 million tons of metals (which includes aluminum, steel, and mixed metals) eliminates greenhouse gas emissions the equivalent of about 25 million metric tons of carbon dioxide. This is the same as removing almost 5 million cars from the road for one year.

JUNK MAIL AND PAPER PRODUCTS

Fifty percent of all paper produced in the United States is used for packaging. Forty-one percent of all the refuse that goes into dumps is paper. Every year

Americans throw away enough office and writing paper for Donald Trump to build a wall twelve feet high stretching from Los Angeles to New York City. Americans use 85 million tons of paper annually—of which 50 to 65 percent is recycled, but still consumes more than 850 million trees and about. It should be noted that most of the paper used these days comes from sustainable forests and pulp woods.

The average American spends eight full months of their life opening junk mail and the amount Americans receive in one day could produce enough energy to heat 250,000 homes. On average, a person in the United States uses more than 700 pounds of paper every year. Burning that paper would create 300 pounds of carbon dioxide.

A ton of recycled paper saves thirteen trees, 2.5 barrels of oil, one thousand gallons of water, four tons of carbon dioxide, and two-and-one-half acres of landfill. The 2.6 billion holiday cards sold each year in the United States could fill a football field ten stories high.

TIRES AND RUBBER

Close to 300 million tires are made in the in United States each year. Because they retain heat, tire piles easily ignite, creating toxins and GHG-emitting, hard-to-extinguish fires that can burn for months. Approximately 300 million tires are scrapped every year, almost one for every person in the United States. Annual waste tire generation composes about 2 percent of municipal solid waste by weight. It takes half a barrel of crude oil and 518 gallons of water to produce the rubber for just one truck tire.

Twenty percent of tires sold in Mexico are imported used tires from the United States. It requires only 29 percent of the energy to produce one pound of recycled rubber versus one pound of new rubber. About 78 percent of all waste tires generated annually in the United States are recovered for recycling or reusing. About 45 percent of all waste tires recovered in the United States are converted to tire-derived fuel, a low-sulfur, high-heating-value fuel.

About 8 percent of waste tires are finely ground into "crumb rubber," which can be produced for roadbed material, road embankment fill, filtration material for landfill and construction, belts, hoses and rubberized mats, and agricultural uses, and can also be incorporated into rubber-modified asphalt, sealant compounds, or back into new tires.

Approximately 70 percent of all rubber for shoes used is made of synthetic petroleum-based polymers.

FOOD AND PACKAGING

One dollar out of every $11 Americans spend for food goes for packaging and as much 10 to 50 percent of the price of food is the combo cost of advertising and packaging. The global food packaging industry is now worth $100 billion a year, growing 10 to 15 percent annually. Americans dump the equivalent of more than 21 million shopping bags full of food into landfills every year, or more than 34 million tons of food waste each year. An estimated 25 percent of food each year is lost to spoilage. The average American family of four ends up throwing away an equivalent of up to more than $2,275 annually in food. Estimates are that as much as 50 percent of all US household waste is packaging.

About 30 percent of the total municipal waste is from packaging, approximately 76,760 thousand tons, and about 7 percent is from retail waste. Only 43.7 percent of that is recycled. If just 5 percent of all discarded food had been recovered (for composting, donations, and animal feed), more than $50 million in landfill costs would have been saved.

GENERAL GARBAGE

Trash production has increased 60 percent in the last thirty years. Los Angeles, the second largest city in the country, dumps more than 10,000 tons each year in landfill dumps. On average it costs $30 per ton to recycle trash, $50 to send it to the landfill, and $65 to $75 to incinerate it.

The highest point in Hamilton County, Ohio (near Cincinnati) is Mount Rumpke. It is actually a mountain of trash at the Rumpke Sanitary Landfill, towering 1,045 feet above sea level. New York City sends more than 10,500 tons of residential waste each day to landfills in places like Ohio and South Carolina.

The covering of America's largest landfill, east of downtown Los Angeles, is underway, and is slated to become a park, of all things, as well as a methane well for producing energy, enough to power about 70,000 homes in Southern California.

Every year, more than 130 million tons of America's trash ends up in landfills. Airports and airlines recycle less than 20 percent of 425,000 tons of passenger-related waste produced each year.

Between Thanksgiving and New Year's, an extra million tons of waste is generated each week. Thirty-eight thousand miles of ribbon are thrown away each year, enough to tie a bow around the Earth.

In a lifetime, the average American will throw away 600 times their adult weight in garbage—a 150-pound adult will leave a legacy of 90,000 pounds

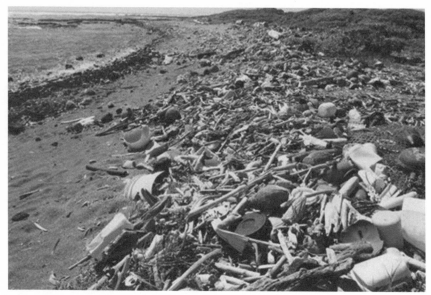

Figure 36.2.   **Hawaii's plastic beaches.**
Source: greenhome.com

of trash behind. The methane gas produced daily at a large landfill is enough fuel to heat 50,000 homes. For every pound of waste you eliminate or re-cycle, you save energy and reduce emissions of carbon dioxide by at least one pound. Each day American families produce an estimated four million pounds of hazardous household waste (chemicals, batteries, etc.). That would fill the Superdome in Louisiana more than 1,500 times.

Edward Humes, author of *Garbology: Our Dirty Love Affair with Trash*, says constantly covering up our trash means we never fully understand how much garbage we generate. "You notice what we call our trash companies, waste 'management.' Think about that," Humes says. "They're managing our waste; they're not reducing our waste, they're not disappearing our waste. And what that means is they're really good at picking it up and getting it out of sight making garbage mountains out of it."

GET INVOLVED

If you wish to become involved in a public or private recycling program, contact your local, state, or federal government. Many states offer programs, grants, and loans to assist public and private entities in the safe and effective management of the waste stream.

37

The Home Energy Audit

Do-It-Yourself "Sherlock Homes!"

If you could fly across the United States and see the energy losses of communities via an infrared camera, it would look as if the whole country was ablaze in a red inferno of wasted energy. According to the DOE, the cost of all the energy consumed annually for buildings in the United States is about $400 billion. Approximately one-third is used to heat, cool, and light our homes and operate home appliances, totaling approximately 15 to 20 percent of total greenhouse gases emitted annually.

At present we are in a semi-embryonic state of researching and marketing new ways to clean up fossil fuels and to power our country with alternative, sustainable, and nonpolluting fuel sources. Now is the time for the rest of us to step up by practicing what experts are calling the best way to decrease toxic gases, conserve resources, and save money—conservation in the home.

A home energy audit analyzes your home's structural "envelope" and insulation, appliances, and use of resources—as well as your family's lifestyle—in order to get a gauge on how resource- and energy-efficient your house is. You can hire a professional for $450 (the national average) to conduct an energy audit, or you can be your own "Sherlock Homes" and conduct a simple but conscientious walk-through to spot problems. This do-it-yourself home energy audit will not be as thorough as a professional home energy assessment, but it can help you pinpoint some of the areas to address and change.

FACTS AND FIGURES AND PRACTICAL SUGGESTIONS

An analysis published by the Berkeley Lab, Lawrence Livermore National Laboratory (LLNL), suggests that the USA is just 39 percent energy-efficient, meaning that 61 percent of our energy is wasted annually.

Making standard efficiency improvements on an inefficient home can save as much as 30 percent in utility bills, or $570 a year on average, and can help an average household find simple ways to reduce its carbon dioxide emissions by 15,000 pounds annually.

An energy audit and subsequent substantial weatherization and upgrades will pay for itself in two to three years. Some utility companies will do a free basic audit for customers, and if you qualify for financial assistance they will provide various products and labor free of charge. You may also qualify for further discounts on products and labor at the state and federal level (see chapter 34, "More Power to Power More People").

When assessing your home, keep a list of areas you have inspected and problems you have found, making notes of areas to fix or that need a more comprehensive analysis. This list will help you prioritize your efforts for energy efficiency upgrades.

Ask your utility company for a cost calculator (or use the DOE's at: http://energy.gov/energysaver/maps/appliance-energy-calculator) to determine the energy use of your appliances. Check the ages of your appliances; they may be ready for replacement. Examine your monthly utility bill when finished with your audit and see if you can find areas for improvement. Ask yourself these questions before and after an energy audit:

- How long do I plan to own my current home?
- How much money do I spend on energy?
- Where are the greatest energy losses?
- How long will it take for an investment in energy efficiency to pay for itself?
- Do the energy-saving measures provide additional benefits that are important to me?
- Can I do the energy-saving projects or will I need to hire a contractor?
- What is my budget—in time and money?
- Do the energy-saving measures provide additional benefits that are important to me?
- How much time do I have for maintenance and repairs?

WHAT TO LOOK FOR IN A
PROFESSIONAL HOME ENERGY AUDITOR

Professional energy audits can go into great detail. The energy auditor should do a room-by-room examination of the residence, as well as a thorough examination of past utility bills. Before contracting with an energy auditing company, we suggest you take the following steps:

Ask for their experience and testimonials. Check the Internet for rating sites. Get several references and ask if they were satisfied with the work. Call the Better Business Bureau and inquire about any complaints against the company. Make sure they conduct thermographic inspections (infrared scanning to detect heat loss). Ask about any special education, certifications, or professional groups they belong to.

Ask if they will conduct a calibrated blower door test. This uses a powerful fan which mounts into the frame of an exterior door. The fan pulls air out of the house, lowering the air pressure inside. The higher outside air pressure then causes air to flow in through all unsealed cracks and openings to show where it is possible to:

- Reduce energy consumption due to air leakage.
- Prevent moisture condensation problems.
- Avoid uncomfortable drafts caused by cold air leaking in from the outdoors.
- Determine how much mechanical ventilation might be needed to provide acceptable indoor air quality.

Also, ask if they will conduct a carbon dioxide test and a ventilation test. Find out if the report will prioritize improvements based on their cost-effectiveness, and how it will be organized. You'll want to be sure it's intelligible, contains a concrete inventory of measures, prioritizes improvements needed based on cost-effectiveness, and provides clear instructions for those things you can take of yourself. Ask if the auditor is also a contractor.

DIY—TESTING FOR CRACKS AND GAPS

First, close all exterior doors, windows, and fireplace flues. Turn off all combustion appliances, such as ovens and ranges, gas burning furnaces, and water heaters. Turn on all exhaust fans (generally located in the kitchen and bathrooms) or use a large window fan to suck the air out of the rooms. The fans pull air out of the house, lowering the air pressure inside. The higher outside air pressure then pushes air back into the house through all unsealed cracks and openings.

Use incense sticks or smoldering material and look for fluttering smoke indicating a leak, or your wet hand that will feel cool to a breeze when locating these leaks inside.

EXAMINE THESE SPACES AND PLACES

Inspect all areas where two different building materials meet—such as cement/wood framing, wood floor/drywall, and roof material/bricks—and look for cracks and gaps, also check around pipes and wires, electrical outlets, foundation seals, switch plates, recessed lighting, and mail slots. Find out what type of insulation was used in your home. One of the best ways is to look at exposed areas such as in your garage, attic, or basement. When making improvements, be sure to keep notes on materials used. Look for cracks and holes in the mortar, foundation, and siding, and seal them with the appropriate material designed for cement or mortal, wood or stucco.

Black & Decker has created a new tool called the Thermal Leak Detector. It's a very simple device that allows you to detect temperature differences between different points in your house. Test air conditioning (AC) in the same manner as a heat test, measuring temperature in reverse (see chapter on HVAC). To confirm the AC system has the correct airflow and refrigerant charge, professional assistance is recommended.

SAFETY

Crawl spaces may contain dusts, insects, vermin, and animal droppings. You will want to wear appropriate clothing and safety equipment as well as making sure you are physically up to inspection tasks. Asbestos is still common around pipes, air ducts, old heating equipment, and in vermiculite insulation. It may look like a light gray or white fibrous material. Asbestos is dangerous, but particularly so when particles become airborne. Do not touch, vibrate, or disturb anything you suspect contains asbestos, except to remove it while wearing a dust mask. Fiberglass insulation is very irritating; use goggles, a dust mask, gloves, and long sleeves to protect lungs and skin from particles. Turn off electricity at the breaker before probing for insulation or checking near any wiring, and secure ladders and stepstools.

THE HOME AUDIT

Attics and Ceilings and Roofs

- Attic hatches should make a tight seal.
- Attics and ceilings should be insulated to R-38.
- Skylights should have a tight seal.
- Make sure attic fan is working properly.

- Check insulation for proper thickness.
- Check roofing material for age and wear.
- Check for places where snow dams can occur.
- Ceilings should be light-colored for better illumination.
- Use a plastic barrier between wall and roof.

Bathroom

- Check faucets and showerheads for leaks.
- Each bathroom should have an exhaust fan ducted outside (not into the attic, basement, or crawl space).
- Check windows for tight seals.
- Examine toilets for leaks.
- Fixtures should be rated for efficiency.
- Check fan and venting for obstructions.

Basement

- Crawl spaces should be insulated with a minimum of R-12.
- Check vented crawl spaces that can be associated with moisture and mold problems.
- All crawl spaces require a layer of 6-mil (or heavier) polyethylene plastic spread over the floor of the crawl space to help keep moisture and soil gases from getting in.
- Vapor barriers should be placed on walls.
- Corners of foundation should be closed off.
- Basement ceilings are your floor's insulation, use a minimum of R-12.

Doors and Windows

- Double-pane windows are most effective for conserving heat and cool air.
- Search windows for cracks.
- All windows should be caulked and weather-stripped and be sure that the window glazing is in good shape.
- Inspect windows and doors for air leaks. If you can rattle them, it is a sign of possible air leaks.
- Windows should be rated U-0.35 or better.
- Use insulating drapes or other window treatments for better insulation.
- Wall or window-mounted air conditioners should have a tight fit.
- Check caulking and weather-stripping, especially around doors and windows, for gaps, cracks, and weathering.

- If you can see daylight around a door or window frame, seal these leaks by caulking or weather stripping.
- Check the storm windows to see if they fit snugly and are not broken. They should be tight and sealed. Check them for inside condensation and frost.
- Consider replacing old windows and doors with newer, high-performance ones. If new factory-made doors or windows are too costly, you can install low-cost plastic sheets over the windows.
- Install insulated, solid, exterior doors.

Ducts

- Check ductwork with a good digital thermometer if the ductwork is metal and located in the subfloor.
- The best way to identify leakage is with a duct pressure test, or to crawl around and physically look at every piece of duct in your system for indications of leaks—discolored joints, tape or joint deterioration, and any mold (for more info check chapter 13, "Air Ducts").
- The range hood should be ducted outside (not into the attic, basement, or crawl space).
- The clothes dryer should be ducted efficiently to the outside.
- Professionals use various tools to conduct duct pressure tests that are used by HVAC contractors.
- If you have access to the type of tape used for ducting for the fans, check it (smooth or flex), and the diameter, length, and condition.
- If there are ducts in unheated areas, they should be insulated with a minimum of R-8 insulation.
- When sealing any home, always be aware of the danger of indoor air pollution and combustion appliance "backdrafts." An exhaust fan may pull cooking or heated gases back into the living space—a dangerous and unhealthy situation.
- Seal any duct leaks you may have found.

Electronic Appliances

- List what appliances are left on when not in use (many will have their LED lights on). Plug all electronics and appliances into power strips that you turn off when not in use (turning off power strip completely shuts off electricity).
- Check appliances older than ten to twelve years for their working condition and power needs. Think about replacing the older, inefficient ones.

Fireplace

- Fireplace dampers should be closed and sealed if not in use.
- Check any seals around glass doors.
- Check any gas connections to ensure they are tight and will retain heat.
- Check dampers for thickness of ash or creosote.
- Check for any obstructions by removing cap on chimney or by visual inspection.
- Make note of how much wood a stove burns to keep the house at a set temperature.

Floors

- Are the top (attic floor) and bottom (basement ceiling) and floors between home levels insulated with at least R-30?
- Check any corners for gaps and leaks.
- Add insulation and/or floor coverings to mitigate the cold.

Furnace

- How old is it?
- Check burners or heating elements.
- Check the flue and make certain that it is venting properly.
- Is it efficiently delivering heat with reasonable costs?

Garden

- Use trees for windbreaks and plant them in strategic locations to mitigate weather conditions. For optimum use of shade, they should be planted on north and east sides of buildings and should be planted away from air conditioners and toxic gas vents.
- Make sure all sprinkler systems are working properly for each season and for correct times.
- Check the pool heater, cover, and filters.
- Check the spa heater, water connections, cover, and the condition of the water.

Heating and Cooling Systems

- Check for dust.
- Check filters monthly, especially in seasons when heavily used, and change if needed. Keep all parts clean.

- Check all insulation where possible for type and thickness.
- Check for vapor barrier on the indoor side of insulation.
- Check all openings where drafts may enter (pipes, outlets, etc.).
- Add, upgrade, or replace wherever necessary due to age and wear.

Kitchen

- Ensure that all appliances are energy-efficient and are running efficiently.
- Keep the refrigerator away from appliances with a heat source.
- Check stove doors and seals for a tight fit.
- Be sure microwave seals are tight.
- Check dishwasher doors and seals for a tight fit.
- Check refrigerator doors and seals for a tight fit. Check running parts and clean and remove dust and dirt that inhibit proper operation.

Laundry Room

- Clean washer with proper washer cleaner.
- Check seals for leaks on front-loading washers.
- Check seals on clothes dryer doors. Clean filters after each load. Check vents for obstructions and proper venting outside.
- Be attentive to your water use.

Lighting

- Check all lighting fixtures for incandescent, halogen, or light-emitting diode (LED) bulbs. Switch to compact fluorescent light bulbs or LEDs.
- Remind family members to turn off the lights when not in use. Part of your daily routine should be making sure that everyone complies.

Walls

- Check for leaks, such as gaps along the baseboard or edge of the flooring and at junctures of the walls and ceiling.
- The wall caps and roof jacks (used to flash around and cover pipes or stacks such as sewer or furnace ventilation pipes that penetrate the roof) should be sealed or caulked.
- Outside walls should be completely protected from the weather.
- Interior attic walls and ceiling should be insulated with at least R-19.
- Ensure that attic fans are working properly and have some sort of vent.

Water Heater and Piping

• Install insulation around water heater.
• Insulate pipes with pipe insulation.
• Check the anode rod in water heater for condition.
• Check water heater thermostat setting at 120°F.
• Water heaters should be flushed every one to three years depending on the model and water source, which helps to control the build-up of mineral deposits.

Programmable Thermostat

• Your thermostat should be programmable and use programmable settings and automatic thermostat for maximum efficiency.
• Keep aware of settings especially with manual thermostats as many families' members play dueling temperatures.

Standby and Miscellaneous Power

• List each appliance.
• Determine if they are energy-efficient and replace if not.
• Determine whether the appliance can be completely turned off and put in "sleep" mode when not in use.
• When purchasing new equipment, be certain that it has a "completely off" switch and is EnergyStar-rated.
• Use strip plugs to turn off connected appliances completely off.

The home energy audit will give you plenty of places and proposals where to begin saving energy and money. It might not seem like a lot to do for Mother Earth, but how we handle our refuse on the planet—in the water, land, and air—might mark a new beginning and not the end of our world as we know it. Good luck.

Index

About the Author

Jeff Dondero has a diverse background and experience in writing, ranging from web content, B2B, books, hard news, to interviews to feature writing. He began his career as a stringer and freelancer for the *San Francisco Examiner*, worked as a reporter and editor for several suburban newspapers, was the entertainment editor for *The Marin Independent Journal*, was a writer and editor of various magazines, wrote for KTVU-TV in the San Francisco Bay Area, toiled in a trade magazine mill, and created a website dedicated to sustainable construction industries (http://www.greenbuildingdigest.net/). He was invited to be a writer-in-residence at an art colony in Rancho Vista, Arizona, in 2014, where he wrote a slim volume of poetry. He continues to expand his national readership with books, social media, various writers' blogs and websites, and radio and television appearances.